The Healthy Pregnancy Book

The Healthy Pregnancy Book

Month by Month,
Everything You Need to Know
from America's Baby Experts

**William Sears, MD, and Martha Sears, RN,
with Linda Holt, MD, and BJ Snell, PhD, CNW**

LITTLE, BROWN AND COMPANY
New York   Boston   London

This book is intended to supplement, not replace, the advice of a trained health professional. If you know or suspect that you have a health problem, you should consult a health professional. The author and publisher specifically disclaim any liability, loss, or risk, personal or otherwise, which is incurred as a consequence, directly or indirectly, of the use and application of any of the contents of this book.

Little, Brown and Company
Hachette Book Group
237 Park Avenue, New York, NY 10017
littlebrown.com

First Edition: September 2013

Little, Brown and Company is a division of Hachette Book Group, Inc. The Little, Brown name and logo are trademarks of Hachette Book Group, Inc.

The publisher is not responsible for websites (or their content) that are not owned by the publisher.

The Hachette Speakers Bureau provides a wide range of authors for speaking events. To find out more, go to hachettespeakersbureau.com or call (866) 376-6591.

Drawings by Deborah Maze

ISBN 978-0-316-18743-5
LCCN 2013946521

10 9 8 7 6 5 4 3 2 1

RRD-C

Printed in the United States of America

Contents

A Note to Pregnant Mothers: How We Birthed This Book,
and How to Use It   *xv*

Planning to Become Pregnant: Eleven Habits to Increase
Your Chances   *3*

PART I: THE HEALTHY PREGNANCY PLAN

Chapter 1: Get Motivated to Get Healthy   *11*

The Fetal Effect • F.O.O.D. for Thought • Placenta Power — Not So
Perfect • Why Babies Are Vulnerable • Scientists Detect Chemicals in the
Cord • How to Build a Brighter Baby Brain

Chapter 2: How to Eat: Graze, Sip, and Dip   *20*

Why Grazing Is Great • Our Rule of Twos • The Hormonal Harmony
of Pregnancy • Snack Smart • Pregnancy Eating Tip: One Fistful of
Food • Enjoy the Sipping Solution • How to Choose the Prenatal
Supplement That's Right for You • Dr. Bill and Martha's Pregnancy
Supersmoothie • Nutrition Questions You May Have

Chapter 3: What to Eat: The Top Twelve Pregnancy Superfoods   *28*

What's in a Pregnancy Superfood? • The Nourishing Nine Nutrients You
Need for a Healthy Pregnancy • Go Fish! • Traffic-Light Safe Seafood
Eating • Go Nuts! • During Pregnancy, Give Yourself an Oil Change • Go
Greens! • Martha's Pregnancy Salad • Awesome Avocados • Eat
Eggs • Yummy Yogurt • Blueberries, the Brain Berries • Big on Beans and
Lentils • Fabulous Flaxseeds • Go Organic! • Shape Young Tastes — in

the Womb! • Oh, Olive Oil! • Drink Up! • Terrific Tofu • Outstanding
Oatmeal • "White Out" Your Diet • Try Dr. Bill and Martha's 5-S
Diet • Traffic-Light Eating for a Healthy Pregnancy • Pregnancy Nutrition at a
Glance

Chapter 4: Gain the Weight That's Right for You and Baby   *51*

What Is a Healthy Weight Gain? • Where Your Extra Weight Goes • Why
Excess "Mommy Fat" Is Hard to Shed • Why Is Gaining Too Much Weight
Not Healthy for Baby? • Eighteen Strategies to Curb Your Cravings and Gain
Optimal Weight • A Healthy Online Resource while Pregnant

Chapter 5: Exercise Right for Two   *59*

How Exercise Benefits Both Mommy and Baby — New Research • Twenty
Pregnancy Perks of Exercise • Eight Tips for Exercising Right for You and
Baby • Exercise Precautions while Pregnant • No-No Exercises while
Pregnant • Anytime-Anywhere Exercises • Safe and Fun Swimming while
Pregnant • Don't Get Overheated • Exercises for an Easier Birth

Chapter 6: Don't Worry, Be Pregnant   *73*

Can Baby Feel Mommy's Stress? • "Pregnancy Brain" Prepares You for "Mommy
Brain" • Ten Stressbusters Every Pregnant Mother Can Learn

Chapter 7: How to Sleep Peacefully while Pregnant   *79*

Why You Wake Up So Often • Why Pregnant Mothers Need More Sleep • The
Pregnancy Sleep Prescription • Snooze Foods • Sleeping Comfortably

Chapter 8: Go Green!   *87*

Go Greenest Earlier in Your Pregnancy • Thank You for Not Smoking •
Advance Warning: "Birth Defect Control" • How Smoking Harms Babies and
Mothers • Thank You for Not Taking Illegal Drugs • Thank You for Not
Drinking Alcohol • Food Chemicals to Limit • The Dirtiest Dozen • Caffeine
Concerns • Eleven More Ways to Go Green • Cell Phone Safety while
Pregnant • Make Your Personal Care Products Safe for Baby

Chapter 9: Practice the Pills-and-Skills Model of Self-Care   *102*

Self-Help Skills for Common Pregnancy Ills • Popular Pills while Pregnant: Be
Cautious • Resources for Medication Use during Pregnancy

PART II: YOUR PREGNANCY: MONTH BY MONTH

Chapter 10: First Month: Newly Pregnant — 107

How Your Baby Is Growing, 1–4 weeks — 107

Week 1: Fertilization • Week 2: Implantation • Week 3: Placenta and Baby Grow Together • Week 4: Baby's Body Takes Shape

How You May Feel — 110

Joyful • Confused • Anxious • Moody • Fatigued • Guilty • Early Signs of Pregnancy • Nausea and Morning Sickness • Questions You May Have about Morning Sickness • How Husbands Can Help • Fifteen Stomach-Friendly Tips • Stomach-Soothing Favorites • Food Cravings

Concerns You May Have — 125

Due Date • Pregnancy Tests • Early Spotting • "We're Pregnant!" — Sharing the News • Assembling Your Birth Team • Choosing Dr. Right • Questions to Ask Your Doctor • How to Get the Most out of Your First Prenatal Checkup • Obstetrician or Midwife? Consider Both! • Choosing a Midwife • Choosing Where to Birth Your Baby • Journal Your Baby's Womb Life • My Pregnancy Journal: First Month

Chapter 11: Second Month: Feeling More Pregnant — 146

How Your Baby Is Growing, 5–8 weeks — 146

How You May Feel — 148

Aware of Breast Changes • Beyond Tired • Nauseated • Heart Beating Faster • Mouth Watering • Urinating More Frequently • Thirsty • Constipated • The Chocolate Compromise • Bloated and Gassy • Heartburn • Cramps • Listening to Your Hormonal Symphony Orchestra

Concerns You May Have — 153

Touchy and Hypersensitive • Impatient with Husband • Feeling Dependent • Itchy Skin • Difficulty Sleeping • Bleeding and Spotting • Genetic Screening: If, When, and How Much? • My Pregnancy Journal: Second Month

Chapter 12: Third Month: Almost Showing   160

How Your Baby Is Growing, 9–12 weeks   160

Preventing Prematurity • Hearing Baby's Heartbeat

How You May Feel   162

Breasts Go Through a Growth Spurt • Clothing Doesn't Fit • Getting the
Support You Need: Choosing a Bra • Pelvic Discomforts Even Before You Start
to Show • Don't Worry, Be Happy

Concerns You May Have   164

Enjoying Sex while Pregnant • Chiropractic Care during Pregnancy • Fear of
Miscarriage • The Myth of the Deprived Man • My Pregnancy Journal: Third
Month

Chapter 13: Fourth Month: Feeling Better   174

How Your Baby Is Growing, 13–16 weeks   174

Feeling Your Uterus Grow

How You May Feel   175

Time to Tell? • Hello There! • Re-energized • Fewer Trips to the Bathroom
• Increased Vaginal Discharge • Bleeding Gums • Nosebleeds • Congestion

Concerns You May Have   179

Dizzy and Feeling Faint • Feeling Warmer • Skin Changes • Caring for Skin
during Pregnancy • Working while Pregnant • Telling Your Employer • How
to Best Negotiate Your Maternity Leave • What the Laws Allow • Resources
for Working Women's Rights • My Pregnancy Journal: Fourth Month

Chapter 14: Fifth Month: Obviously Pregnant   197

How Your Baby Is Growing, 17–20 weeks   197

How You May Feel   198

More Steady Emotionally • Enjoying the Perks of Being Pregnant • Overwhelmed
with Advice • Introspective and Meditative • Staying Near Your Nest • "Mommy
Brain" Begins • Feeling First Kicks

Concerns You May Have   **201**

Vision Changes • Unhappy Feet • Happy Hair and Nails • Belly Button Changes • Breast Changes • Not Feeling Motherly • Pregnant while Mothering Other Children — Help! • We're in This Together: Involving a Distant Dad • Girl or Boy? Do You Want to Know? • Testing for Gestational Diabetes • My Pregnancy Journal: Fifth Month

Chapter 15: Sixth Month: Feeling Baby Move   **217**

How Your Baby Is Growing, 21–25 weeks   **217**

How You May Feel   **218**

Enjoying More Kicks • Feeling Your Uterus "Move" • Need to Slow Down • Sleepier • New Aches and Pains • Leg Cramps • Numbness and Tingling in Your Hands • Shooting Pains in Your Lower Back and Legs • Ten Ways to Prevent Backache

Concerns You May Have   **225**

Enlarging Veins • Hemorrhoids • Leaking Urine • Abdominal Muscles Separating • Men: Feeling Pregnant • Traveling while Pregnant • Air Travel • Help! I'm Pregnant • Pregnancy Travel Records • Cruising while Pregnant • Taming Traveler's Diarrhea • Car Travel • Choosing a Childbirth Class That's Right for You • "Natural" Childbirth • Choosing a Hospital • Choosing a Birth Center • Choosing a Home Birth • Why Some Expectant Mothers Choose a Home Birth • My Pregnancy Journal: Sixth Month

Chapter 16: Seventh Month: Bigger and Loving It   **253**

How Your Baby Is Growing, 26–29 weeks   **253**

How You May Feel   **254**

More Curvy • The Pregnancy High • Resourceful • Forgetful • Heart Working Harder • Breathing for Two • Thirstier • More Swelling • Clumsy • More Baby Movements • Baby Hiccups

Concerns You May Have   **258**

Aching Hips and Back • Groin and Pelvic Pains • More Vaginal Discharge • More Practice Contractions • Enjoying Late-Pregnancy Sex • Worried about the What-Ifs • Will I Be a Good Enough Mother?

More Choices to Make 260

Choosing a Professional Labor Coach • Questions You May Have about Labor Coaches • Choosing a Pediatrician for Your Baby • Choosing the Right Medical Insurance for Your Baby • Cord Blood Banking • Composing Your Birth Wish • Why Are So Many Women Having Cesarean Births? • Seven Reasons for Needing a Cesarean • Our Birth Wishes • How to Increase Your Chances of a Vaginal Birth • Wanting a VBAC • Scheduled C-Section • Is Labor Good for Baby? • Healing after C-Section • Making the Best out of a C-Section • My Pregnancy Journal: Seventh Month

Chapter 17: Eighth Month: Almost There 288

How Your Baby Is Growing, 30–33 weeks 288

How You May Be Feeling 289

Impatient • Needing to Rest and Nest • Replaying a Previous Birth • Feeling Bigger • Stronger Practice Contractions • Stronger Kicks • Sleepless while Pregnant

Concerns You May Have 291

Managing Pain in Childbirth: Know Your Options • Pain Has a Purpose • Ten Pain Management Strategies That Work • Putting Childbirth Pain in Perspective • Hypnobirthing • Narcotic Pain Relievers • Epidural Anesthesia • Epi-Lite • Questions You May Have about the Safety of Epidurals • My Pregnancy Journal: Eighth Month

Chapter 18: The Hormonal Symphony of Birth 323

Grow-and-Prepare Hormones • Power-and-Progress Hormones • Relieve-and-Relax Hormones • Performance-Enhancing Hormones • Produce-Milk and Bond-with-Baby Hormones • The Next Movement of Labor: Baby Meets Mommy • The Encore: Birth Bonding • Supportive Birthcare Providers • The Less-Synchronous Symphony of a PharmaTech Birth • An Expert's Finale of Birth Music

Chapter 19: Ninth Month: This Is It! 338

How Your Baby Is Growing, 34–40 weeks 338

How Labor Hormones Work 339

How You May Feel   339

Ready! • Wanting to Get Back to "Normal" • More Need to Rest and Nest • Baby Dropping, Feeling Better — Sort of • More Pelvic Pressures • Feeling Different Kicks • Feeling Bigger and Off-Balance

Concerns You May Have   342

Continuing to Work • Packing and Preparing for Birth • Sleepless in the Homestretch • Small Changes in Weight • What to Do When You're "Overdue"

From Labor to Birth   346

Thirteen Ways to Help Your Labor Progress • Love Your Laborade • How Far Along Am I? • Working Out Your Best Birthing Positions • Have a Ball!

Stages of Labor and Birth   355

Prelabor: What You May Experience • Best Laborsaving Ideas and Devices • Labor Begins: How to Tell • The First Stage of Labor: Early Phase • The First Stage of Labor: Active Phase • When to Go to the Hospital or Birth Center • When You May Need Extra Help in a Vaginal Birth • Transition Phase of Labor • The Second Stage of Labor: Pushing Baby Out • The Third Stage of Labor: Delivery of the Placenta • My Pregnancy Journal: Ninth Month

Chapter 20: The Week After   382

How You May Feel   382

Thrilled • Overwhelmed • Need to Rest • Ups and Downs • "Beat Up" • Afterpains • Painful Perineum • Bleeding and Vaginal Discharge • Feeling Faint • Difficulty Urinating • Leaking Urine • Profuse Sweating • Constipation • Painful Hemorrhoids • Gas and Bloating • Feeding the Postpartum Mother • Making Milk for Your Baby: Breastfeeding Starter Tips

Concerns You May Have about Breastfeeding   389

Engorged Breasts • Sore Nipples • Tongue-Tie • Breastfeeding after Surgical Birth • Breastfeeding Special Needs Babies in Special Circumstances

How to Help Your Body Heal from Childbirth   393

Making the Transition into Motherhood   394

PART III: IF YOU HAVE A CHALLENGING PREGNANCY

Chapter 21: Special Pregnancies   *399*

Having a Baby after Age Thirty-Five • Having a Baby with Down
Syndrome • Genetic Testing • Mothering Multiples

Chapter 22: If You Have Medical Complications   *406*

Anemia • Bed Rest Prescribed • Eleven Top Tips to Make the Best of Your
Rest • Beta Strep Infection • Fifth Disease • Genital Herpes • Gestational
Diabetes • Type 1 Diabetes • HELLP Syndrome • Hepatitis B • High-Risk
Pregnancy • Hyperemesis Gravidarum • Incompetent Cervix • Intrauterine
Growth Restriction (IUGR) • Miscarriage: Fearing and Grieving • Placenta
Problems: Placenta Previa, Placenta Accreta, Placenta Abruptio • Preeclampsia
• Premature Labor: Birthing a Preterm Baby • Rh Incompatibility

Resources for a Healthier Pregnancy   *425*

Acknowledgments   *429*

Index   *431*

About the Authors   *445*

A Note to Pregnant Mothers: How We Birthed This Book, and How to Use It

Welcome to the Sears Parenting Library! Because pregnancy is one of the most important events in a mother's life, this could be the most important book you will read.

Assembling the right birth book team for you. In planning this book we interviewed expectant mothers, asking them, "What do you most expect from the authors of a book on pregnancy?" We found out that what they want most is authors with experience and credentials.

Naturally, readers want the advice of an experienced *mother*. We have just the person: Martha Sears, mother of eight (seven of whom she gave birth to), childbirth educator, and registered nurse. Martha has been there — and done that — a lot.

Next, expectant mothers want advice from an experienced obstetrician. So, our team includes Dr. Linda Holt, mother, obstetrician, University of Chicago professor of obstetrics, and birth attendant at some three thousand deliveries during her thirty-one years as an obstetrician.

The ultimate goal of a healthy pregnancy is a healthy baby, so we have Dr. William Sears, a pediatrician of forty years, former director of a university hospital newborn nursery, and specialist who has attended more than a thousand challenging births.

To complete this team, we have a certified, experienced midwife. Dr. BJ Snell, mother of two, has been a certified nurse midwife for twenty-five years and has experience delivering and caring for more than three thousand babies. We believe that she is one of the most credentialed and experienced midwives in America. We love having Dr. BJ's contribution to this book since midwives offer a balanced approach: they regard pregnancy not as a disease full of fear, but rather as a normal physiologic process.

What expectant mothers want to read. We also asked expectant mothers, "What do you most want to read in a pregnancy book?" They told us that they want the most up-to-date information on what they can do to enjoy a healthy pregnancy and deliver a healthy baby. So we begin this book with a strong focus on health tips and then follow with the usual month-by-month format of what you should expect on your way to having a baby.

And because mothers told us they really don't understand or appreciate the beautiful hormonal happenings going on inside their bodies while giving birth, we orchestrated a must-read section: "The Hormonal Symphony of Birth" (page 324).

Pregnancy is not the time for textbook-type reading. Mothers want to keep it simple and make it fun. As you will see, our goal is to make you smile on every page. We hope you enjoy our frequent "baby bubbles," as you imagine your little pregnancy coach inside nudging you with health tips.

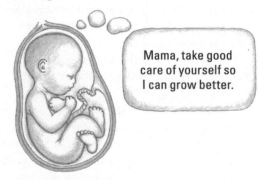

Finally, we asked obstetricians, "What type of pregnancy book do you most want your expectant mothers to read?" They replied, "A book that shows mothers how to better care for their pregnant bodies and increase their chances of having healthier pregnancies, easier deliveries, and healthier babies."

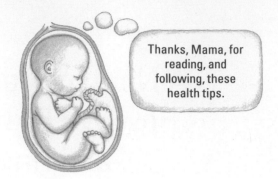

We begin our journey by taking you inside the womb to watch a baby grow. We show you what's happening inside your body and inside your baby, and tell you what you can do to increase the chances of your birth wish coming true: delivering a healthy baby.

Over the past ten years new research has revealed that the health habits of the mother, for better or worse, can influence not only the health of her newborn baby but the lifelong health habits of her adult child. In putting together our maternal health program, we wondered why so many books and childbirth classes had left out some of these new insights on what a mother could do to safeguard her child's health.

A common worry among authors is "We don't want to increase a mother's guilt by telling her that her pregnancy habits might harm her baby." We believe this is old-fashioned — and baby-unfriendly — thinking. In our experience, mothers want to have science-based health tips and tools showing them what they can do to increase their chances of being healthy and giving birth to a healthy baby. We have included solid science revealing the amazing biological connections between mother and baby — not to worry you, but rather to educate and empower you.

We are entering a new wave of better

birthing. During the first wave (from the 1960s to the 1980s), mothers became awake and aware and began to believe in their bodies' ability to *give* birth instead of someone else *taking* birth. The second wave occurred when birthing practices caused babies to come out via a different route: surgically instead of vaginally. The use of technology increased, the use of pharmacological births increased, and surgical birth rates tripled. In the current wave, mothers who understand the natural hormonal harmony of pregnancy and birth are "standing up" (back-birthing is what started this whole mess in the first place) for their right to physiological births instead of pharmacological births. We believe that the next twenty years will be the golden age of birthing, with more certified midwives and more certified birth centers adjacent to hospitals. This birth movement will be primarily directed by mothers who understand that their body is wired for the hormonal symphony of birth and choose birthcare providers and a birth place that enable them to conduct their own personal symphony of birth.

What expectant mothers don't want to read. Not only did we ask expectant mothers what they most wanted to read in a pregnancy book, we also asked what bothered them most when they read some of the popular pregnancy books. Their reply? A focus on all the things that can go wrong. We do address the "what ifs" of pregnancy and acknowledge that challenges can occur even for the most prepared and health-diligent mother. Throughout the book we discuss that even though things can go wrong, mothers can learn strategies to increase their chances

SHOW ME THE SCIENCE

With more and more medical studies appearing online, pregnant mothers are becoming scientifically savvy. Many of our "mom advisers" told us they want to read a pregnancy book based on scientific studies in addition to our professional experience. We listened. You will find "Science Says" boxes sprinkled throughout the text.

of giving birth to a healthy baby. We want this book to inform, not alarm; to empower expectant mothers, not worry them.

How to use this book. Since the 1997 publication of the popular guide *The Pregnancy Book: Month-By-Month, Everything You Need to Know* (William Sears and Martha Sears), new and exciting studies have proven that a mother's health habits not only have profound effects on her pregnancy but can greatly influence the intellectual, physical, and emotional development of her baby and child. For this reason, we have written *The Healthy Pregnancy Book* to replace that older book.

To help you get started, in Part I we explain eleven health tools you can use even before you get pregnant, and certainly during your pregnancy. While unforeseen circumstances may cause some pregnancies to be difficult and some babies to be less than perfectly healthy, we promise that using as many of these tools as possible will greatly increase your chances of having a healthy pregnancy and giving birth to a healthy baby.

After you have learned about — and begun practicing — your health plan, Part II will take you on a tour of the changes that occur in each month of your pregnancy, including information on why they occur and how you can influence them for the better. You will learn why you have certain feelings and how to handle them. In each chapter you will learn how your baby is growing that month and discover the marvelous changes going on inside of you — specifically, your health habits that influence the health of your baby.

In Part III, we list common complaints, illnesses, and other quirks that mothers may experience. We purposely put these at the end of the book because most mothers don't experience them. The last thing you need to read while you're pregnant is a description of what could go wrong. In fact, one of the top health tips of this book is to worry less during your pregnancy.

Let's get started on your healthy pregnancy! As you're reading the next few chapters, keep clearly in your mind the amazing opportunity and privilege you have to prepare your body and mind for the journey we call motherhood, from the moment of conception onward.

The Healthy Pregnancy Book

Planning to Become Pregnant:
Eleven Habits to Increase Your Chances

Give your baby the healthiest start possible: preconception planning is just what the doctor ordered. Is your body ready to birth a baby?

New insights into child development reveal that the healthier the mother is during her pregnancy, the healthier her baby is likely to be as an infant, child, and adult. Here's another incentive for you to start our Healthy Pregnancy Plan — now! There is a high correlation between mother's prenatal health and her ability to conceive. The sooner you start to follow the health tips in our book, the sooner you are likely to conceive.

WHY YOU SHOULDN'T WAIT TO GET PREGNANT

If you wait for the "perfect time" to get pregnant, you're less likely to get pregnant. From our experience, and after studying what science says about fertility, we have concluded that waiting is risky for the following reasons:

- According to the American Society for Reproductive Medicine, infertility rates increase with age, from less than 10 percent for women in their twenties to nearly 20 percent for women in their thirties, and 30 percent for women in their forties.

- The chance of miscarriage nearly doubles from age twenty to forty.

- Women who spend their most fertile years using chemical contraception methods that interfere with their natural hormones are more likely to have problems conceiving later on.

- The longer you wait, the harder and more complicated your pregnancy is likely to be.

- The longer you wait, the higher your chances of birthing a baby with a genetic abnormality.

In his book *The Fertility Guide,* Dr. Walter Willett, renowned professor of medicine and chairman of the Department of Nutrition at the Harvard School of Public Health, emphasizes that the longer a couple waits to have a child, the greater their chances of fertility problems.

Women expecting to get pregnant underestimate the overwhelming changes that will occur in their minds and bodies when they become pregnant. Every organ system will change. Every hormone will change. Your body will work harder than it ever has, 24/7. Take a look at one organ: your heart. When you are pregnant, your blood volume increases by 50 percent, and your heart has to work that much harder to nourish you and that growing little person inside. The awesome thing is that a woman's body is designed to pull that off, gradually and gracefully.

Are you fit for this feat? Waiting to get fit until you get pregnant is unfit timing. That's when your energy reserves will be used up by your growing baby, so it's the hardest possible time to make major lifestyle and habit changes. *Now* is the time to make healthier choices. Here's our preparing-for-pregnancy health plan:

1. Is Your Body Fit to Birth a Baby?

Are there L.E.A.N. (**l**ifestyle, **e**xercise, **a**ttitude, and **n**utrition) issues that need to be resolved, or at least worked on, before you get pregnant?

❑ Do you have dietary habits that may affect your fertility and your likelihood of having a healthy pregnancy?

❑ Are you taking medications that need to be tapered or changed?

❑ Do you have a chronic illness that needs to be better controlled, such as diabetes?

❑ Do you have harmful lifestyle habits that could affect fertility and pregnancy? (See page 88.)

❑ Do you have emotional issues that need to be stabilized before the hormonal havoc begins? (See page 73.)

❑ Do you have harmful habits, such as the use of illegal drugs, tobacco, or excessive alcohol, that need to be handled before becoming pregnant? (See page 88.)

❑ Are you using chemical birth control? If so, it's time to toss the pills. Discuss with your healthcare provider how to get off them immediately and switch over to natural family planning to learn about your fertility peaks. It's important to give your body at least three months before conceiving so that the effects of chemical contraception can wear off.

It's not necessary to wait for the best time, best lifestyle, best health to get pregnant. Many mothers with less-than-ideal lifestyles and severe chronic illnesses have gone on to birth healthy babies. Yet, the better you care for yourself now, the better your baby-growing and baby-birthing are likely to be.

2. Make Health Your Hobby

Pregnancy may just be the motivation you need to get off the couch, visit the produce section of the supermarket, eat in and not out, and do all the other good things for your body that your mother preached and medical talk shows highlight. Put up this reminder throughout your home and workplace:

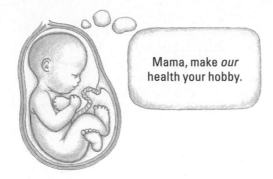

Mama, make *our* health your hobby.

3. Schedule a Preconception Checkup

Consider having a thorough checkup with either your healthcare provider or a newly selected OB/GYN and/or midwife. Besides a general physical examination, your healthcare provider will:

- Review your medical history and family genetics history to see whether there are issues that might affect your pregnancy. Come prepared with your medical and family history.

- Review previous miscarriages or pregnancy-attempt history for clues on how to increase your chances of conception and birthing this time.

- Order a complete profile of laboratory tests to be sure you enter pregnancy with a stable biochemistry and an optimal balance of hormones.

- Give you advice on getting a chronic condition under control. Unless advised by your healthcare provider, don't let a chronic illness — such as an autoimmune disease, diabetes, or a mood disorder — put you off from

getting pregnant. Often the hormonal and biochemical changes that take place in a pregnant woman's body become therapeutic for existing ailments, leading some women to conclude: "My health was never better once I became pregnant!"

- Check your immunizations. Your healthcare provider may do various antibody titers to see whether you need boosters. Be sure to bring your immunization record, especially if you have had any immunizations in the past ten years. (See "Getting Vaccines Safely While Pregnant" on our website: AskDrSears.com/topics/vaccines.)

Not only is a checkup by your medical doctor necessary for proper preconception planning, but one by your dentist is important, too. You want to enter pregnancy with healthy gums and healthy teeth for two reasons: Pregnancy hormones are going to mess with your mouth anyway, making already sore gums sorer. And gingivitis, or periodontal disease, can cause harmful inflammatory biochemicals and germs to enter your bloodstream and perhaps harm your pregnancy.

4. Preload Your Body with Nutrients

Now is the time to eat more of what you and your little one need and less of what you don't. Besides preloading with prenatal supplements (see "How to Choose the Prenatal Supplement That's Right for You" on page 23), eat more foods containing the nourishing nine:

- Omega-3 fats

- Folic acid

- Iron

- Calcium

- Vitamin B$_{12}$

- Vitamin D

- Vitamin C

- Zinc

- Iodine

(See page 48 to learn why you and baby need more of these nutrients, and which foods are highest in them.)

The reason we call this "preloading" is because now is when you can best stomach dietary changes. Those early pregnancy months of queasiness and picky eating are not the most tummy-friendly time to make significant dietary changes. So, store up those needed nutrients now.

5. Eat More of the Twelve Pregnancy Superfoods

In chapter 2, you'll learn what you should eat more of while you're planning to become pregnant and why. In a nutshell, you will now be eating, very simply, the Real Food Diet. You will need to become a "picky eater," selecting food based on quality and nutrient density — that is, the most nutrition in the smallest volume. This may be the first time in your life that you have to be scientifically selective about what you eat. Certainly this does not mean that you have to take all the fun out of eating and make it a mathematical exercise. In fact, calorie counting is just what the pregnancy doctor *doesn't* order. It's quality of calories rather than quantity that's important. In chapter 3 you will learn to eat a right-fat, right-carb diet rather than a low-fat, low-carb diet.

Reshape your tastes. Pre-pregnancy is the time to begin getting your body accustomed to the foods you and your baby need, not just those you want. Try this exercise in taste reshaping: Eat a diet of primarily the twelve pregnancy foods. Follow the "how to eat" and "what to eat" healthy pregnancy tips in chapters 2 and 3 at least 90 percent of the time. Over a few months you will experience metabolic reprogramming (simply put, taste reshaping), in which your food cravings and gut feelings change toward preferring real food over fake food. Then, by the time sperm meets egg and baby starts growing, your body is already craving those foods and a way of eating that is not only friendly to your more selective intestines but provides the best "grow foods" for your baby. It's as if that little motivator inside continues to prompt you to eat as you should have been eating all along anyway.

6. Get Used to Grazing

In chapter 2 you'll discover the three magic words of pregnancy cuisine: *graze, sip,* and *dip.* This way of eating is healthiest for people at all ages and stages, but is especially gut-perfect during pregnancy.

7. Get Lean

"Lean" means having the right amount of body fat for your body type, and the right amount of body fat for your health needs and those of your baby. "Lean" does not mean skinny. In fact, a woman needs a certain amount of body fat to produce the hormones that help her ovulate. This is why teen athletes, such as gymnasts, often have delayed menstruation: they have too little body fat.

On the other hand, too much body fat increases your chances of complications during pregnancy (see page 53), in addition to lowering your chances of getting pregnant in the first place. Getting your weight under control increases your chances of getting pregnant and lowers your chances of having a complicated pregnancy, gestational diabetes, and an unhealthy newborn. (See page 54 for more on optimal weight control during pregnancy and page 58 for our L.E.A.N. Expectations Program.)

8. Go Green to Get Pregnant

The cleaner and greener the air you breathe, the food you eat, the lotions you use, and even the lipstick you wear, the greater your chances of conceiving and birthing a healthy baby. Begin going green now to prepare for growing baby in a "green" house. (See chapter 8 for tips and strategies on how to go green during pregnancy. To increase your motivation for going green, turn to page 18 to read about recent scientific breakthroughs showing how a green environment increases your chances of growing a healthy baby.)

9. Don't Worry, Get Pregnant!

If you suffer from stress or mood instabilities, now is the time to get help and get stable. In chapter 6 you will learn about new research showing that unborn babies and mommies share the hormonal effects triggered by thoughts, for better or worse. Learning natural stressbusters (see page 75) is especially important if you are now on mood-altering medications, many of which are not safe to take while pregnant.

> ### PRACTICE THE PILLS-SKILLS MINDSET
>
> If you are the type of patient who enters the doctor's office with a problem and opens with, "Doctor, what can I *take?*" now is the time to change your mindset to "Doctor, what can I *do?*" This means developing self-help skills that are safer for you and baby than pills. On page 59 you will learn that your body is like a giant walking pharmacy, and you can make your own "internal medicines," dispensed in the right dose at the right time, without harmful side effects. Of course, don't toss the pills without first discussing safe medication weaning with your doctor, since many medications, especially mood mellowers, blood sugar regulators, and blood pressure regulators, need to be gradually tapered.

10. Move!

If you're habitually sedentary and planning to get pregnant, now is the time to get moving. It is certainly easier to be mobile now than when you're heavily pregnant and off-balance. We're often surprised to learn how few people really understand the power of movement to help you make your own internal medicines (see page 59 for more on this). The right exercise program for you is one that you will stick to. While you're still in the pregnancy planning stage, start an exercise routine that helps you feel so good you'll want to continue it.

11. *"We're* Pregnant!"

Long before you wow your mate with that little blue line on the pregnancy test, keep in mind that your baby needs happy parents. While making a baby, growing a baby, and then parenting a baby can strengthen a marriage, the sooner your partner learns to share the responsibility, the better. It's important for him to make preconception lifestyle changes with you, especially if he has habits like smoking, excessive drinking, or illegal drug use. Secondhand smoke, for instance, can be nearly as harmful to baby as mommy's own smoking — for example, it doubles the risk of sudden infant death syndrome (SIDS).

Following these strategies to increase your chances of getting pregnant will hopefully reward you with one of the greatest privileges of womanhood — growing a human being. In the following chapters you will learn habits that will increase your chances of having a healthy pregnancy and birthing a healthy baby.

I

The Healthy Pregnancy Plan

What's going on in there? Every mother wonders how her habits affect how her baby is growing. Once upon a time it was thought that a baby in the womb grew according to a predetermined genetic blueprint, and as long as a mother took reasonably good care of herself, her baby would grow according to that genetic blueprint. Genes were believed to be so powerful that they determined growth, and that there was not much that nurturing could change. In other words, it was thought that nature was much more important than nurture in regards to prenatal development.

New research shows that how the genes behave and how they affect your baby's growth, for better or worse, are very much influenced by what a mother eats and does, and even by her level of unresolved stress. And research in the new field of epigenetics shows that a baby's womb environment can set up a baby for health, or disease, for the rest of her life. Does diabetes or heart disease begin in the womb?

You are your baby's first filter. The brain grows the fastest during pregnancy, especially during the last three months, and it is the organ most susceptible to toxins. The mother, as well as the placenta, acts as a filter for these toxins. What goes into your mouth, your gut, even possibly your thoughts conceivably could pass into your baby. In this section, you'll learn how this happens. Following are the nine top tips for a healthy pregnancy and baby:

1. Learn about the fetal effect.
2. Graze for good health.
3. Eat the top twelve pregnancy superfoods.
4. Gain the weight that's right for you.
5. Exercise right for two.
6. Don't worry, be pregnant.
7. Sleep peacefully.
8. Go green; avoid environmental pollutants.
9. Practice the pills-and-skills model of self-care.

1

Get Motivated to Get Healthy

For many mothers, pregnancy is just the jump start they need to finally take up the health habits they've been putting off. Pregnant mothers who follow our Healthy Pregnancy Plan are more likely to:

- Enjoy more comfortable pregnancies

- Have their babies go to term

- Have an easier transition into parenthood

- Have babies who are smarter

- Have babies who are healthier

- Become emotionally and physically healthier themselves

THE FETAL EFFECT

This is a phrase we coined in our medical practices to help an expectant mother appreciate the healthful effects her baby feels because of the healthful habits she practices. Our goal in this book is to help you give your growing baby the best possible "fetal effect."

Our health topics are intended to show you that pregnancy is a privilege that enables you to translate what you do for yourself over nine months into increasing your chances of delivering a healthy baby who grows into a healthy child and adult. After reading Part I, we want you to be both motivated to make these changes and empowered with the tools to do so.

F.O.O.D. FOR THOUGHT

Fetal origins of diseases — F.O.O.D. — is the theme of this chapter. Once upon a time preventive medicine pundits preached: "Adult diseases begin in childhood. Let's raise healthier children." New insights reveal that preventive medicine needs to go one step earlier — fetushood. This new science of F.O.O.D. teaches that a healthy society begins with healthy pregnant mothers. The healthier the mother during her pregnancy, the more likely her baby will be born with a healthy blueprint for life.

The "fetal origins" belief proposes that disturbances in fetal nutrition and endocrine balance can result in permanent changes in organ structure, physiology, and metabolism, which can predispose these babies to cardiovascular, metabolic, and endocrine disease in adult life. This "programming" means that a chemical insult in a sensitive or critical period of development can have long-term effects. The fetal origin of cardiovascular disease, especially high blood pressure, seems to present the strongest case. The endothelium — the lining of the blood vessels — is most affected, causing these kids to grow up with stiffer arteries.

Opponents of the fetal origin theory counter that lifestyle and diet influences after birth may account for these differences. Yet, in analyzing the data, researchers have taken this theory into consideration and concluded that the fetal origin effect is still an important factor. On the other hand, there is no question that postnatal lifestyle and diet can greatly lower the magnitude of any fetal programming effects. Studies have shown that animals that suffer from both an unhealthy intrauterine and postnatal health environment experience a double whammy. Children who have both of these unhealthy starts in life are even more prone to adult diseases than if they had just one or the other.

SCIENCE SAYS: A HEALTHIER WOMB ENVIRONMENT LEADS TO A HEALTHIER ADULT LIFE

Numerous studies have validated the fetal origin theory that nearly every system can be affected by the pregnant mother's health habits:

- Cardiovascular system: impaired endothelial function and stiffness of arteries, which predisposes these arteries to high blood pressure in adults

- Endocrine system: unstable insulin and blood sugar metabolism

- Reproductive system: increased incidence of polycystic ovarian syndrome

- Skeletal system: reduced bone mineral content

- Digestive system: problems with liver metabolism, such as cholesterol abnormalities

- Immune system: allergies and "itis" illnesses

How F.O.O.D. Happens

The most common example of how a mother's prenatal habits can cause lasting health changes in her baby is that excess baby fat becomes excess adult fat. If a baby in utero is not given enough of the right nutrients or is exposed to too much of the wrong nutrients, a strong adaptation mechanism clicks in so that baby's tissues are programmed to conserve sugar and fat. That baby is born a calorie storer instead of a calorie burner, which predisposes the child and adult to obesity.

Blame baby's brain. Remember, the brain is the fastest growing and most energy-consuming organ of the developing baby. It gets first dibs on fetal nutrition. If there isn't enough to satisfy the brain, it steals the nutrients from other organs, such as the liver, resulting in fetal programming of the liver to have abnormal metabolism.

It's more than just genetics. It was once thought that a baby's birth weight was determined primarily by genes. Fetal origin researchers argue that nutrition may have an even more influential role than genes. A clue to the predominant role of intrauterine nutrition over genetic influence came from studies in which a fertilized egg from a donor mother was transferred into a surrogate mother's uterus. It was found that the intrauterine health and nutrition of the recipient, or birth mother, had more of an influence on baby's later development than the genes from the donor mother. What goes on in the womb is at least as important to the baby's predisposition to disease as genes are.

One of the earliest clues to F.O.O.D. was the finding that during World War II, women who were exposed to famine tended to give birth to babies who had a higher incidence of abnormalities in glucose metabolism as adults. This is one of the first studies to downgrade the baby-as-a-perfect-parasite theory — that when there isn't enough nutrition to go around, baby gets enough and mother suffers. The truth is, the health of both mother and baby suffer.

Another possible explanation for these long-term effects is that if babies don't get the right nutrition in the womb, some protective switch clicks on so that their tissues lower their demand for nutrition, with two consequences: babies are born undernourished, and their tissues are programmed not to get the most out of nutrition for the rest of their lives, so they tend to remain underdeveloped. It's almost as if their tissues are programmed to survive, but not thrive, with fewer nutrients. While the majority of babies can catch up in growth with good nutrition after birth, some may still have that life-long tendency to not take advantage of available nutrients.

Undernutrition at certain times during intrauterine development is more likely to affect the organs that have their highest growth spurt during that time. For example, a critical period for reproductive organs occurs early in pregnancy, yet the critical period for kidney development occurs later, between twenty-six and thirty-four weeks. The good news is that the fetal demand for nutrients is lowest in early pregnancy, when mother's gastrointestinal upsets may cause her to be a picky eater.

The grandchildren effect. Some research has even suggested that the fetal effect can continue on for successive generations, from undernourished mother to undernourished baby and so on. So, expectant moms, give your grandchildren a healthy head start.

Get into the Genes You Are Growing

Let's go into the genes of a growing baby and learn how F.O.O.D. works. Every baby's genes have "family quirks," such as a genetic tendency for diabetes. This quirk may be thought of as a dial on the genes. Mother's L.E.A.N. (lifestyle, exercise, attitude, nutrition) habits while pregnant can either turn up this dial and increase the tendency for the child to later become diabetic, or turn down the dial and reduce the child's risk even into adulthood. How does what happens in fetushood affect health in adulthood? Read on.

You are what you eat—and so is baby. You've heard the nutrition wisdom "You are what you eat." A new and revealing field called *nutrigenetics* is proving what mothers have long suspected: food affects the genes. Here's how. Suppose your baby, through absolutely no

DIABETES GENE

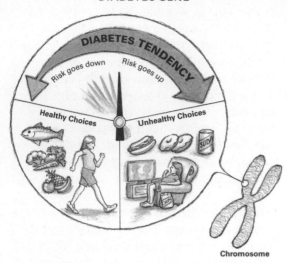

Chromosome

decrease her child's later tendency toward diabetes. Say a mother, through unwise L.E.A.N. habits, has a high average blood sugar and develops gestational diabetes. If unchecked, her baby's blood-sugar–regulating genetic machinery is dialed up, increasing his tendency toward high blood sugar and consequent diabetes. This new science matches patterns we are now seeing. Gestational diabetes is on the rise. Childhood and adult diabetes are on the rise. Here's a shocker: the Centers for Disease Control and Prevention (CDC) predicts that unless American families change the way they eat and live, one-third of children are destined to become diabetic. Is that scary stat enough to get expectant mothers to toss the soda and begin exercising?

fault of yours, is carrying genes for diabetes or heart disease. The good news is that whether those genes are turned on ("expressed") or turned off is partially under your control. We all have genetic on/off switches. Our diet and lifestyle can play a major part in whether the genetic switch is flipped.

Keep in mind that the genes of rapidly multiplying cells and growing tissues (the unborn baby's cells multiply and tissues grow faster than at any other time in her life) are more affected by health habits than adult tissues.

What Science Says

F.O.O.D. science is in its infancy, but here are some fascinating early results of what science suspects:

The diabetes dial. Mother's blood sugar levels during pregnancy can increase or

---

SCIENCE SAYS: DIABETES BEGINS IN THE WOMB

Fetal undernutrition can lead to a reduced number of insulin-making beta cells in the pancreas, leading to what we call the diabetes effect. Furthermore, chronically high insulin from mother's overeating seems to program baby's developing body to be born with higher insulin and blood sugar levels, increasing the chances of baby becoming diabetic. An unfortunate new fact of American life is that many babies are born prediabetic.

The heart disease dial. Want to help your baby-child-adult build a healthier heart? Consider this: the epidemic of high blood pressure (currently afflicting approximately 25 percent of adults) can begin in the womb. What causes most high blood pressure is low arterial elasticity, cardiology-speak for how flexible the arteries are. Stiff arteries lead to higher blood pressure. Persistent high blood pressure weakens the heart, which has to pump blood more forcibly into stiffer arteries. If a mother's diet is healthy, the nutritional building blocks that travel from the placenta into baby's developing arteries can foster the growth of more elastic arteries, which increases baby's chances of having a stronger, longer-lasting heart.

The cancer dial. If a pregnant mother is undernourished, her baby is more likely to be born premature or "small for date," meaning that his organs are smaller than they should be for his maturity. The undernourished baby enters the world metabolically different from an optimally nourished infant. Back to those metabolic dials: In order to enjoy "catch-up" growth, baby's growth hormone is dialed up, enabling him to grow faster. Sounds good? Not so fast. The increased growth hormone, called IGF-1 (insulin growth factor 1), has a tendency to stay high instead of automatically getting lower after catch-up growth happens. A sustained higher blood level of IGF-1 increases a child's chances of developing adult diseases such as diabetes, cardiovascular disease, and even cancer.

Cancer cells develop when cells get their genetic code mixed up and keep growing out of control. Healthy cells have a built-in genetic timer that tells them to grow and multiply and then self-destruct to make room for younger, healthier cells. IGF-1 is like a cell-growth fertilizer. When it stays too high for too long, it can disturb the normal cell replication process, increasing a cell's chance of becoming a cancer cell.

The allergy dial. The United States is seeing an epidemic of food allergies and "itis" illnesses: arthritis, bronchitis, colitis, dermatitis, and so on. Could there be a F.O.O.D. relationship to allergies and inflammatory conditions? We believe there is. Perhaps this epidemic is due to a hypersensitive immune system. When a baby's developing immune system is presented with a lot of chemical substances, the immature immune system has to make a judgment: Is this "natural" and okay for the body, and therefore we'll let it alone? Or, is it harmful or foreign to the body and therefore we'll attack it? A baby's immune system is easily confused, especially if overloaded with these foreign invaders, and can't always make the wisest decision. So, baby may be born with a supersensitive immune system that has trouble distinguishing between foods and other chemicals that are good or bad for the body, and it winds up attacking some of the body's own tissues. This wrongly programmed immune system can cause babies and children to grow up with an increased tendency to the "itises."

The metabolism dial. Not surprisingly, if a mother has a healthy metabolism, her baby has a greater chance of having a healthier metabolism. This is called fetal metabolic programming. If, however, Mom is a metabolic mess, with blood sugar swings and unhealthy fat metabolism, baby begins life with a higher risk of suffering metabolic difficulties in controlling weight, blood sugar, cholesterol, and appetite. Clues to this fetal effect come from studies revealing that young animals fed a junk-fat diet grow up to show abnormalities in cholesterol metabolism and in insulin receptor sites on the cell membrane, causing them to be more likely to develop type II diabetes. This metabolic programming, for better or worse, is evident in childhood obesity. If a mother gains excessive fat during pregnancy, her baby is predisposed to a lifelong struggle with weight control.

Does F.O.O.D. affect mood? Not only can physical illnesses originate in the womb, so might mental illness. Theoretically, chronic, unresolved high levels of maternal anxiety hormones may turn up baby's stress-hormone regulating dial. As a result, baby could enter the world with dialed-up difficulties in managing mood-mellowing hormones. Researchers are divided on this "worry too much" fetal effect. Some believe the placenta can disassemble stress hormones that reach excessively high levels, thus shielding baby from the physical and psychological stresses of the outside world. Other researchers believe an undernourished placenta may be unable to metabolically turn down excess stress hormones, such as cortisol.

A word of caution: remember, this science is still young and imperfect. Preliminary studies suggest a statistically increased risk, not a life sentence to mental strain. A child's body is very resilient. Even kids who had a less than healthy womb environment can grow up to be healthy adults. L.E.A.N. habits after birth can usually lessen or even overcome an unhealthy fetushood. But it makes sense to do your best to give your baby the best metabolic start from the beginning — in utero.

PLACENTA POWER — NOT SO PERFECT

The placenta is a remarkable organ that provides a connection between the mother and her developing baby. Just like the baby, the placenta needs nurturing so that it can provide the best environment for the growing baby. The old and unscientific teaching was that the placenta is a perfect filter and that baby nestles securely in mother's womb protected from harmful chemicals in the atmosphere and pollutants in food. New insights into the mother-baby hormonal connection show that much of what's in the air mother breathes, the food she eats, and the habits she has in some large or small way pass through into baby.

This new research calls into question the concept that the womb is a perfect hiding place from the health hazards of the world.

How does maternal nutrition in pregnancy relate to placental and therefore fetal growth? The conclusion from some studies was that a high-carbohydrate, low-protein diet in early pregnancy can lead to lower placental growth and lower birth weight. Studies show that the higher the amount of protein in a mother's diet, the higher the placental weight. Empower yourself with the tools necessary to make your womb a healthier environment for baby.

WHY BABIES ARE VULNERABLE

There's something going on in there that makes a baby's growing tissues more vulnerable to toxins in the blood. In the first trimester, your baby has lots of stem cells, which have the potential to change into cells specific to the different organs, like the heart, lungs, and brain. These multitasking cells are highly vulnerable to hormone disrupters, or biomutagens. As the name biomutagen implies, these chemicals can change the biological direction that stem cells take, so that development of, say, a certain organ may not fully take place, resulting in a cleft palate, only one kidney, or a missing chamber in the heart, for example.

Babies' brains are more vulnerable. Because the brain is the most vulnerable organ in the body, nature has provided the blood-brain barrier, a protective layer of cells strategically located between blood vessels and brain tissue. That's the good news. The bad news is that the blood-brain barrier is underdeveloped in babies. In fact, a growing number of pediatricians and infant behavior specialists suspect that this is one of the reasons that learning and behavior problems, such as ADD (attention deficit disorder) and a lot of other "Ds," have been shown to begin during fetushood. In addition to a "leaky" blood-brain barrier, other quirks within baby's growing brain can make it more vulnerable to food chemicals collectively known as neurotoxins.

Your baby's body and brain are only as healthy as each cell in them. The cell membrane, especially the brain cell membrane of growing tissues, is like a flexible bag designed to protect all the energy and growth structures, such as genes, inside the cell. Nutrients and chemicals from the food mother eats that pass into baby's blood through the placenta seep through these cell membranes and feed the genes and the microscopic "energy storage batteries," or mitochondria, inside the cell.

A healthy cell membrane has a biochemical perk called selective permeability, meaning that it lets in the nutrients the cell needs and keeps out the harmful stuff. A cell membrane can be damaged by undernourishment or by an overdose of neurotoxins, or what preventive-medicine specialist and neurosurgeon Dr. Russell Blaylock calls excitotoxins.

Baby's garbage disposal system is underdeveloped. Toxins that get into the blood are normally filtered by the liver and excreted by the kidneys. Yet the fetal liver and kidneys, baby's main garbage-disposal organs, are immature, which can allow toxins to build up to harmful levels.

Babies have more fat. Babies have proportionally more body fat than adults, and pesticides and other harmful chemicals are stored mainly in fat tissue.

Growing tissues are more vulnerable. The genetic machinery of rapidly growing and dividing cells, which happens fastest in the womb, is more vulnerable to the possible effects of toxins.

Chemicals are never proven safe for babies. Many of the chemicals added to the food you eat and the household supplies you use have never been proven safe for babies. If only there were a trusted government label on additives, such as SPS — scientifically proven safe. The best government agencies can do is to give their stamp of approval on chemicals as GRAS — **g**enerally **r**ecognized **as s**afe. Notice that even government testing agencies hedge by saying "generally," which you could interpret as "we're not really sure." The chemical in question is usually tested on rats. If an acceptable percentage of the rats survive and don't get sick, this chemical can get GRAS approval. Government watchdog agencies operate on the principle of "maximum acceptable levels," estimates that are based upon what might harm adults. For obvious reasons, no studies have been done to prove that they are safe on babies in the womb. To translate adult studies into "OK for baby" conclusions is unscientific and unsafe.

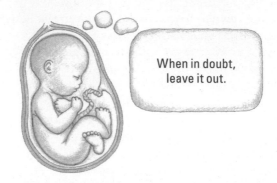

When in doubt, leave it out.

SCIENTISTS DETECT CHEMICALS IN THE CORD

Once upon a time it was thought that the placenta provided the perfect hiding place from environmental pollutants. Research continues to expose this myth. How many food and environmental chemicals actually do cross the placenta and get into baby? A lot!

- A 2004 study of ten babies detected 232 possibly toxic chemicals in their cord blood.

- An analysis of the cord blood in ten infants born between 2007 and 2008 revealed an average of 200 toxic environmental pollutants, including bisphenol A (BPA) used in some plastics, polychlorinated biphenyls (PCBs), and perfluorochemicals (PFCs) used on nonstick and stain-resistant surfaces.

- A 2009 study of the maternal and cord blood of sixty-two mother-infant pairs found that the higher the mother's blood levels of potentially toxic chemicals, the higher the levels in the cord blood of their newborns.

- A 2011 study of thirty pregnant women revealed the presence of chemicals used in GMO plant production in their baby's cord blood.

- A 2011 study analyzing data from the CDC showed that the pregnant women studied had at least eight types of toxic chemicals in their urine.

Researchers conclude that while the placenta may detoxify some chemicals by binding them so they can't cross into baby's circulation, they are concerned that an overworked placenta may lead to it underperforming as a baby growth–promoting and baby-protecting organ.

HOW TO BUILD A BRIGHTER BABY BRAIN

Research shows that the better a woman takes care of herself during pregnancy, the better her baby's brain is likely to develop. Ponder these brain facts every expectant mother must know:

- Above all other organs, your baby's growing brain is most affected, for better or worse, by the health habits you have, especially the food you eat.

- By the third month of pregnancy, baby's growing brain is using 70 percent of the food energy that goes through your placenta into baby.

- Your baby's brain grows fastest (it more than triples in size) in the last three months of pregnancy.

- Research on experimental animals shows that mother animals whose diets were deficient in the brain-building fats (discussed on page 29) were more likely to deliver offspring with smaller brains.

- The unborn baby's brain gets first dibs on nutrition, even when mother's diet may be insufficient. Pediatricians have observed that even in babies with low birth weights, the head size is disproportionally larger than the rest of the body, as if the most important organ, the brain, steals nutrition from the less important ones, especially during these critical windows of opportunity. It's as if the brain says to the muscle, "You can put on more muscle at any time in your life, but I need the nutrition now!"

- Baby's brain is 60 percent fat, which is why you need to eat a right-fat diet, not a low-fat diet during pregnancy (read more about the right fats on page 33).

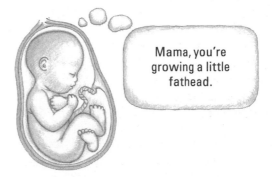

Mama, you're growing a little fathead.

- The fetal brain can grow as many as 250,000 nerve cells each minute. Seventy percent of the total number of brain cells that will be present throughout life are there before birth. At six weeks the fetus's developing brain is almost as big as the rest of the baby's body. By birth your baby's brain will have grown around 100 billion neurons, or nerve cells, and each one connects with thousands of other neurons. Each of these brain cells grows thousands of tiny branches that connect with the branches of other nerve cells. In a nutshell, building a brighter baby brain means helping baby's brain make the right connections.

What helps build brain cells and connections? How and what you eat, which you will learn about in the next two chapters.

2

How to Eat: Graze, Sip, and Dip

Intestinal and hormonal changes during pregnancy can make it a challenge to get the nutrition you and baby need. A growing baby pressing on an already queasy tummy may change the way you eat. Try these simple tips: graze, sip, and dip.

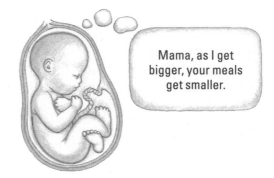

Mama, as I get bigger, your meals get smaller.

WHY GRAZING IS GREAT

Grazing is good for Mommy and baby. Many mothers find that as their pregnancy progresses, a way to satisfy the "always hungry" feeling is to nibble throughout the day. You may find that you don't have to make a conscious decision to become a grazer — your body naturally prompts you. As part of this mysterious internal wisdom of the body, your gut brain will start talking to your head brain, advising you what foods are most friendly to your increasingly sensitive digestive system, and how much and how often to eat. Here's why grazing is good for you and your baby:

It relieves reflux. Your growing uterus pushes on an expanding stomach, which pushes acids up into a sensitive esophagus, contributing to "pregnancy heartburn," especially after a big

meal. (Learn more about heartburn on page 23.) You will soon find that there is less room in your stomach for big meals.

It relieves constipation. When you wolf down a huge meal, a large amount of undigested food stays in the intestines, leading to indigestion and constipation. You will find your gut brain talking to you more during pregnancy, as if to say "Don't feed me so much so fast or I will have to work too hard!"

I tended to be a fast eater. To slow down my eating while pregnant, I retired the fork and used chopsticks, which also forced me to take smaller bites.

Eating for two means eating twice as well, not twice as much. When we mention this

OUR RULE OF TWOS

- Eat *twice* as often.

- Eat *half* as much at a time.

- Chew *twice* as long.

- Take *twice* the time to dine.

very simple yet practical rule of thumb for eating while pregnant, mothers in our medical practice react: "Oh, that's so simple. It makes sense. I can do that." With grazing, the intestinal tract does more work at the top end, which saves discomfort at the lower end, the one most affected by your enlarging uterus. Another grazing perk: it reduces the chance of hemorrhoids.

It steadies blood sugar. One of the reasons you will have the urge to nibble constantly is that there are days that you should. A steady blood sugar leads to steadier moods, which are usually a bit out of balance during pregnancy. (See page 60 for why steady blood sugar is important for baby's health.)

It helps keep you lean. Another pregnancy perk of grazing is that you tend to gain less excess body fat. Obesity researchers have long noticed that grazers tend to be leaner than gorgers. The reason seems to be that grazers can burn more calories.

THE HORMONAL HARMONY OF PREGNANCY

During your pregnancy you'll get tired of hearing everything blamed on hormones, yet they are the culprit of so much. At no time in your life will your hormones be in such a state of flux. Hormones are biochemical messengers that travel all over your body to give instructions. As your baby and your body change, your hormones change to meet those growing needs.

Knowing how to achieve hormonal harmony is important for maintaining a healthy pregnancy. Imagine that your hormones are players in a symphony orchestra. During pregnancy, these players are called upon to perform at their best. Insulin is the master hormone and the conductor of this symphony orchestra. When your insulin is stable, the other hormones are in tune. As a result, beautiful music, or a feeling of well-being, occurs during your pregnancy.

Exaggerated fluctuations of insulin are under your control. The more stable your insulin levels, the more stable your moods and weight gain. Insulin is a fat-storage hormone. If it is too high, as it is when you gorge (especially on junk sugar foods), it prompts your body to store the extra calories you consume as excess fat. Continual oversecretion of insulin, mainly from unsteady blood sugar, is a common cause of gestational diabetes.

What's good for Mommy is also good for baby. Remember that "diabetes dial" on your baby's genes you learned about on page 14? Hormonal harmony helps baby's maturing endocrine system achieve its own hormonal harmony and lowers the risk of baby becoming diabetic as she gets older. By keeping blood sugar stable, grazing on good foods helps your endocrine system, and your baby's, play harmonious music. (See "Listening to Your Hormonal Symphony Orchestra," page 152.)

SNACK SMART

During pregnancy, a smart snack is one that contains at least 3 grams of fiber, 3 grams of protein, and healthy fats. It should not contain antinutrients, such as high-fructose corn syrup, artificial dyes and colorings, and unhealthy additives. Try these smart snack suggestions:

- Baby carrots dipped in hummus

- Apple slices dipped in peanut butter

- Whole-grain cereal with yogurt

- String cheese and a piece of fruit

- Cottage cheese and fruit

- Pita bread spread with hummus

- Rice cakes with peanut butter and banana

- Parmesan cheese melted on a slice of whole-grain bread

- Celery sticks with peanut butter

- Cherry tomatoes with cheese cubes

- Homemade oatmeal-raisin cookies

- Raw almonds

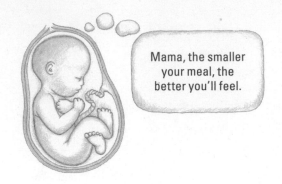

Mama, the smaller your meal, the better you'll feel.

ENJOY THE SIPPING SOLUTION

Try our supersmoothie (recipe below). In formulating this recipe, we made sure it contains most of the extra nutrients you need for you and your baby, and it's an intestine-friendly way to eat during pregnancy. Sip on the supersmoothie all day as your breakfast, lunch, and snacks. Then, have a normal, healthy dinner, like our pregnancy salad (see recipe, page 38).

The "sipping solution" is a particularly comfortable way to eat early in your pregnancy, when blended food is more stomach-friendly, and later on, when your growing baby and uterus push on your stomach so there is less room for a plateful of food. We have recommended the sipping solution in our medical practice for many years. Pregnant mothers report that when they sip on a smoothie all day long, they suffer less indigestion, constipation, heartburn, mood swings, and fatigue.

Dr. BJ notes: Many women come in for their preconception visit or first prenatal visit with a bag full of supplements. They have the best of intentions and believe that more is better. I try to help them recognize that supplements cannot take the place of balanced nutrition. Unfortunately, many women in our culture

---

PREGNANCY EATING TIP: ONE FISTFUL OF FOOD

As a general guide, limit the size of your meals to the size of your fist, which is roughly the size of your stomach. Especially in the later stages of pregnancy, more than one fistful of food at each of your eight minimeals is likely to, shall we say, be a pain in the gut. Shoot for at least eight of the twelve superfoods daily (page 28).

Pregnancy Digestive Problems	How the Sipping Solution Helps
Reflux and heartburn Indigestion Constipation	Blended, liquefied food empties faster from the stomach, the nutrients are absorbed more efficiently, and the high-fiber liquid is a natural laxative.
Inflammation, "itises"	The antioxidants in the smoothie boost immunity.
Blood sugar and mood swings	Blood sugar and insulin levels are steadier, as are moods.
Excessive weight (fat) gain	Grazers and sippers tend to be leaner, probably because their stomach and intestines get used to feeling satisfied with smaller volumes.
Fatigue	A steady supply of healthy nutrients gives you a steady supply of energy.

HOW TO CHOOSE THE PRENATAL SUPPLEMENT THAT'S RIGHT FOR YOU

While ideally it's better to get your nutrition from real foods rather than from packaged supplements, during pregnancy this may be more challenging. This is why most obstetricians recommend that pregnant women take prenatal supplements. In choosing your prenatal supplement, consider the following:

• Be sure it contains the big three: folic acid, omega-3s, and iron. Your levels of these must go way up during pregnancy. Levels of most of the other vitamins need to go up only slightly during pregnancy.

• If you can't eat the recommended 1,200 to 1,600 milligrams of calcium through foods, your supplement should contain 400 to 800 milligrams of calcium.

• Consider a supplement containing potassium iodine to avoid iodine deficiency.

• Consider a probiotic, which can help alleviate some of the intestinal ailments.

• Don't megadose. This is mainly true for vitamin A, which in high doses (greater than 10,000 IU a day) has been shown to increase the risk of birth defects — such

(continued)

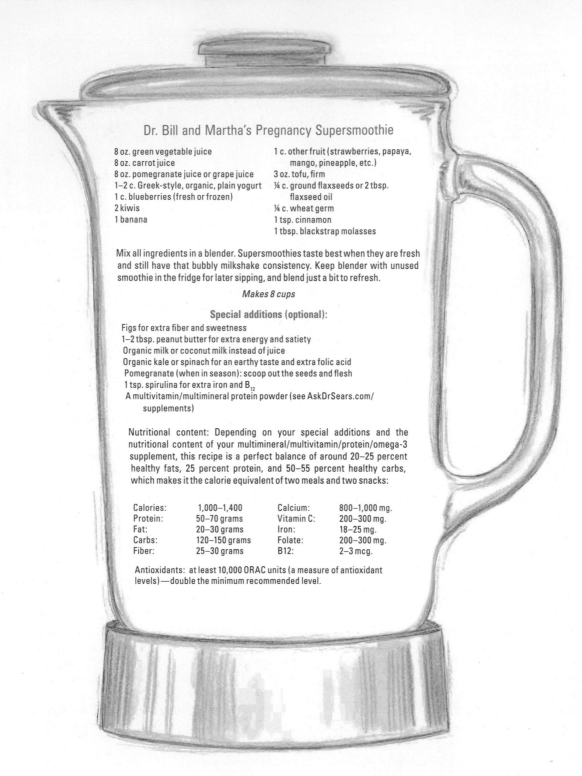

Dr. Bill and Martha's Pregnancy Supersmoothie

8 oz. green vegetable juice
8 oz. carrot juice
8 oz. pomegranate juice or grape juice
1–2 c. Greek-style, organic, plain yogurt
1 c. blueberries (fresh or frozen)
2 kiwis
1 banana

1 c. other fruit (strawberries, papaya, mango, pineapple, etc.)
3 oz. tofu, firm
¼ c. ground flaxseeds or 2 tbsp. flaxseed oil
¼ c. wheat germ
1 tsp. cinnamon
1 tbsp. blackstrap molasses

Mix all ingredients in a blender. Supersmoothies taste best when they are fresh and still have that bubbly milkshake consistency. Keep blender with unused smoothie in the fridge for later sipping, and blend just a bit to refresh.

Makes 8 cups

Special additions (optional):

Figs for extra fiber and sweetness
1–2 tbsp. peanut butter for extra energy and satiety
Organic milk or coconut milk instead of juice
Organic kale or spinach for an earthy taste and extra folic acid
Pomegranate (when in season): scoop out the seeds and flesh
1 tsp. spirulina for extra iron and B_{12}
A multivitamin/multimineral protein powder (see AskDrSears.com/supplements)

Nutritional content: Depending on your special additions and the nutritional content of your multimineral/multivitamin/protein/omega-3 supplement, this recipe is a perfect balance of around 20–25 percent healthy fats, 25 percent protein, and 50–55 percent healthy carbs, which makes it the calorie equivalent of two meals and two snacks:

Calories:	1,000–1,400	Calcium:	800–1,000 mg.
Protein:	50–70 grams	Vitamin C:	200–300 mg.
Fat:	20–30 grams	Iron:	18–25 mg.
Carbs:	120–150 grams	Folate:	200–300 mg.
Fiber:	25–30 grams	B12:	2–3 mcg.

Antioxidants: at least 10,000 ORAC units (a measure of antioxidant levels)—double the minimum recommended level.

as cleft lip, cleft palate, and heart defects — by fivefold. The reason vitamin A is more easily overdosed is that it is fat-soluble, meaning it is stored in body fat. Other vitamins, such as vitamin C and the B vitamins, are water-soluble, and therefore any excess is easily excreted through the urine. It's safest to stick with the dosage of vitamins recommended by your healthcare provider.

(Go to AskDrSears.com/supplements to see what supplements we recommend.)

claim they "don't have time" to work on their nutrition, so they turn to supplements to make them feel more balanced.

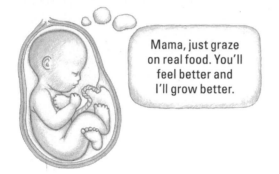

Mama, just graze on real food. You'll feel better and I'll grow better.

NUTRITION QUESTIONS YOU MAY HAVE

I'm a vegan, but I wonder if it's a safe diet while pregnant?

You're right to wonder. The stricter your vegan diet, the riskier it is for baby. While vegetarian mothers are less likely to gain excess weight, being a vegan or a strict vegetarian while pregnant is a nutritional challenge. It just so happens that some of the top extra nutrients you need — namely, omega-3 fats, vitamin D, vitamin B_{12}, and iron — come mainly from seafood and animal sources. Some vegans even note that during pregnancy, they crave certain animal-based foods they previously shunned. Nine meatless months are possible, yet pregnancy may be a good time for you to consider healthier alternatives:

• Become a pesco-vegetarian. Adding 12 ounces of safe seafood per week would increase your chance of getting more of those nourishing nutrients you and baby need, especially omega-3 fats, vitamin B_{12}, and vitamin D.

• During your pregnancy become a flexitarian. Listen to your body. If you crave animal-based foods, such as yogurt, eggs, or salmon, give in to these healthy cravings.

• To beef up your iron, eat more of these meatless pregnancy superfoods: beans, lentils, tofu, figs, prune juice, spirulina, and blackstrap molasses. Plant-source iron, such as that from spinach and kale, is not absorbed as well as meat-source iron, so you'll need to eat more citrus fruits (vitamin C increases the absorption of iron from your veggies). As a general guide, 1 cup of beans, lentils, or firm tofu will give you almost as much iron and protein as 3 ounces of meat.

• Care about your calcium. The best vegetarian sources are calcium-fortified foods such as orange juice, tofu, blackstrap molasses, figs, beans and greens, and sesame seeds.

• For nutritional insurance, be sure to take a prenatal supplement that contains the nutrients that are most difficult to get from a vegan diet, namely omega-3 DHA, vitamin B_{12}, and iron. (See "How to Choose the Prenatal Supplement That's Right for You," page 23.)

• Adding a daily serving of spirulina powder to your smoothie (see page 24) gives you two of the nutrients you miss by avoiding animal foods: vitamin B_{12} (9 micrograms) and iron (7 milligrams).

How many extra nutritious calories do I need while pregnant?

Most mothers need only 100 extra nutritious calories a day during the first trimester and 300 to 500 additional calories a day during the rest of the pregnancy. But instead of counting calories, just eat more real foods. Instead of trying to consume "300 extra calories," think of adding two extra servings of protein and two extra servings of fruits and vegetables. This is a more accurate, more doable, and healthier approach. Or, just think: each day for the health of myself and my baby, I need to eat four to five extra servings of the pregnancy superfoods daily. (Review the list of superfoods on page 29.)

Here's the real meaning of "eating for two": You become twice as picky, and you need to consume twice the amount of protein and omega-3s. This is not a green light to indulge — you certainly don't need twice the number of calories. Really you're eating for 1.2, especially in the first trimester. For most mothers, extra fat stores will supply the extra calories.

Shoot for a balanced week rather than a balanced meal or balanced day. Your gut feelings and your appetite are going to fluctuate from day to day, so just make sure you are getting what you need over the course of a week.

Even though your daily caloric need rises by around 15 percent, your daily need for nutrients such as iron, folate, omega-3s, and other nutrients may increase by 50 percent. It's a good idea to start eating these extra micronutrients early in pregnancy.

I hear a lot about vitamin D deficiency. How much vitamin D do I need?

Vitamin D helps build strong muscles and bones, for both you and your baby. Recent research reveals that 94 percent of pregnant African American mothers, 60 percent of Hispanic mothers, and 50 percent of Caucasian mothers have vitamin D deficiency. Low levels of maternal vitamin D are associated with:

• Increased C-section rates

• More allergies in baby

• Weaker bones in baby and mom

Consider these guidelines:

• Ask your healthcare provider to measure your vitamin D blood level.

• Depending on your diet, sun exposure, and blood levels, your healthcare provider may recommend a supplement containing 1,000 to 4,000 IU daily.

• The best two sources of vitamin D are salmon and sunshine. So, eat fish and go outside for around fifteen minutes a day, with bare arms and legs exposed to the sun, weather permitting. (See page 49 for other sources of vitamin D.)

I suffer from food allergies. What can I do to protect my baby from allergies?

You'll be happy to know that new studies show that you can make several health changes to protect your baby from allergies. First, of course, limit foods you are allergic to. It used to be thought that if mother ate less of the foods most likely to cause allergies, such as dairy, wheat, shellfish, soy, nuts, and eggs, her baby would be less likely to be allergic to these foods. Since there is no scientific proof of this, allergists now advise mothers to eliminate only the foods they are certain they are allergic to. This sensible advice lowers your risk of undernutrition. Omega-3 fish oil, vitamin D, and probiotics have been shown to lower your baby's chances of getting allergies such as asthma and eczema. Be sure to consume plenty of these. And breastfeeding is one of the best ways to reduce later allergies in your child.

3

What to Eat: The Top Twelve Pregnancy Superfoods

Eating right while pregnant has different challenges at different stages of pregnancy. In the first trimester, you may be more interested in your stomach feeling right than in eating right. So, undernutrition could be a concern. During the feel-better phase of the second trimester, mothers tend to overeat and therefore overgain. That's when the previous food aversions change to food cravings. In the third trimester, the pressure on your stomach from that growing little person inside may prompt you to graze on minimeals instead of gorging on big meals.

One of the perks of pregnancy is that many mothers who have been putting off making healthier eating choices are finally motivated to change now that there is a little person inside. Realistically, the Healthy Pregnancy Diet isn't much different from how every woman should eat anyway. We've just added some do's and don'ts.

Eating for two is not complicated. Simply put:

- Eat more nutrient-dense foods.

- Eat fewer foods that interfere with the health of you and your baby.

- Eat smaller, more frequent meals, as you learned in the previous chapter.

You can do that!

WHAT'S IN A PREGNANCY SUPERFOOD?

The best food for you and your baby should be:

- Nutrient-dense, providing more nourishment per calorie

- Filling without being fattening

- Rich in nutrients mother and baby most need

- Friendly to queasy stomachs

- Versatile and tasty

- Able to boost the immune system

- Free of harmful additives

Our picks for the top twelve pregnancy superfoods are:

1. Seafood

2. Nuts, raw

3. Greens

4. Avocados

5. Eggs

6. Yogurt

7. Blueberries

8. Beans and lentils

9. Flaxseeds, ground

10. Olive oil

11. Tofu

12. Oatmeal

THE NOURISHING NINE NUTRIENTS YOU NEED FOR A HEALTHY PREGNANCY

To best nourish your growing baby and your changing body, each day you need to average *an extra:*

1. 500 milligrams of omega-3 DHA

2. 25 grams of protein

3. 800 milligrams of calcium

4. 400 milligrams of folic acid (folate)

5. 12 milligrams of iron

6. 1,000 IU of vitamin D

7. 2 micrograms of vitamin B_{12}

8. 220 micrograms of iodine

9. 300 to 500 extra healthy calories (during the second and third trimesters)

These twelve superfoods are our top choices for supplying the extra nutrition you and your baby need each day.

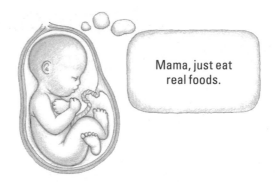

Mama, just eat real foods.

1. GO FISH!

"Eat more safe seafood" is our first prescription for what you can do during your pregnancy to help your baby's brain grow. As you learned on page 19, baby's brain is 60 percent fat. It just so happens that the top fats in fish are also the top fats your baby's brain needs. Over the past ten years there have been thousands of scientific articles proving the health benefits to mother and baby of sufficient omega-3 fats (DHA and EPA) during pregnancy.

Research shows that mothers who eat more safe seafood or take omega-3 fish oil supplements during pregnancy and for three months after delivery:

- Are less likely to suffer pre- and postpartum depression

- Have a lower chance of delivering a premature baby or one with a less-than-optimal birth weight

- Have babies who are more likely to have better visual acuity, especially if baby was premature

- Have children who are less likely to develop skin and respiratory allergies

- Have children who are more likely to have higher IQs

This one simple "oil change" can have a profound effect on the emotional and intellectual health of you and your baby.

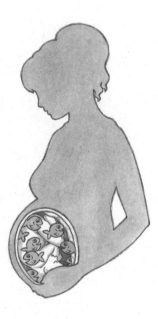

of every organ of the body, especially the brain, is "you're only as healthy as each cell in your body." In a nutshell, your goal is to help each cell in your baby's growing body multiply trillions of times a day without any "mistakes." Omega-3s help this happen.

Omega-3 DHA/EPA is called "the membrane molecule" because it makes the cell membrane healthier. Each cell is surrounded by a fatty bag. Just as hair conditioner makes hair soft and flexible, omega-3s condition cells, making these flexible bags selectively permeable, meaning that they let only good nutrients into the cell and keep the bad stuff out. Omega-3s are the prime structural and functional components of the cell membrane.

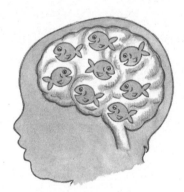

"My brain is going through a growth spurt."

How Omega-3s Build Brighter Baby Brains

Research reveals that a baby's growing brain extracts the most omega-3 DHA from mother's blood during the last three months of her pregnancy. This makes sense since this is the time when baby's brain grows most rapidly. One of the basic health principles

---

HEALTHY PREGNANCY TIP

Omega-3 DHA/EPA is to the brain what calcium is to the bone.

Omega-3s make myelin. Coating the nerve-cell fibers is a fatty sheath called myelin, the white matter of the growing brain that acts like insulation on electrical wires and makes the electrical messages in the brain travel faster. Myelin is mostly fat. The more myelin your baby's brain cells make, the faster and more efficient these electrical messages are. Omega-3s feed the myelin-making cells, which have some of the highest nutrient requirements of any cell.

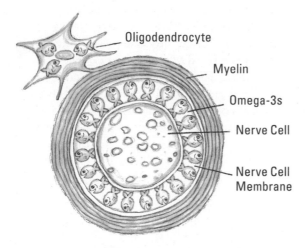

Oligodendrocyte

Myelin

Omega-3s

Nerve Cell

Nerve Cell Membrane

Omega-3s make brain connections. Your baby's brain grows by making trillions of connections. At the end of each nerve fiber are tiny gaps called synapses. A nerve fiber fires neurotransmitters, which are biochemical messengers that carry information like a high-speed ferryboat from one brain cell to another. On the receiver brain cell are receptors, like locks, into which these neurotransmitter "keys" must fit. Omega-3s make these brain messengers travel faster and more efficiently, and they fashion the receptor sites so the keys fit perfectly.

SCIENCE SAYS: EAT OMEGA-3s, GROW HEALTHIER BABIES

Want to feed your baby in the womb the top grow food? Go fish! Studies have found that mothers who eat sufficient omega-3 DHA during their pregnancies are likely to give birth to more mature babies. Investigators noticed that mothers who live on islands where lots of seafood is consumed are more likely to have babies whose gestation lasts between four and eight days longer and who tend to be a bit heavier. In 2003 researchers from the Department of Obstetrics and Gynecology at the University of Missouri and the Department of Dietetics and Nutrition at the University of Kansas Medical Center studied 291 pregnant women (between twenty-four and twenty-eight weeks) whose dietary intake of omega-3 DHA was low. They divided these mothers into two groups. One group ate an average of 100 extra milligrams of DHA (in the form of a DHA supplement added to eggs) a day than the other group. They analyzed the blood concentration of omega-3 at the start of the study and again from the umbilical cord after birth. They discovered that the DHA-supplemented women did indeed enjoy better baby growth. Specifically, babies whose mothers were supplemented with DHA showed:

- Three to six days longer gestation

- A 100-gram increase (a little less than a quarter pound) in mean birth weight

(continued)

- A higher level of DHA content in infant red blood cells

- A slightly higher placental weight

- Less premature delivery

- Less preeclampsia or high blood pressure

Why do omega-3s act like intrauterine grow food? These researchers theorized that omega-3s could slightly delay the appearance of labor-triggering hormones called prostaglandins.

Another study published in 2000 in the *British Journal of Obstetrics and Gynecology* showed that Danish women who consumed 2,700 milligrams of omega-3 DHA/EPA daily from the twentieth week of pregnancy to birth had a lower incidence of delivering preterm, an eight-day increase in the duration of gestation, and nearly a half pound (209 grams) increase in mean birth weight. Researchers also concluded that these effects were found mainly in women who were omega-3 deficient, since a study of Norwegian women who already consumed sufficient omega-3s during pregnancy showed no increase in the length of gestation or birth weight.

We conclude, as did these researchers, that omega-3 supplements in women who already have a dietary insufficiency of omega-3s can help babies who ordinarily would be born with less-than-optimal maturity and birth weight.

Omega-3s help moms be happier. Not only do growing baby brains like omega-3s, so do tired mommy brains. One of the newest and most exciting therapeutic findings on the medical benefits of omega-3s is that mothers who eat more omega-3s during pregnancy experience less depression before and after birth. While not all studies come to this conclusion, many do. A dietary omega-3 deficiency contributes to mood disorders such as depression and anxiety at all ages. As you've learned, babies need extra omega-3s for growing brains and bodies. Research shows that many pregnant women have lower blood levels of omega-3 DHA in the third trimester, when baby's brain grows the most. During pregnancy and breastfeeding, baby literally sucks the omega-3s out of mom, possibly leaving her with an omega-3 deficiency and resulting depression. A healthy pregnancy diet means having an omega-3 sufficiency — enough for both baby and mother.

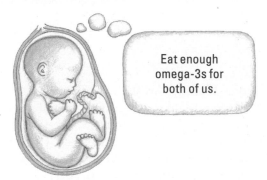

Eat enough omega-3s for both of us.

The new field of psychoneuroimmunology reveals another reason that omega-3 insufficiency during pregnancy may lead to depression. Imagine what's going on inside your body. During the last trimester your immune system perks up to protect both mother and baby from infection and prepare mother's body for birth. Your body goes into what is called a proinflammatory state, with higher levels of protective biochemicals called cytokines. One of the main biochemical perks of omega-3s is that they act as inflammatory regulators, keeping the inflammatory system balanced. Excessive inflammation can cause wear and tear on mother's nervous system and result in depression, as well as rob mom of much-needed energy and sleep.

Don't Eat Dumb Fats

Above you learned that "smart fats" make proper-fitting locks on the nerve cell membranes so the keys — the neurotransmitters — can fit into them to grow more brain connections. "Dumb fats," like hydrogenated oils and other factory-made fats, cross the placenta and clog the locks on the cell membranes so the keys don't fit. Also, hydrogenated oils — trans fats — can block the enzyme needed to upgrade the omega-3s in plant oils to omega-3 DHA in baby's brain. When you're pregnant, your baby needs you to make a smart oil change. For smarter baby brain growth, eat a right-fat diet, not a low-fat diet.

How much omega-3 should I eat daily?

Nutritional researchers reveal that the average American woman eats only 150 milligrams of omega-3 DHA/EPA per day. Although you may read that the current recommendation is 500 milligrams of omega-3s a day for pregnant and breastfeeding mothers, we believe you should eat at least 1,000 milligrams (1 gram) of omega-3 DHA/EPA daily. To be sure you get 1,000 milligrams of omega-3 daily:

- Pregnant and breastfeeding mothers should eat 12 ounces of safe seafood per week. Six ounces of wild salmon twice a week would average around 600 milligrams of DHA/EPA daily.

- Take 500 milligrams of omega-3 DHA/ EPA fish oil supplements daily.

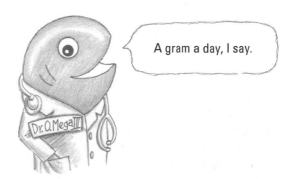

A gram a day, I say.

Dr. O. Mega III

Here's how we arrived at the 1,000 milligrams a day recommendation. The International Society for the Study of Fatty Acids and Lipids and the National Institutes of Health both recommend 500 milligrams a day as "the minimum preventive medicine requirements for all adults." If 500 milligrams is the recommendation for all adults, then certainly a pregnant woman must need more than 500 milligrams. Baby's brain is growing faster than at any other time during life and omega-3s are one of the prime essential fats for brain growth. The rest of baby's body is also in a continual growth spurt. (Omega-3 authorities agree that there are no safety issues with 1,000 milligrams of omega-3 a day for any adult, including mothers during pregnancy and lactation.)

(For more information on how much omega-3 to take during pregnancy and why, read *The Omega-3 Effect* by William Sears and James Sears.)

If I really don't like fish or it's hard to get safe seafood where we live, should I take a fish oil supplement, and how much?

Absolutely! Take at least 1,000 milligrams of omega-3 DHA/EPA daily. Look on the nutritional label of your fish oil supplement to be sure that the DHA and EPA omega-3s add up to 1,000 milligrams, with at least 600 milligrams being omega-3 DHA. You don't have to worry about taking too much, yet there is no current evidence that taking more than 1,000 milligrams a day is beneficial. However, if you do want to take 2,000 milligrams a day it is certainly safe. (See AskDrSears.com/safeseafood for updates on dosages and safe seafood.)

Especially in the first trimester, some mothers will get a queasy stomach when they sniff seafood. It helps to overcome this temporary nuisance by getting fresh or fresh-frozen seafood, which smells less "fishy." You might also try having someone else cook it for you, and then you can enjoy the finished product. Camouflage the fish taste with your favorite healthy sauce or mix fish into a veggie stir-fry. Try what we call taste reshaping. First, convince yourself how good seafood is for you and your baby by reading *The Omega-3 Effect.* Many mothers find that the motivation of having a healthier pregnancy and smarter baby upgrades their taste from "Don't like fish" to "Must eat fish" to "Like fish."

Still insist you don't like fish? Ponder this research. In addition to being high in omega-3s, seafood is also high in vitamin D. A 2008 study published in the *Journal of Clinical Endocrinology and Metabolism* revealed that mothers who were deficient in vitamin D were twice as likely to need a cesarean birth, presumably because vitamin D deficiency could impair uterine muscle strength. Conclusion: to build up enough uterine strength to push that baby out, go fish!

I'm worried about mercury and other pollutants in seafood. What fish are safest for me and my growing baby?

All consumers, especially pregnant mothers, are confused about safe seafood. These guidelines should clear up the confusion. In a nutshell, medical authorities who have thoroughly researched seafood conclude that 12 ounces per week of any fish, except those in the red-light column in the chart below, can be safely eaten by pregnant mothers because the health benefits of the seafood outweigh the worry. (The red-light fish are large, older predatory fish that are more likely to be contaminated.)

Which fish is the safest and healthiest and the one you most recommend for pregnant women?

Our vote for the safest and most nutritious seafood is Alaskan sockeye or king salmon. Wild Pacific salmon is our top choice for several reasons: Alaskan seafood is grown in the wild in pristine waters, and Alaskan fishery authorities enforce regulations to ensure safe seafood. These fish also have some of the highest levels of omega-3. Furthermore, the nutrient that makes wild salmon pink is called astaxanthin, and it is one of nature's most powerful antioxidants for boosting your immune system.

(For the safest seafood sources we have personally researched, see AskDrSears.com/safeseafood.)

TRAFFIC-LIGHT SAFE SEAFOOD EATING

Green-Light Fish (Safe — enjoy without limit.)	*Yellow-Light Fish* (Safe — enjoy but limit to 12 ounces per week.)*	*Red-Light Fish* (Don't eat!)**
Anchovies	Halibut, Atlantic	King mackerel
Arctic char	Lobster	Marlin
Catfish (U.S.)	Mahi-mahi	Shark
Cod, Pacific	Orange roughy	Swordfish
Halibut, Alaskan	Sea bass	Tilefish
Herring	Shrimp, Atlantic	
Rainbow trout	Snapper	
Sablefish, Alaskan	Tuna, fresh albacore, yellow fin	
Salmon, preferably Pacific (fresh, frozen, or canned)		
Sardines		
Shrimp, Pacific		
Tuna, canned light		
Tuna, fresh Pacific***		

Source: U.S. Department of Agriculture, *Dietary Guidelines for Americans,* 2010.

* The Environmental Protection Agency (EPA) recommends limiting intake of these fish to 12 ounces per week, especially for pregnant and breastfeeding mothers.

** These large, older predatory fish are more likely to be contaminated.

*** Troll- and pole-caught tuna tend to be smaller and contain fewer contaminants than long-line, deep-water tuna, which tend to be larger and therefore more contaminated.

I'm a vegetarian. How can I get enough omega-3s?

Vegetarians and vegans must be prudent while they're pregnant. Studies show that omega-3 DHA levels are lower in the blood of infants born to vegetarian mothers, and DHA blood levels of breastfed infants of vegetarian mothers is only about one-third that of the level of nonvegetarians. Levels are even lower for vegans. While the following statement may surprise vegans and is controversial among some nutritionists, we've consulted the world's experts in omega-3 scientific research, who unanimously conclude that *pregnant mothers should not rely only on plant sources of omega-3s,* such as flax. The reason is that the omega-3s in seafood are the two fats babies and mothers need most, DHA and EPA. The omega-3 fats in plants, such as flaxseeds, are different; and the process of converting them to DHA and EPA may not be efficient in mothers.

NUTRIENT PROFILE OF WILD ALASKAN SOCKEYE SALMON (6-OUNCE FILLET)

		Percent Daily Value*
Calories	287	—
Protein	43 grams	40–50%
Omega-3 EPA and DHA	1,000 milligrams EPA; 1,200 milligrams DHA	200%**
Vitamin B$_1$ (thiamine)	0.37 milligram	25%
Vitamin B$_2$ (riboflavin)	0.26 milligram	14%
Vitamin B$_3$ (niacin)	16.5 milligrams	83%
Vitamin B$_6$	1.18 milligrams	60%
Vitamin B$_{12}$	9.6 micrograms	100%
Vitamin D	894 IU	100%
Sodium	112 milligrams	5%
Potassium	694 milligrams	20%
Iron	0.8 milligram	3%
Zinc	1 milligram	7%
Iodine	100 micrograms	50%
Choline	191 milligrams	35%
Selenium	62 micrograms	90%
Astaxanthin	8 milligrams	***

Source: USDA Nutritional Nutrient Database for Standard Reference, 2011. Notice that most of the nutrients found in a salmon fillet are the ones you need to have a healthy pregnancy.

* This column refers to the U.S. government's recommended daily *minimum* value for adults, not necessarily the value for optimal health, especially for pregnant women.

** The government's recommended daily value is not yet available. Most authorities recommend 1,000 milligrams daily for pregnant and breastfeeding mothers.

*** Studies suggest an average of 6 to 8 milligrams daily. The USDA recommended daily value is not yet available.

Our recommendation: eat both fish oil and flaxseed oil during pregnancy, or take 1,000 milligrams per day of *vegan omega-3 DHA supplements from algae,* such as Neuromins by Martek. (Learn why flaxseed oil is also a healthy food during pregnancy, page 40.)

2. GO NUTS!

Just as you should "go fish" during your pregnancy, you should also "go nuts"! Nuts are one of the most nutrient-dense foods, rich in protein, healthy fats, fiber, vitamin E, calcium,

DURING PREGNANCY, GIVE YOURSELF AN OIL CHANGE

To get the most benefit from eating more nutritious oils, it's also important to eat less health-harming oils, ones that can biochemically compete with and lessen the good effects of the healthy oils. Learn more about why this happens in *The Omega-3 Effect* (William Sears and James Sears).

Eat these oils	*Not these oils*
• Fish oil • Flaxseed oil • Nut oils • Olive oil • Virgin coconut oil	• Partially hydrogenated oils, also known as trans fats • Cottonseed oil*

* Cottonseed oil, besides being one of the most pesticide-laden oils, is very low in omega-3s. Because it is relatively stable and cheap, it's become the darling of the food industry.

Quirks pregnant mothers have	*How omega-3s can help*
Moodiness	Steadies mood swings
Vision changes	Promotes clearer vision
Dry eyes	Lessens evaporation from tears
Dermatitis	Smooths scaly skin
High blood pressure	Lowers blood pressure
Delayed tissue healing after delivery	Promotes tissue healing
Blood clots in leg veins	Lessens dangerous blood clots

and many other vitamins and minerals you and your baby need. And nuts are a favorite with vegetarians and vegans. "Aren't nuts high in calories?" you may ask. Yes, but they're healthy calories. Nuts are one of nature's perfect foods, containing the right balance of healthy fats, protein, and fiber, with a calorie-saving perk known as *high satiety factor,* meaning that a palmful of nuts fills you up faster than a larger volume of high-carb foods containing the same number of calories. The result: you're unlikely to overeat nuts.

Make your own pregnancy trail mix. Because different nuts offer different nutrients, combine a variety of nuts (such as raw almonds, Brazil nuts, walnuts, and pistachios) and your favorite dried fruit and seeds in a homemade trail mix. This allows you to tap into a valuable nutritional principle called synergy — when you eat a lot of nutrients together from different sources, each one helps the body process the others better. Whenever possible,

purchase raw nuts, because roasting not only adds fats but can also destroy some of the nutrients.

3. GO GREENS!

For a healthier pregnancy, "go greens"! Dark green vegetables such as spinach, broccoli, kale, chard, arugula, collard greens, and asparagus are a good source of all the vitamins and minerals pregnant mothers need, especially folate, the "brain-vitality

---

Martha's Pregnancy Salad

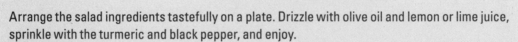

One 4-ounce grilled salmon fillet

4 ounces nonfat cottage cheese
  or 1 ounce grated parmesan cheese
  or crumbled goat cheese

4 ounces cooked or canned kidney
  beans

3 cups spinach

1 serving nori, chopped

¼ cup chopped tomatoes

1 tablespoon raw sunflower
  or sesame seeds

1 egg, hard-boiled and sliced

1 tablespoon extra-virgin olive oil

Juice of half a lemon or lime

½ teaspoon ground turmeric

¼ teaspoon ground black pepper

Arrange the salad ingredients tastefully on a plate. Drizzle with olive oil and lemon or lime juice, sprinkle with the turmeric and black pepper, and enjoy.

This balanced-nutrition salad is so filling that you may prefer to cut the recipe in half, eat it at two different meals, or graze on it throughout the afternoon. It is so nutrient-dense that it contains at least 50 percent of your total daily needs of most nutrients in a mere 600 calories.

Nutrients	Daily Requirements while Pregnant
Omega-3 fats: 500 milligrams	1,000 milligrams
Protein: 60 grams	100 grams
Calcium: 350 milligrams	1,400–1,600 milligrams
Iron: 10 milligrams	30 milligrams
Folate: 500 milligrams	600–800 milligrams
Vitamin D: 800 IU	1,000 IU
Vitamin B$_{12}$: 5 micrograms	2.6 micrograms
Iodine: 70 micrograms	220 micrograms
Choline: 320 milligrams	450 milligrams

vitamin." Greens are a good nondairy source of calcium and are packed with fiber to help pregnancy-prone constipation. And they are good for your eyes, as they contain the eye-building nutrients lutein and zeaxanthin. Whenever possible, look for organic greens.

4. AWESOME AVOCADOS

Avocados are the most nutrient-dense fruit, rich in vitamins A, B, and E, folic acid, and healthy fats, in addition to the nutrients lutein and zeaxanthin. As another nutritional perk, avocados, like nuts, enjoy a high satiety value. And avocados are one of the most versatile foods for the ever-changing tastes of a pregnant mother. They make a perfect accompaniment to other superfoods, such as omelets and salads, and can be made into guacamole to be enjoyed with raw vegetable dippers.

5. EAT EGGS

Eggs are one of the most nutrient-dense superfoods. For a mere 75 calories you enjoy 6 grams of protein and many of the vitamins and minerals pregnant mothers need. Eggs contain choline, a valuable brain-building nutrient, and egg yolks contain the antioxidants lutein and zeaxanthin, which help build healthy vision. (Unless advised to the contrary by your doctor, skip the "egg white only" omelet and enjoy the whole egg.) Another bonus: because eggs are high in the sleep-inducing amino acid tryptophan, an egg before bed may help pregnant mothers who have difficulty sleeping.

Here's a chicken and egg story that pregnant women should enjoy. Remember we previously said that baby becomes what mommy eats? You can get a clue to this nutritional fact by looking at the yolk of different eggs. The yolk of an egg from a farm-fed, free-range chicken is a deeper orange because it's higher in nutrients, especially omega-3 DHA. Contrast that with eggs from the usual commercial-fed hens packed in a coop, sitting around eating factory food. The yolk is pale because it contains fewer nutrients. Which yolk do you want your baby to be like?

By now you are probably wondering why the first five superfoods are so high in fat. Your baby's brain utilizes more energy than any of his other organs. It bears repeating: the brain of your growing baby is mainly fat. So, if we had to pick one time in a woman's life that low-fat diets are risky, it would be during pregnancy. Remember, a right-fat diet, not a low-fat diet, is what you and your baby most need.

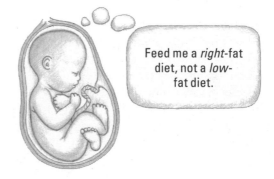

Feed me a *right*-fat diet, not a *low*-fat diet.

6. YUMMY YOGURT

We hope you have a yen for yogurt during your pregnancy. Besides being packed with two of the top nutrients pregnant mothers need, protein (10 to 20 grams per cup) and calcium

(300 to 400 milligrams per cup), this superfood is rich in probiotics, which are good for the gut. Yogurt gives you healthy slow-release carbs for energy, and the culturing process enables both the protein and the lactose sugars to be more easily digested than those nutrients in regular milk, a perk for pregnant mothers who may experience indigestion from lactose or casein intolerance. For the health of you and your baby, choose organic yogurt. And go Greek! Calorie for calorie, Greek yogurt contains around twice the amount of protein of regular yogurt. Some of the whey and much of the lactose is strained out, leaving higher-protein, lower-lactose yogurt, which some pregnant mothers find more friendly to their queasy stomachs.

A HEALTHIER SWEETENER DURING PREGNANCY

Instead of "added sugar," and certainly instead of the factory-made sweetener high-fructose corn syrup, try a healthier alternative: blackstrap molasses. The nutrient profile of blackstrap molasses seems to be just what the pregnant body ordered. One tablespoon of this sticky sweetener contains 170 milligrams of calcium and 3.5 milligrams of iron, in addition to traces of many other vitamins and minerals, all for only 47 calories.

---

7. BLUEBERRIES, THE BRAIN BERRIES

Remember your mother telling you, "Put more color on your plate"? Double mother's nutritional wisdom during your pregnancy.

The blue skin of the blueberry is full of the flavonoid anthocyanin, a potent antioxidant that protects tissues, especially the brain, from damage and inflammation. The list of health effects of blueberries is growing. Blueberries have been called the "brain berry" because studies have shown that they act as a neuroprotectant against damage to nerve tissue. They have been called the "repair berry" because they help heal tissue. Finally, blueberries are dubbed the "belly berry" thanks to studies from Japan showing that the blue pigment somehow works its way into the fat cells in the belly and reduces the number of cells that grow into excess belly fat. They taste good and can be added to many of the other superfoods, such as yogurt, oatmeal, smoothies, and salads. Whenever possible, purchase organic blueberries.

8. BIG ON BEANS AND LENTILS

Legumes are loaded with nutrients. Like many of the other superfoods, they have a high satiety factor, so they fill you up for fewer calories. Beans are high in B vitamins, protein, fiber, folic acid, calcium, and iron. Like eggs, they also are a good source of the sleep-inducing nutrient tryptophan.

9. FABULOUS FLAXSEEDS

We recommend mixing 2 tablespoons of freshly ground flaxseeds into a daily smoothie, adding them to your muffin batter, or sprinkling them on salads or oatmeal. Two tablespoons of this superseed contains 100 healthy calories, 4 grams of protein, and

GO ORGANIC!

Is going organic worth the extra price for a healthier pregnancy? Absolutely. We've already discussed why "chemical food" can be harmful to baby, but it's worth summarizing here:

- Baby's brain, the organ most vulnerable to harmful chemicals, grows fastest in the last three months of pregnancy and the first two years after birth. The brain is 60 percent fat, and fat tissue is the most vulnerable to damage by toxins.

- The blood-brain barrier, the protective coating that blocks some toxins from seeping from blood into brain tissue, is not well developed until after birth. This makes baby's brain more vulnerable while in the womb.

- Baby's "garbage disposal system," namely, the liver and kidneys, are immature, especially prenatally.

- The genetic machinery of rapidly growing and dividing cells is susceptible to the possible toxic effects of pesticides and harmful chemicals.

- Proportionally speaking, babies have more body fat than adults, so baby bodies store more toxins.

- The "maximum acceptable limits" of chemicals stated by government agencies are unknown for babies. Babies do not metabolize and detoxify chemicals as easily as adults do. And they eat more food in proportion to their body weight than adults do. Basically, the USDA doesn't know how these chemicals affect babies.

Here are our top tips for going organic:

- **Go organic for the dirty dozen.** Go organic on fruits and vegetables, especially those that you don't peel. If you don't have access to organic, buy a fruit and vegetable wash that will remove surface pesticides, waxes, and oils that water alone can't easily get rid of. These are the latest dirty dozen and clean fifteen (lowest in pesticides) as analyzed by the Environmental Working Group, a consumer advocacy group that guides people to wisely go organic:

THE DIRTY DOZEN (buy only organic and wash carefully)	THE CLEAN FIFTEEN (nonorganic is fine, as long as you wash carefully)
1. Celery	1. Onions
2. Peaches	2. Avocados

(continued)

THE DIRTY DOZEN (buy only organic and wash carefully)	THE CLEAN FIFTEEN (nonorganic is fine, as long as you wash carefully)
3. Strawberries	3. Sweet corn*
4. Apples	4. Pineapples
5. Blueberries	5. Mangos
6. Nectarines	6. Sweet peas
7. Bell peppers	7. Asparagus
8. Spinach	8. Kiwis
9. Cherries	9. Cabbage
10. Kale and collard greens	10. Eggplant
11. Potatoes	11. Cantaloupes
12. Grapes (imported)	12. Watermelons
	13. Grapefruits
	14. Sweet potatoes
	15. Honeydew melons

* Much sweet corn is genetically modified but not labeled GMO. If this is a concern to you, go for organic corn.

- **Go organic for dairy.** The last thing you and your growing baby need is a bunch of "endocrine disrupters," the term now used to describe the possible harmful effects of hormones and other pharmaceuticals given to commercial dairy cows.

- **Go organic for meat and poultry.** Try to eat meat and poultry that are free-range and not given chemical additives or hormones. Ditto for eggs; there is some suspicion that animals tend to excrete chemicals in their milk and eggs. Choose lean cuts of meat and poultry since chemical additives tend to concentrate in fat tissue.

- **Go organic for fats.** Because chemical additives are most likely to be stored in fats, it's smart to choose organic high-fat foods such as oils, butter, and nuts.

SHAPE YOUNG TASTES — IN THE WOMB!

When your baby is around six months old you will learn the secret of infant feeding: shaping young tastes. Also called metabolic programming, early taste-shaping means that the foods your baby's taste buds and gut get used to are the ones your baby is most likely to prefer and even crave later on. Could this taste shaping begin in the womb? New research suggests so. Since baby's taste buds and sense of smell are developed by around the sixth or seventh month in the womb, researchers wondered whether the flavors from the foods that mother ate that passed into the amniotic fluid baby swallowed could affect baby's taste preferences later on. In what has become known as the Carrot Juice Study, pregnant women who were asked to drink carrot juice during the last three months of pregnancy were more likely to have babies who liked the flavor of carrot juice than mothers who drank only water. The same taste shaping was found in studies on experimental animals. It's as if the baby in the womb becomes programmed to enjoy the flavors of the food in mother's culture, prompting baby to crave the healthy foods that mom ate.

6 grams of fiber, and is a rich source of healthy fats. Grind your own flaxseeds, since calorie for calorie, ground flaxseeds provide more health benefits than flaxseed oil.

10. OH, OLIVE OIL!

Olive oil is a nutritious and delicious pregnancy superfood. Made from the flesh of olives, virgin and extra-virgin olive oil can be processed using less pressure and lower temperatures, thus preserving more of the olive's natural nutrients. Ninety percent of the fats in olive oil are healthy monounsaturated fat, which is heart-healthy and cholesterol-lowering. When added to salads it increases the absorption of the nutrients from the other vegetables, such as carrots and tomatoes. It's a nutritious replacement

DRINK UP!

While you don't eat for two, you do drink for two, because the fluid in your body (extra blood volume, amniotic fluid, etc.) increases much more than the amount of extra tissue. While the weight of extra tissue (baby tissues, uterus, breast tissue, etc.) may increase by only around 15 percent, accounting for the 15 percent higher need of extra calories, your fluid requirements during pregnancy may increase by as much as 50 percent, or a few extra cups of water daily. Try to drink ten 8-ounce glasses of water a day. The color of your urine gives you a clue to your hydration. Clear or pale yellow urine is a sign that you are probably drinking enough fluids. Dark-colored, ammonia-smelling urine definitely signals that you are underhydrated.

for butter — dip whole-grain bread in a bit of olive oil and balsamic vinegar instead of spreading it with butter. But as with all oils, don't overdo it. A tablespoon a day drizzled on salad is a healthy 125 calories.

11. TERRIFIC TOFU

Try tofu while you're pregnant as a good source of protein, calcium, vitamins, and minerals. Tofu is bland on its own, but when blended with other foods it takes on the flavor of those foods. This is why it's a favorite nutritious addition to stir-fries and smoothies. For a mere 60 calories you get 8 grams of protein, 200 milligrams of calcium, 5 to 7 milligrams of iron, and lots of other vitamins and minerals. Go with firm tofu, which is more nutrient-dense.

12. OUTSTANDING OATMEAL

Opt for oatmeal as a healthy pregnancy breakfast. The special fiber in oatmeal, called beta-glucans, is particularly gut-friendly because it steadies the absorption of carbs and thereby steadies blood sugar swings. It is rich in protein, fiber, iron, zinc, vitamin E, and B vitamins. Use real oatmeal, not the instant stuff. A favorite breakfast during Martha's pregnancies was Crock-Pot oatmeal. Prepare steel-cut oatmeal in a slow cooker and let it simmer slowly overnight, then awaken to the aroma of fresh oatmeal. Add a dollop of yogurt and a handful of blueberries, sprinkle with cinnamon, and enjoy! For mothers who are very gluten sensitive, try breakfast cereals made from other supergrains, such as millet, amaranth, quinoa, and buckwheat.

"WHITE OUT" YOUR DIET

Put more color on your plate by trying a "no-white" diet. If you are a bread lover, make the switch from white to 100 percent whole-grain bread, which is much more dense in protein, fiber, vitamins, and minerals. Next time you're in the supermarket try the same bread test we do with kids. Pick up a loaf of white bread and compare it to a loaf of whole-wheat bread. You'll notice that the white bread is lighter and squishier because many of the nutrients have been removed. Compared with white bread, whole-wheat bread contains one-third more protein, three to four times more fiber, four times more zinc, and more folic acid and iron.

While we're on the subject of colors, wild and brown rice are more nutritious than white rice. Dark pink fish (such as salmon, trout, and Arctic char) is more nutritious than white fish. Dark chocolate contains more nutrients than milk chocolate. Sweet potatoes contain more nutrients than white potatoes. You get the idea! Make your pregnancy diet more colorful — your health and your baby will thank you.

TRY DR. BILL AND MARTHA'S 5-S DIET

Our 5-S diet is especially healthful to get your body ready for birth, and to heal after birth.

It's also the one we use in our medical practice to help heal "itis" illnesses:

- **S**eafood: primarily Alaskan salmon

- **S**moothies: multiple dark-colored fruits and berries, organic yogurt, ground flaxseeds, and cinnamon

- **S**alads: organic arugula, kale, spinach, and tomatoes

- **S**pices: ginger, turmeric, black pepper, rosemary, cinnamon (whatever spices are the most stomach-friendly)

- **S**upplements: the three that we recommend are the ones most supported by science:

- Omega-3 fish oils, primarily salmon oil from Alaska

- Juice Plus+, a concentrate of many fruits and vegetables

- Prenatal supplements recommended by your healthcare provider

These supplements fill in the gaps on weeks you don't eat 12 ounces of seafood and nine to twelve servings of fruits and vegetables daily. And, let's add two more S's: homemade soups and stews, which, like smoothies and salads, enjoy the nutritional perk called synergy: Blend many nutrients together and each one becomes more healthful.

TRAFFIC-LIGHT EATING FOR A HEALTHY PREGNANCY

Green-light foods	*Yellow-light foods*	*Red-light foods*
Good for you and baby — enjoy!	Slow down, not too much! Enjoy as an occasional treat.	*Do not* eat these foods. They are not good for you and baby.
• Beans and lentils	• Butter	• Beverages sweetened with corn syrup, such as cola*
• Chocolate, dark	• Cakes and cookies, made with 100% whole-grain flour	• Foods containing artificial dyes (e.g., red #40) in the ingredient list
• Cinnamon		
• Cocoa powder	• Fast food/fatty meats	
• Eggs	• French fries	• Foods containing artificial sweeteners
• Fish, especially wild salmon	• Frozen yogurt	

(continued)

TRAFFIC-LIGHT EATING FOR A HEALTHY PREGNANCY *(continued)*

Green-light foods	*Yellow-light foods*	*Red-light foods*
• Flaxseeds, ground, and flaxseed oil • Fruits, all • Garlic and onions • Meat, lean • Milk, low-fat • Nuts and seeds • Nut butters • Nut oils • Olive oil • Poultry, skinless • Rice, wild or brown • Soybeans, edamame • Sweeteners: honey, blackstrap molasses • Tofu • Turmeric • Vegetables, all • Wheat germ • 100% whole-grain bread, pasta, cereal • Yogurt: Greek, plain or fruit-added	• 100% fruit juice, without added sweeteners • Ice cream, whipped cream, and sour cream • Pasta made from white flour • Pastries and pies, made with healthy fats and whole-grain flour • White bread • White rice	• Foods containing cottonseed oil, hydrogenated oils, or shortening • Gelatin desserts containing artificial flavors and colors • Marshmallows, candy bars, and hard candy • Nitrite-containing cold cuts and hot dogs • Packaged high-fat, low-fiber bakery goods

* Drinking sweetened beverages during pregnancy increases the risk of gestational diabetes.

PREGNANCY NUTRITION AT A GLANCE

Eating healthy while pregnant isn't all that different from how you should eat when you're not pregnant. You'll notice that even though your daily calorie intake may increase by only 10 to 20 percent while pregnant, certain nutrients may increase by as much as 50 percent. The conclusion you can draw is that while pregnant you need to upgrade the *quality* of your food rather than increase the *quantity*. While you need more of just about every nutrient, focus most on the nourishing nine:

Average daily nutrients you and your baby need	Richest food sources	Why you and baby need it
Omega-3 fats: 1,000 milligrams	Salmon, 6 ounces: 2,000 milligrams	Baby's brain development; mommy's mood stability, vision acuity, immunity regulator.
Folate/folic acid*: 600–800 micrograms	Spinach, 1 cup: 260 micrograms Enriched whole-wheat bread, 1 slice: 250 micrograms Lentils, ½ cup: 200 micrograms Asparagus, ½ cup: 134 micrograms Edamame, ½ cup: 100 micrograms Wheat germ, 2 tablespoons: 85 micrograms	Development of baby's spinal cord. Be sure to take this supplement early in the first month (or, better yet, before becoming pregnant), since the neural tube in the spine closes during the third or fourth week of pregnancy. Folic acid deficiency also increases the risk of prematurity and behavior problems.
Iron: 30 milligrams	Spirulina powder, 1 teaspoon: 7 milligrams Blackstrap molasses, 1 tablespoon: 5 milligrams	Extra red blood cell volume for mommy and baby. Deficiency can lead to fatigue.

(continued)

Average daily nutrients you and your baby need	Richest food sources	Why you and baby need it
	Cereal (whole-grain, such as All-Bran), 1 serving: 4–8 milligrams	
	Firm tofu, ½ cup: 4–7 milligrams	
	Lean meat/poultry, 4–6 ounces: 4–5 milligrams	
	Lentils, 4 ounces: 3 milligrams	
	Prune juice, 8 ounces: 3 milligrams	
	Salmon/tuna, 4 ounces: 2 milligrams	
	Kidney/black beans, ½ cup: 2 milligrams	
	Dried figs, 5: 2 milligrams	
Calcium: 1,400–1,600 milligrams	Yogurt, 1 cup: 400 milligrams	Strong bones. Growing baby bones drain mommy bones, so build up your calcium bank.
	Low-fat milk, 1 cup: 300 milligrams	
	Cheese, 1 ounce: 200 milligrams	
	Canned salmon (with bones), 3 ounces: 180 milligrams	
	Tofu, ½ cup: 100 milligrams	
Vitamin B_{12}: 2.6 micrograms	Spirulina powder, 1 teaspoon: 9 micrograms	Baby's brain development.
	Salmon, 3 ounces: 4 micrograms	
	Lean beef, 3 ounces: 2 micrograms	
	Yogurt, 1 cup: 1.4 micrograms	
	Milk, 1 cup: 1 microgram	
	Egg, 1: 0.5 microgram	

Average daily nutrients you and your baby need	Richest food sources	Why you and baby need it
Vitamin D: 1,000 IU	Salmon, 6 ounces: 1,000 IU Fortified milk, 1 cup: 100 IU Egg, 1: 23 IU Sunshine: varies with exposure	Boosts immune system and uterine muscle strength; bone development.
Vitamin C: 200 milligrams	Bell pepper, 1 cup: 175 milligrams Strawberries, 1 cup: 84 milligrams Broccoli, 1 cup: 82 milligrams Papaya, 1: 180 milligrams	Immune strength protection for growing tissues.
Zinc: 11 milligrams	Alaskan king crab, 3 ounces: 6 milligrams Lean grass-fed beef/turkey, 4 ounces: 5 milligrams Spinach, 2 cups: 3 milligrams Pumpkin/sesame seeds, ¼ cup: 3 milligrams Tofu, ½ cup: 2 milligrams Wheat germ, 2 tablespoons: 2 milligrams	Boosts immune system.
Iodine: 220 micrograms	Salmon, 6 ounces: 100 micrograms Nori (seaweed): 100 micrograms per serving Yogurt, 1 cup: 80 micrograms Iodized salt, ½ teaspoon: 75 micrograms Egg, 1: 24 micrograms	Optimal thyroid function.

(continued)

Additional Considerations		
Protein: 100 grams	Salmon, 6 ounces: 43 grams Greek yogurt, 1 cup: 23 grams Black beans: ½ cup, 7.5 grams Egg, 1: 6 grams	Growth of extra tissue for mommy and baby.
Choline: 450 milligrams	Salmon, 6 ounces: 191 milligrams Egg yolk, 1: 125 milligrams Soy beans, ½ cup: 100 milligrams Broccoli, 1 cup: 62 milligrams Wheat germ, ¼ cup: 50 milligrams	Baby's brain development.

*"Folate" is the term used for this nutrient in foods. "Folic acid" is the term used for the synthetic form of this nutrient, such as found in prenatal vitamins or added to foods.

Gain the Weight That's Right for You and Baby

Pregnancy may be the only time in your life when you can be happy about gaining weight. As you watch the scale, smile — you're growing a baby! All mothers understand that they need to gain weight, yet most wonder how much.

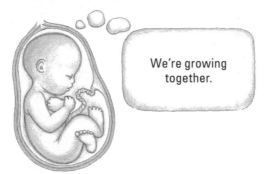

We're growing together.

WHAT IS A HEALTHY WEIGHT GAIN?

Besides baby's weight, just add up all the extra pounds you need to grow a healthy baby (see the chart on page 52). Obstetricians currently recommend that most women gain 25 to 35 pounds. Whether you gain at the low end or the high end of this range depends upon your body type and whether you were overweight or underweight initially. Here are some guidelines:

- The weight gain in the first trimester for a woman of medium build should be 3 to 6 pounds.

- Weight gain during the next six months should average 1 pound per week. Gaining more than 4 pounds in one week could be an unhealthy sign.

Special guidelines for special situations. New guidelines from the Institute of Medicine and the American Medical Association have changed the recommendation for healthy weight gain in pregnancy in special situations:

- Mothers who are already obese at the beginning of their pregnancy should gain only 10 to 20 pounds during pregnancy. (Some recent research suggests that obese mothers who follow a healthy diet and lifestyle during their pregnancy do not have to gain any weight to birth a healthy baby.)

- Mothers of multiples need to gain 35 to 45 pounds during pregnancy.

(A useful resource for the latest advice on pregnancy weight gain can be found online at iom.edu/pregnancyweightgain.)

For moms who are underweight initially, it is important to understand that your body *needs* extra body fat. A healthy pregnant body needs fat reserves, insurance that there's enough energy for your baby to grow and for sufficient supporting tissue.

Don't worry if you have a few weight gain spurts that don't go according to the book. As long as you're eating the right diet and following the rest of these healthy pregnancy tips, your weight gain is probably right for you and your baby. Your healthcare provider will be alert to anything problematic with weight gain when certain measurements are made (blood pressure, urinalysis, and so on) at your regular checkups.

What goes up will soon come down. Guess what? Along with your baby, you'll "deliver" nearly half the weight you gained. Be prepared to retain a bit of extra body fat postpartum as a milk-making energy reserve, and know that breastfeeding can actually help you shed the extra pounds faster.

WHERE YOUR EXTRA WEIGHT GOES

Your weight gain is lavished on the star of the show, your baby, and the supporting cast that this blooming star depends on. The following amounts are averages, as each mother-baby pair is unique:

Baby	7½ pounds
Enlarging uterus	2 pounds
Placenta	1½ pounds
Amniotic fluid	2 pounds
Breast enlargement	2 pounds
Extra blood and fluid volume	8 pounds
Extra fat reserves*	7 pounds
Total:	**30 pounds**

* The "increased fat" is the only part that is mostly under your control.

WHY EXCESS "MOMMY FAT" IS HARD TO SHED

It's hard to lose excess weight if you gain too much during pregnancy because, as we discussed earlier, excess fat cells produce hormones such as leptin and adiponectin, which slow your metabolism and fat burning. After delivery, your body is still in a state of conserving fat, prompting you to hold onto it. The more excess fat cells you put on during pregnancy, the longer it will take to lose them. Women who are "burners" seem to have the pounds melt off effortlessly. Others, whose metabolisms are more typical, find that no matter what they do, the "baby fifteen" just won't go away. For them, it is important to do the hard work of returning to their pre-pregnant weight before the next pregnancy. If they don't, the 30 pounds left from these two pregnancies may very well stay with them. With another pregnancy, weight concerns could be overwhelming.

WHY IS GAINING TOO MUCH WEIGHT NOT HEALTHY FOR BABY?

Excess weight means excess health problems—for mother and baby. The closer you are to your optimal weight gain, the healthier you and your baby are likely to be, and the less complicated your delivery is likely to be. Women who gain excess weight during pregnancy are prone to:

- Have a longer, more painful labor

- Need a cesarean section

- Develop toxemia

- Deliver baby preterm

- Deliver a heavier baby (greater than 9 pounds)

- Experience more birth complications

- Double their risk of delivering a baby with a birth defect

- Greatly increase their child's risk of being obese and developing diabetes

- Feel more joint pains (back, pelvis, knees, ankles)

- Become more depressed

- Experience leg and ankle swelling

- Sleep poorly

- Take longer to get back to pre-pregnancy weight

Baby is born with a "weight problem." As discussed on page 14, it seems that excessive maternal weight gain during pregnancy changes the baby's developing genes for appetite control, metabolism of fats and carbohydrates, and insulin metabolism.

"Prediabetic"—a more change-motivating term. Don't be shocked if your healthcare provider tells you you're "prediabetic" instead of the wimpy, less-motivating diagnosis "overweight." Besides being unhealthy for baby and mother, excess weight gain makes medical care more difficult for the doctor — for example, ultrasound detection of prenatal problems can be compromised and deliveries more difficult.

Consider the amazing changes that your body goes through to grow another human being, and embrace those changes. If you dread being admonished for your "weight gain," request that your healthcare provider check your weight at the very end of your appointment so that you start your visit on a positive note. And then let that "dread" motivate you to be healthier for the next visit. Many healthcare providers believe that if a mother eats a healthy diet and has adequate exercise, there is little need to worry about what the scale shows.

EIGHTEEN STRATEGIES TO CURB YOUR CRAVINGS AND GAIN OPTIMAL WEIGHT

Some of the "diets" recommended for weight loss are downright dangerous during pregnancy. They're either too restrictive, too complicated, or too unhealthy. Here are the simplest and most effective weight-control strategies to use while you're pregnant:

1. Eat Real Foods

What diet keeps you lean? The *real food diet*. What diet makes you fat? The *fake food diet*. It's as simple as that. The real food diet contains food that goes from sea, tree, or farm to your plate, and spends little time, if any, in a food-processing factory. Remember, real food has a crave-control perk called a high satiety factor, while fake food is less filling and has an addictive factor, prompting you to overbuy and overeat.

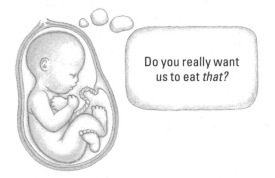

Do you really want us to eat *that*?

Throughout your pregnancy, especially in the first trimester, focus more on eating right than eating more. In the second half, you will need to eat right *and* eat more as baby goes through growth spurts.

2. Graze!

As discussed earlier, grazing (see page 20) and the sipping solution (see page 22) are two time-tested ways of resetting your body's expectation of how much food you need. Grazing and sipping on minimeals throughout the day stabilize your blood insulin levels, let you refuel your body and burn calories as needed, and allow you to still store a bit of extra body fat — if you need to. As you graze, your baby grazes, too. If you have wide swings in eating, then your baby might as well, causing her to produce more insulin to take care of the spikes in blood sugar.

> The leanest explanation of the best pregnancy diet:
>
> **Graze on real foods.**

Another good reason to graze is that it helps you naturally increase your calorie-burning — and excess-fat-burning — rate. Science has shown that this is the reason grazers tend to be leaner.

After a few weeks of grazing, your body will reset its food expectations so you'll be satisfied with less. With your previous overeating habits, your body believed that this was the normal way of eating. You should make changes slowly, so you can fool your body into being satisfied with less. Eventually, your body will have a lower "set point," the level of eating that satisfies your body.

Martha notes: Sometimes you need to eat whatever will stay down, but try to balance that with good nutrition. While "I'm pregnant" is sometimes a valid excuse, try to be honest with yourself about needs versus wants. If you crave sweets, try eating some protein with it, such as honey-sweetened Greek yogurt.

3. Don't Go Hungry

The sensation of hunger aggravates nausea and stimulates reactive overeating. The body misinterprets hunger pains as: "It's famine time, I better store up like a hibernating bear." Your appetite increases, and you'll tend to overeat. You're more likely to give in to unhealthy cravings when you're hungry. Ditto for shopping trips. Veteran pregnant shoppers have found that if they're hungry while they stroll around the supermarket, they're more likely to grab the red-light foods listed on page 45. Grazing is good for you because it keeps you from getting hungry.

4. Resist Temptation

The temptation to overeat is usually highest in the second trimester. In the first three months you're more likely to just want your supersensitive stomach to settle rather than be full. In the last three months your big baby presses on your intestines and stomach, dampening your desire to overeat. So, that leaves the middle trimester as the time to indulge. Be vigilant during this time in curbing your cravings. (See page 124 for some tips on curbing cravings.)

Try to switch your cravings to something you can happily indulge in. Instead of potato chips, grab a handful of raw almonds or walnuts, or at least buy chips that are "popped" instead of fried or baked. This takes planning and being aware of your weaknesses. Ginger snaps or vanilla wafers can be just as satisfying as Oreos. A granola yogurt parfait is much less guilt producing than full-fat premium ice cream. Unless you have nerves of steel when it comes to portion control, save the Häagen Dazs for treat days.

DON'T DO DIET SODA

Artificial sweeteners in diet soda fall in the category of "when in doubt, leave it out." The safety of these substances has never been proven, especially for babies and pregnant mothers. An interesting study in one of the most reputable health and nutrition journals, the *American Journal of Clinical Nutrition,* showed that women who drank at least one diet soda per day were 38 percent more likely to deliver a premature baby. Mothers who drank more than four daily were 80 percent more likely.

---

5. Make Every Calorie Count

Nutrient-dense foods tend to be more satisfying and more filling, making it less likely that you will overeat. Somewhere inside your body is a built-in calorie counter that automatically registers the number of calories you consumed that day, and prompts you when you've eaten enough. (Admittedly, this calorie controller sometimes falls asleep on the job.) Nutritional scientists have discovered that the calories from sweetened

beverages don't register on your internal counter, thus warranting the term "empty calories." Make sure every calorie counts.

6. Enjoy "Free" Foods

"Free" foods are "eat all you want anytime, in any amount" foods. Vegetables are free foods for two reasons: They fill you up with fewer calories, and you burn many of the calories in vegetables just by digesting them. Lightly dressed salads are truly a pregnant mother's leanest food. (See Martha's recipe for Pregnancy Salad on page 38.)

7. Eat Fill-Up Foods First

The time-honored dietary custom of "salads first" is especially useful for pregnant mothers. Begin your meal with high-protein, high-fiber foods, which are more filling. You will be satisfied sooner and less likely to overeat. Even more important, high-protein, high-fiber, and healthy-fat meals actually lower your craving for junk carbs. Here are some of our favorite fill-up foods for snacks or meals:

• Avocados	• Nuts
• Beans and lentils	• Oatmeal
• Eggs	• Salads
• Figs	• Salmon
• Greek yogurt	• Tofu
• Hummus	• Whole grains

8. Use Chopsticks

Besides eating more real foods and less processed foods, one reason Asians tend to stay leaner during pregnancy might be that they use chopsticks. This encourages them to take smaller bites and to take longer to dine. Forget the fork and choose chopsticks as a simple weight-control tactic.

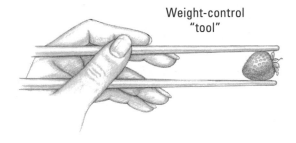

Weight-control "tool"

9. Chew-Chew Times Two

Besides taking smaller bites, chew twice as long as you are used to, say 20 to 30 chews per mouthful, depending on the texture. Prolonged chewing, besides helping you eat less and become satisfied sooner, has some pregnancy perks: extra chewing secretes extra saliva, which buffers irritating stomach acids, lessening heartburn, and it prompts the upper end of the intestines to do more work on digestion, sparing the discomforts at the lower end.

10. Begin the Day with Breakfast

Breakfast eaters tend to be leaner. Known as "front-loading," when you start the day with a breakfast of real food, you program your body to crave real food the rest of the day. Breakfast skippers and those who eat junk food for breakfast tend to overeat, especially junk carbs, the rest of the day.

11. Move!

Movement not only helps keep you lean, it also mellows your mind during pregnancy. Along with controlling excess fat gain, and even losing excess mommy fat, movement has many other health benefits, as you will learn in chapter 5.

12. Stress Less

As we've discussed, excess stress hormones, such as cortisol, stimulate the storage of excess fat, particularly around the abdomen. And excess abdominal fat can interfere with normal neurochemical balance, resulting in moodiness. In chapter 6 you'll learn how to lower your stress while pregnant.

13. Give in, Occasionally

Some cravings may be your wisdom-of-the-body voice prompting you to eat more of what you need. You may like, even crave, foods you previously disliked, perhaps because your changing body has nutritional needs it didn't have before. Even confirmed vegans may crave meat, which could be their gut voice telling them that their body needs more iron. Consider two common pregnancy cravings: pickles and potato chips. These foods are high in salt, which your body needs, and they stimulate thirst so you drink more water. Perhaps your body is telling you that it needs a lot of extra fluid to fill up baby's amniotic swimming pool.

Dr. Linda notes: I noticed severe cravings for steak and hamburger early on in pregnancy. My husband was shocked, since he had rarely seen me eat any meat other than lean chicken or fish. I'm sure it was my body's way of getting extra minerals and iron, since my diet tended to be somewhat low in these. And I would look at sweets in magazines and actually start drooling. My big craving was gummy bears. I didn't think it was healthy for my two-year-old to see mommy wolfing down gummy bears and then telling her they're not good for her. So I looked for healthier "sweets," like figs and homemade oatmeal raisin cookies.

14. Make an "Instead of" List

Write down your most common cravings. Cross off the least-healthy ones and replace them with healthier alternatives. For example, instead of a hot fudge sundae, have a frozen Greek yogurt with honey and blueberries.

15. Try a Healthy Treat a Day

A few squares of dark chocolate or a homemade cookie or two may be just what your body needs to keep food cravings at bay. Martha insisted we upgrade dark chocolate to a green-light food (see page 45). If you crave nutritious, nutrient-dense foods, give in to your cravings and enjoy. Eventually, you will train your cravings to be satisfied by what is good for you and baby.

16. Out of Sight Is Out of Tummy

If you don't buy it, it's easier to avoid it. Try to stock your kitchen full of mainly green-light,

a few yellow-light, and no red-light foods. The hardest craving to curb is the one within easy reach — you have to put your body through all kinds of stress to say no to it. Avoid looking at junk food ads in magazines, too. Even a photo of junk food can trigger a "got to have it" reaction.

17. Walk Away

When your cravings are getting out of control, fill up a container of water and take a walk. Sometimes just changing where you go and what you look at gets your brain focusing on things other than what to indulge in. Nibble on a piece of fruit while you walk.

18. Consult a Craving Counselor

Consult your healthcare provider or a nutritionist to analyze whether there are surprise nutrients in your cravings that your body needs, and help you substitute healthier alternatives.

A HEALTHY ONLINE RESOURCE WHILE PREGNANT

L.E.A.N. Expectations is a series of online interactive workshops that teach expectant mothers the best health and nutrition habits for their family. This course focuses on the four pillars of health for the pregnant mother: lifestyle, exercise, attitude, and nutrition. See DrSearsWellnessInstitute.org.

5

Exercise Right for Two

Just as growing a baby prompts you to change your eating habits, that little mover and shaker (literally) inside is a reason to up your commitment to exercise. You're training for one of the most body-challenging marathons of your life — childbirth. It's not necessary to build more muscle, but you do need to tone the muscle you have. Toning or increasing your muscle mass during pregnancy increases your bone density and bone strength. It also helps stabilize your blood sugar, part of that hormonal harmony you will learn about on page 324, which prevents high blood sugar problems and gestational diabetes. Insulin levels naturally drop low when you're active, so you store less excess fat.

HOW EXERCISE BENEFITS BOTH MOMMY AND BABY—NEW RESEARCH

New studies confirm what pregnant women have long suspected: the more you move, the healthier you are. During one of our health talks, Martha confided to the audience, "I'm allergic to exercise." I quipped, "Martha's favorite exercise is *childbirth!*" What motivated Martha to move more began with a dinner conversation at our home. Our guest was Dr. Louis Ignarro, who won a Nobel Prize in medicine for what you are about to learn: the science behind how movement makes you healthier.

Like Martha, you may not be motivated to move and you may not like exercising. But movement helps you make your own "internal medicines," natural health-promoting substances that help you have a healthier pregnancy.

The lining of your blood vessels, called the endothelium, is like the surface pavement on a highway. Once upon a time the endothelium was thought to be nothing more than tissue lining the muscular and fibrous walls of the blood vessels. Yet, thanks to research by Dr. Ignarro, we now know that the endothelium is your body's largest endocrine organ. If you open all your blood vessels and spread them out flat, your endothelium would cover the surface area of several tennis courts.

Each cell of the endothelium is its own endocrine organ, filled with microscopic "medicine bottles" that release

Pregnancy Pharmacy OPEN

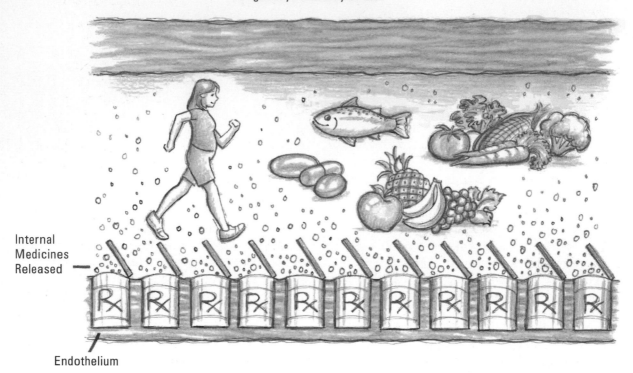

Internal
Medicines
Released —

Endothelium

health-promoting substances into the bloodstream at just the right time, in just the right amount, with no harmful side effects — and they're free!

Your endothelium is constantly sensing the needs of your body and responding to those needs by dispensing these substances into your bloodstream. There are medicines to lower your "highs," such as high blood pressure. There are medicines to raise your "lows" and mellow your moods, just like antidepressants; and medicines to heal your hurts, like anti-inflammatories. There is a lot going on in your pregnant body, and this amazing endothelium helps supply the internal medicines you and baby need.

How do you get these millions of microscopic bottles to release your internal medicines? The answer: move! Brisk movement causes blood to flow faster over the surface of the endothelium. The fast-moving blood creates an energy field called shear force, which releases a natural biochemical called nitric oxide (NO). NO acts as a biochemical key to open your pharmacy and dispense the medicines you need.

The more you exercise, the more your endothelium gets used to the extra blood flow. In research lingo this is called up-regulation of the endothelial cells, a sort of upgrade of the quantity and quality of the substances that can be released. For the habitual exerciser — the physically fit person — the endothelium is more responsive to NO.

Another motivation for you to move more while pregnant: Studies show that women who exercise more during pregnancy have higher levels of endorphins (natural pain relievers) during their pregnancy and labor and tend to report less painful labors and less need for pain-relieving drugs during labor (read more about endorphins on page 297).

EIGHT TIPS FOR EXERCISING RIGHT FOR YOU AND BABY

1. Consult your healthcare provider first. Before you embark on an exercise program, work in partnership with your healthcare provider to determine the exercise program that is right for you and safe for your baby. The following conditions will affect choices that you make about an exercise routine:

TWENTY PREGNANCY PERKS OF EXERCISE

Here are some of the many ways exercise improves your physical and mental well-being:

1. Mellows mother's moods, lifts depression.

2. Prepares body for easier birth, strengthens and stretches muscles and joints.

3. Prepares body to rely less on medication during labor.

4. Boosts immune system.

5. Optimizes weight gain.

6. Facilitates excess fat loss postpartum.

7. Stabilizes insulin levels, promoting hormonal harmony.

8. Lowers risk of gestational diabetes.

9. Lessens constipation.

10. Lessens joint pain, especially in the back and pelvis.

11. Reduces risk of birth complications and cesarean delivery.

12. Leads to shorter labors.

13. Reduces leg swelling.

14. Eases morning sickness and tummy queasiness.

15. Helps you appreciate your pregnant body's abilities.

16. Improves quality of sleep.

17. Lowers risk of prematurity.

18. Improves bone density.

19. Lowers chances of child becoming obese.

20. Improves balance, lessening falls.

- Anemia

- Heart problems

- Asthma or chronic lung problems

- High blood pressure

- Diabetes

- Thyroid problems

- Seizures

- Significant over- or underweight

- Muscle or joint problems

- History of several miscarriages

- History of premature labors

- Carrying multiples

- Incompetent cervix

- Persistent bleeding

- Placental abnormalities (such as placenta previa)

- A previously sedentary lifestyle (a serious couch potato)

2. Dress for the occasion. Wear loose-fitting pants with a loose elastic waistband. To avoid overheating, remove layers as your body warms up. Your clothes should be loose enough to allow sweat to evaporate, thus cooling the skin. Wear supportive shoes that are large enough to allow for swelling feet. To avoid injury to your heel bones, be sure your shoes are well cushioned under the heels. If they're not, insert a ¼-inch shock-absorbing heel pad. It is best to avoid jogging on hard surfaces. Wear a support bra, or even two if your breasts are very large and heavy. Sport bras that limit bouncing are available in department stores

or sporting goods stores. If your clothing rubs and irritates your newly sensitive nipples while exercising, wear a nonconstricting top or a special runner's bra, or coat your nipples with a protective emollient such as Lansinoh or a cooling pad such as Soothies.

3. Start low, go slow. Especially if you're an exercise newbie, don't overdo it. You may not realize that just being pregnant itself is a built-in "exercise routine." Because your heart rate increases by 20 percent even in the first trimester, pregnancy increases your metabolism and causes your body to perform a low level of aerobic exercise. As you and your baby grow, your blood volume eventually increases by at least 40 percent, and your cardiac output (the amount of blood pumped by your heart) increases by 30 to 40 percent. In effect, your cardiovascular system is "exercised" just by being pregnant.

It used to be thought that if a woman exercised too much she would rob the uterus and baby of blood supply. We now know that as long as you exercise sensibly and don't overdo it, your muscles won't divert blood flow from your baby.

If you enter pregnancy already fit, and you already have an exercise routine that works for you, continue it; just modify it as your changing body dictates. If, however, up until now you've never felt compelled to join the "sweat set," be sure to begin with light muscle- and joint-friendly exercises and gradually build up the time and intensity of the exercises. Your main goal for exercise is to feel good and prepare your body for birth, not to lose weight. For the newly pregnant beginner, many obstetricians recommend exercising for thirty minutes three times a week, gradually increasing the duration and intensity. Short, frequent, consistent exercise routines are healthier than sporadic bursts. Even if you've enjoyed indoor workouts before, you may find outdoor exercises, such as swimming or brisk walking in a park, to be much more mentally relaxing than the gym scene of smelly, sweating bodies and clanking machines.

Martha notes: Balance increased exercise with indulgent rest. Make your movements full of fun and joy. Skip the drudgery of a workout if you are dreading it. Instead, dance, hike in nature, or walk to a flower shop, anything to keep you moving and make you smile.

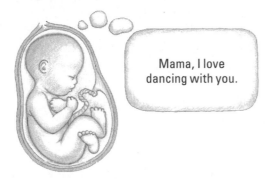

Mama, I love dancing with you.

4. Know your limits. The key to exercising safely while pregnant is to work your body without stressing baby's. As a general guideline, if the exercise is too strenuous for you, it's too strenuous for baby. Your rising heart rate is an indication of how hard your body is working and how fit you are. The more fit you are, the more you are able to do while maintaining the same heart rate. Research has shown that baby's heart rate doesn't go up significantly until the exercising mother's heart rate reaches 150 beats per minute. To know when to slow down, observe these monitors:

- *The pulse test.* Take your pulse on your wrist or your neck just beneath the jaw (count the beats for ten seconds and multiply by 6 to get heartbeats per minute). To avoid accelerating your baby's heart rate, *keep your heart rate below 140 beats per minute.*

- *The talk test.* If you are too winded to carry on a conversation, ease your exercising to a level at which you can comfortably converse.

- *Listen to your body's stop signs.* If you experience dizziness, faintness, headaches, shortness of breath, hard heart pounding or palpitations, abdominal cramping, uterine contractions, pain anywhere, vaginal bleeding, or fluid leaking, stop immediately. (For these last two, notify your healthcare provider!) The key to exercising wisely is to *listen to your body.*

5. As baby grows, mommy slows. In the final months of pregnancy, your baby and your uterus need more of your blood in order to grow, and your heart will have to work harder even when you are resting. There is less reserve blood supply for exercising muscles, so it's time to slow the intensity of your exercise routine. Runners, start walking or swimming. Walkers and swimmers, slow your pace. During the third trimester, the combination of increasing weight, general awkwardness, swelling of legs and ankles, and softer joint ligaments calls for a change from weight-bearing exercises (jogging and dancing) to less weight-bearing ones, such as stationary cycling and swimming.

EXERCISE PRECAUTIONS WHILE PREGNANT

Besides choosing the best body- and baby-friendly exercise, here are some added precautions:

Rehydrate and refuel. Dehydration makes muscles tire more easily. To avoid dehydration, drink two 8-ounce glasses of water before and after exercising. And don't exercise on an empty stomach or when you feel hungry, because exercise uses up blood sugar quickly, and pregnancy already makes you prone to blood-sugar swings. A before-and-after exercise snack protects your body and your baby from hypoglycemia (low blood sugar). Try quick-energy snacks, such as fruit or honey-sweetened yogurt. (Learn more about smart snacks on page 22.)

Keep cool. To keep yourself and your baby from becoming overheated, don't exercise strenuously in hot and humid weather. If you are exercising indoors, be sure to ventilate the room. Wear loose clothing to allow body heat to be easily released.

Warm up and cool down. During pregnancy your body's extra blood supply knows its priorities: your uterus and its resident. It takes time for your cardiovascular system to ramp up to the demands of exercising muscles. Ease into exercise before going full steam ahead. Take five minutes to *gradually* build up to your peak and then, when you are finished, *gradually* wind down the exercise over five minutes, allowing your cardiovascular system to adjust. Abruptly stopping strenuous exercise can cause blood to pool in the exercised muscles. (Of course, it's important to stop abruptly if you notice any of the stop signs listed on page 63.)

What about jogging or running while pregnant? Your baby and your uterus are firmly anchored inside your body. So, if you were previously a jogger, it may be OK to continue; but slow down your pace even during the early months of your pregnancy. Fast running is one of those "when in doubt, leave it out" exercises later in pregnancy for several reasons: it's uncomfortable on already tender joints, and since you're off balance, it's easier to trip while running. If you do run, run on a soft surface, wear heel-cushioned running shoes, and don't run to exhaustion. (Review the precautions on page 63.)

6. Don't jar the joints. Due to the influence of relaxin and other pregnancy hormones, your ligaments loosen, making your joints less stable and more prone to injury if overstretched, especially the joints in your pelvis, lower back, and knees. Avoid sudden hyperextension or hyperflexing exercises, such as back arching and deep knee bends. Gymnastics is out. Five-pound dumbbells are safe for toning arm and shoulder muscles. Avoid joint-jarring moves in sports such as tennis and racquetball.

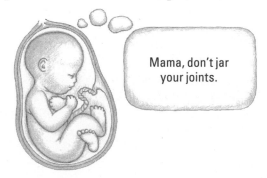

Mama, don't jar your joints.

7. Don't shake the baby. Your baby, safely cushioned in his own pool, is unlikely to be bothered by exercise. Nevertheless, avoid jarring exercises and sudden stops, such as exercises that involve jumping or sudden changes in direction, like basketball or tennis. Avoid running on hard surfaces like cement or asphalt. Swimming and cycling are easier on your body, and baby's.

8. Stay in balance. Your enlarging breasts and uterus change your body's center of gravity, increasing your chances of falling or straining your back muscles during workouts. Avoid exercise that requires precise balance, such as gymnastics or downhill skiing. Dance classes are fun as long as you are willing to grin and bear the fact that your movements may have lost some of their grace.

9. Keep off your back. After the fourth month, avoid exercising while lying on your back. By this stage of pregnancy, your uterus is large enough to compress the major blood vessels that run along the right side of your spine (vena cava and aorta). Allow your body and your baby to rest after exercise. Lie on your left side, a position that prevents your uterus from pressing on the major blood vessels and promotes circulation to your uterus.

NO-NO EXERCISES WHILE PREGNANT

Choose your recreational sports wisely. Because you are carrying an additional 10- to 30-pound load, you just can't do the same sports at the level you are used to. Depending on your stage of pregnancy, some sports may be too risky to both you and baby.

- Tennis should be played with caution, since the sudden stops and pivots may stress your pregnancy-changed ligaments. Ditto for racquetball, which has the added problem of overheating associated with any indoor sport.

- Because of the risk of falling at high speeds, avoid waterskiing.

- Downhill skiing should be avoided during the second and third trimesters, because your changing center of gravity affects your balance. Switch to cross-country skiing on level terrain.

- Because of the risk of falling, put away your ice skates in the second half of your pregnancy.

- Competitive basketball and volleyball are too bouncy and stretchy to be played safely while pregnant.

- Avoid horseback riding. Besides the risk of falling off the horse, straddling and bouncing in the saddle can overstretch the already sensitive pelvic ligaments, leading to pelvic pain.

- Heavy weightlifting is out because of the strain on your muscles and ligaments and the potentially dangerous breath holding that accompanies this sport.

- Because of the possibility of compromising oxygen supply to your baby, scuba diving is an absolute no-no. Try snorkeling instead.

ANYTIME-ANYWHERE EXERCISES

Think of all movement as exercise:

- **Walk while you wait.** As you're standing in line, waiting for a prenatal appointment, or simply standing around, walk around in circles or do some movement.

- **Flex while you stand or sit.** While standing, do a few squats. Go up and down on your toes and flex your knees. While sitting, arch your feet up and down, which flexes the muscles in the front and back of your legs, minimizes ankle swelling, and keeps the blood circulating well in your legs. This is especially important when you are sitting for long periods of time. Take a break from your desk job to get up and move at least once an hour.

- **Walk while you talk.** Walk around instead of sitting while talking on the phone.

- **Enjoy "band aids."** Stretch bands are very muscle- and joint-friendly, especially for a pregnant woman. Leave these bands hanging around your house and flex a few whenever you pass by. Use them as a traveling gym when you're on trips.

- **Work out while you watch.** Do stretch-band exercises while watching TV. During commercials, get up and get a glass of water, let the dog out, or throw in a load of laundry.

SAFE AND FUN SWIMMING WHILE PREGNANT

Take the plunge! Swimming is the ideal pregnancy exercise. Many women find swimming more relaxing and easier on their pregnant body than any other exercise. Swimming is especially helpful in the third trimester, when exercising becomes increasingly uncomfortable. It is actually easier while pregnant because you are more buoyant. Here are other reasons to consider swimming:

- It is easy on the joints. When you stand chest-deep in water, the weight on your overburdened knees, hips, and lower back is lessened. The resistance of water encourages smoother movements that are easier on the joints than the jerky movements of land-bound exercises.

- It is friendly to an aching back and pelvic muscles.

- It mellows moods. Water aerobics, or just plain dancing around in the water, is great exercise for relaxing both mind and body.

- It improves breathing. Swimming the breaststroke expands your chest to inhale more air. (If you get short of breath, use a kickboard to help keep your head above water.)

- It improves circulation.

- It helps relieve ankle swelling.

- Research reveals that mothers who enjoy swimming classes tend to need less pain medication during labor.

Unless your doctor or midwife says otherwise, you can swim right up until your membranes rupture.

Being in water helped me appreciate my pregnant body. I felt so free and floaty when I didn't have to worry about my posture or falling when exercising. It's the only exercise I could do in which I felt being pregnant gave me an advantage.

Take a swim class tailored for pregnant women, often available at your local YMCA or community center. Be sure the instructor is knowledgeable about the special exercising needs of pregnant women.

And now a word about swimsuits. Feeling good about your body in a swimsuit is hard for many women, even when they're not pregnant. Putting on a swimsuit while pregnant may require a strong mental commitment to maintaining a positive body image. You'll feel great once you get into the water, so don't let the swimsuit issue become an insurmountable hurdle.

A maternity swimsuit is one garment you may not be able to borrow. Time and pool chemicals tend to destroy elastic, and an old suit may not keep you covered. If you plan to swim during your pregnancy, invest in a new suit, one that makes you feel good and comfortable.

Safe swimming tips:

- A water temperature of 85°F (29°C) is comfortable for prolonged exercising yet cool enough to be refreshing.

- Be careful getting into and out of the pool and when walking on slippery surfaces. Wearing rubber slip-on shoes in and out of the pool area decreases your chance of slipping.

- Many warm lakes may not be clean enough for swimming. It's safer to stick to pools.

- Don't hyperextend your joints. In the comfort of water you may not realize you are overstretching.

- No diving, please.

- Weather permitting, swim in outdoor pools. The air around indoor pools can get stuffy and humid, and the chlorine odor can cause nausea. With new pool-filtration technology, you can enjoy chlorine-free and cleaner indoor swimming.

- If you swim laps, know when to say when. While water may free the mind of worry, don't forget the precautions listed on page 63. Take the pulse test and the talk test. In water it's easier to be oblivious to exhaustion. If your usual twenty laps becomes too tiring in the final months, slow your pace and do fewer laps.

- Drink water before and after swimming, just as you would for other types of exercise. Even with all that water around you, you can still get dehydrated while exercising in a pool, especially an outdoor pool on a sunny day.

DON'T GET OVERHEATED

While a comfortable hot soak may help you relax and ease the aches and pains of pregnancy, you may have to shorten your time in the tub and lower the temperature a bit. Prolonged elevated body temperatures of 102°F (39°C) or higher in the first trimester of pregnancy can increase the risk of spinal cord defects. Fatty tissue, such as the fat in baby's brain, is the most vulnerable to overheating. Don't worry, bathe warmly. Realistically, women naturally get out of warm baths long before their body temperature ever nears 102°F (39°C). Practice these precautions when enjoying a warm bath, sauna, steam room, or hot tub:

- If the temperature is too hot for you, it is too hot for baby.

- Limit tub time. Enjoy hot baths or hot tub soaks for up to fifteen minutes and keep the temperature no higher than 101°F (38°C).

- Limit visits to steam rooms and saunas to ten minutes with the temperature no higher than 101°F (38°C). Short, frequent dips in a hot tub are safer than prolonged immersion. Sitting in the tub with much of the top of your body exposed will also lessen the risk of overheating.

- Be sure to take extra caution when getting out of a hot bath or hot tub, out of a sauna, or especially out of a slippery steam room. Change positions slowly to avoid fainting. Of course, listen to your body. If you're getting uncomfortable or dizzy, it's time to cool it.

EXERCISES FOR AN EASIER BIRTH

Now let's leave the muscle-toning of hams, glutes, and all that gym jargon, and focus on the muscles "down there." Let's call them "push-out" muscles, those that most efficiently get baby out with the least wear and tear on mommy's pelvis, lower back, and abdominal muscles. Doing exercises that strengthen these muscles will help them better support the pelvic joints that, because of the hormone relaxin, have become looser. Posture will become important as your uterus grows upward into your abdominal cavity, changing your center of gravity. And your bladder will need support as the baby's weight puts pressure downward.

Kegel Exercises

If you do no other conditioning exercises during your pregnancy, do Kegel exercises. Named after the doctor who invented them, Kegel exercises strengthen all the muscles supporting your urogenital tract.

Nature intends the pelvic floor muscles to relax somewhat during pregnancy to prepare for delivery of the baby. But if your pelvic floor is already weak you may find you have trouble with leaking of urine as your uterus grows and strains the muscles that support it and your bladder. Incontinence can continue after pregnancy, since these muscles are stretched to their utmost when you push out the baby.

After childbirth, Kegels will be your ticket to regaining and maintaining a well-toned pelvic floor, thereby avoiding the trouble some women have with drooping pelvic structures. As a side benefit, many women who do Kegel exercises report enhanced sensitivity during intercourse, and many of their partners claim greater pleasure as well.

To locate your pelvic floor muscles, try to stop your urine flow midstream. If you can do it easily and quickly, your pelvic floor is in pretty good shape. If you can't, you'll find that a few weeks of Kegels will work wonders. Another way to locate these muscles is to try to clench them around two fingers inserted into the vagina, or around your partner's penis during intercourse.

There are many different variations on the Kegel, and each one has both a *contract* and a *release* phase. Be sure to practice both. Overemphasizing the contraction part of Kegel exercises conditions women to tighten these muscles, when in fact giving birth requires the releasing of tight and tense perineal muscles. Here are some of the most effective exercises, beginning with the easy ones and progressing to the ones that take a lot of concentration.

Stop and start. Attempt to stop and start your urine flow four or five times as you urinate. It may be a bit tricky because you need to use only the pelvic floor muscles, without assistance from your thigh and lower abdominal muscles.

Reps. Contract and release your pelvic floor muscles. Start with ten repetitions four times a day and work up to fifty reps four times a day. This exercise is great to squeeze in (no pun intended) at stoplights, during TV commercials, or when someone on the phone puts you on hold — another "anywhere, anytime" way to enjoy your changing body.

Holding. Contract your pelvic floor muscles for a count of five, then release. Repeat ten times. Gradually increase the length of time you keep the muscles tensed.

Super-Kegels. The longer you can contract your pelvic floor muscles, the stronger they will be. As you begin your Kegel exercises, you will be in the five- to ten-second range of holding time. Once you get up to fifteen to twenty seconds, you are in the super-Kegel range and are getting the maximum muscle-building power for maximum support of your baby-carrying structures.

Kegel exercises can not only prevent or treat pregnancy incontinence, they can make birth itself easier, because once you have practiced exercising your pelvic floor muscles, you'll know how to release them. Releasing not only makes labor more comfortable, it also helps you avoid tearing these tissues during the birth.

Your main goal in preparing for birth is to train the muscles to go into release mode during birth, when your impulse may be to tense up and resist the passage of the baby's head. Part of this work, then, is to become aware that you have these muscles so you will know them well when you want to let go and let baby come out. Here are three more variations of advanced Kegels to get you on the fast track to well-trained birthing muscles.

The elevator. This exercise takes some concentration, but the results are fantastic. Your vagina is a muscular tube, with the sections arranged like rings, one on top of another. Imagine that each section is a different "floor" of a building, and that you are moving an elevator by tensing each section, getting progressively higher. Start by slowly bringing the elevator up to the second floor and holding for a second, then move up to the third, and so on, until you get to the fifth floor. Hold. Now bring the elevator down, floor by floor, "resting" at each floor, to the first floor (the starting point). Then make a trip to the basement, where your pelvic floor is completely relaxed. As you reach the basement, release and press your pelvic muscles down (childbirth educators call this "bulging to the basement") and hold this "let go" position for a few seconds. This exercise will prepare you to bear down during the pushing stage of labor. Finally, bring the elevator back up to the first floor, your normal stage of vaginal tension (the muscles are naturally somewhat contracted). Try to work up to ten elevator rides four times a day.

The wave. Some of the pelvic floor muscles are arranged in a sort of extended figure-eight pattern (like an "8" with three loops instead of two). One of the loops is around your urethra, one around your vagina, and one around your anus. A good Kegel exercise is to contract these muscles from front to back, and release from back to front. Throw in ten of these "waves" four times a day. There! Now you are really an expert.

Positioning. Once you become proficient at Kegel exercises, try them in a variety of positions — lying down, sitting, squatting, cross-legged sitting, on all fours. This is in anticipation of the various labor and birth positions you will be using.

Stretching Exercises

You'll have no idea what position will be the most comfortable to birth in until the time comes, so you'd be wise to make sure that all your birth-giving muscles are primed and ready to go. Historically, women have used positions that allow gravity to help — squatting or sitting semi-upright with legs apart. Stretching exercises prepare your thigh and pelvic muscles and ligaments for the best birthing positions. But no matter what position you end up giving birth in, spending time in these poses before the big day will help prepare your body by toning the perineal area (the muscle tissue between the vagina and the anus), stretching ligaments, strengthening inner thigh and abdominal muscles, and promoting correct body alignment.

Squatting. Squatting comes naturally to young children, but it is hard work for most of us grown-ups. Squat for one minute, ten times a day, with the goal of being able to squat for longer and longer periods. Squat to clean out the refrigerator. Squat to fold laundry. Squat to change the TV channel — and stay there awhile.

Tailor sitting. Chances are you did a lot of sitting cross-legged on the floor when you were a child. Now you may find it's not as easy as you remember, since it calls for underused abdominal muscles to keep your back straight and maintain good posture. Nevertheless, spend ten minutes in this position, two or three times a day, reading, writing, having dinner — anything that allows you to be aware of your posture. Gradually increase the length of time you sit.

Tailor stretching. With your back against a wall (or against the front of a sofa), uncross your legs and bring your feet together sole to

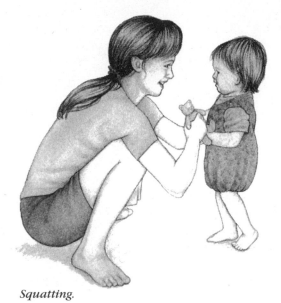

Squatting.

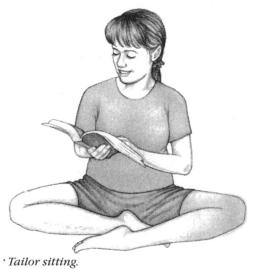

Tailor sitting.

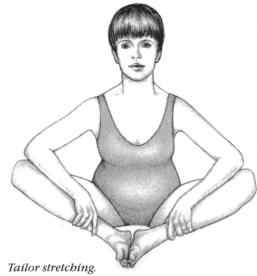

Tailor stretching.

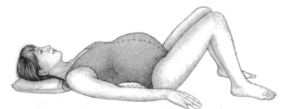

Pelvic tilt position — lying down.

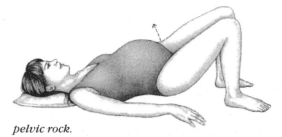

pelvic rock.

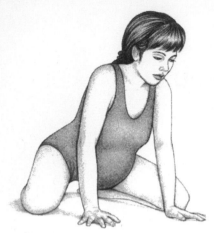

Leapfrog.

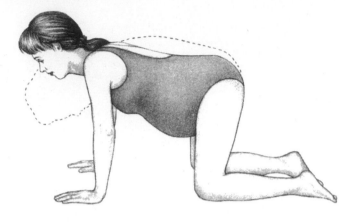

Knees to chest.

sole. Then see how far toward the floor you can get your knees. Don't worry — only the most limber women can get their knees all the way to the floor. But over the course of a few weeks you should be able to improve your flexibility by using your hands and arms to lightly press your knees, one at a time, downward. Don't force them, especially if you have a history of knee problems.

Shoulder rotation. Take the time at the end of a tailor stretch to do a few shoulder circles, bringing your shoulders forward and up, as if to touch your ears, and back around and down. Keep your arms relaxed. The shoulder and neck muscles you stretch with this exercise are the ones that easily get overtensed in labor (and when holding a newborn). Now, ask someone to give you a shoulder/neck massage.

6

Don't Worry, Be Pregnant

How often have you heard "don't get stressed"? Huh? I'm pregnant! So many changes so fast is a recipe for stress. And the "what ifs" add to that stress: Will my baby be okay? Will my pregnancy be complicated? How much will my labor hurt?

The good news is that the health tools you are learning increase the chances that these worries will not become realities. The great majority of babies are born healthy. Feeling empowered will give you the tools to turn your worry into well-being and help you relax, knowing that you are giving your baby the best start.

CAN BABY FEEL MOMMY'S STRESS?

Prenatal scientists disagree about the answer to this question. A growing number of researchers believe there is a correlation between a woman's emotions and her baby's. From six months on an unborn baby can in some manner share mother's emotions through the hormone changes associated with those emotions. A mother's positive and negative feelings do, in fact, appear to affect her baby's state of well-being. One of the most controversial areas of prenatal research is the possible correlation between a pregnant mother's emotional life and the eventual emotional development of her child. Is an anxious mother more likely to produce an anxious child? Science is uncertain how much of this so-called emotional imprinting occurs inside the womb or is affected by parenting practices during the early years after birth. It's probably a little of both. Nearly all prenatal scientists agree that the usual short-term emotional upsets and quickly resolved anxieties do not harm baby emotionally.

Worrying about whether your worry causes baby to worry can impose a heavy burden on an already worried mother. Not only must she abstain from polluted foods and try to avoid polluted air, now she must guard against polluted thoughts. This whole field of psychology is still in its infancy. For the sake of your own mental peace as well as the calm of your baby, don't worry. Ask those around you to do the same.

Why Unmanaged Stress Can Be Unhealthy for Mother and Baby

Unresolved stress can weaken baby's already fragile immune system. Science reveals that persistently high levels of toxic thoughts can be toxic to a baby's vulnerable and growing brain. The effect of high levels of stress hormones on brain tissue is called glucocorticoid neurotoxicity (GCN).

The placenta and the brain may both protect baby from GCN, but don't rely on them. There is some evidence that an enzyme in the placenta deactivates excessively high levels of the stress hormone to keep stressors from affecting baby. The blood-brain barrier, however, is not yet well developed in the baby in the womb, so high levels of stress hormones can get into baby's brain tissue and interfere with brain growth. (See page 30 for information on the protective properties of omega-3s.)

Recent neurological research shows that you can actually change your brain by changing your thoughts. Brain scans reveal that certain regions of the brain actually light up in response to happy thoughts. Cognitive therapists call this "positive self-talk." These switched-on "happy centers" release the

---

"PREGNANCY BRAIN" PREPARES YOU FOR "MOMMY BRAIN"

"Pregnancy brain" or "mommy brain" programs you to be generally supersensitive to everything that helps you care for baby. Neuroscientists at the National Institute of Mental Health have proven what pregnant and new mothers have long suspected — that their brains change on the way to growing and caring for a baby. New mothers actually grow more gray matter (brain cells) in the areas of the brain most involved in caring for their babies. However, there seems to be a neurological trade-off in memory lapses, one of the funny (and sometimes not so funny) things that happen on the way to birthing a baby. For some new moms, mental tasks unrelated to baby care are downgraded to make room for the extra brainwork involved in becoming a mother.

I booked airline tickets online. When we got to the airport I handed the tickets to the agent, who looked at me and the tickets and announced, "Your tickets show you leaving from a different airport." After the shock I started to cry, but in sympathy the nice agent rebooked us on the right flight. Pregnancy brain is real!

Martha believes that all those nuisances that pregnant women experience have a purpose. Perhaps "pregnancy brain" means that mothers are meant to fill their minds with the important aspects of growing a healthy baby and anticipating motherhood, which may not leave room in the memory bank for other thoughts. This prep time for their brains is the reason moms find themselves preoccupied so often with their inner world, even shutting out their husbands. There is indeed a lot to ponder in the journey toward being a parent.

happy hormones serotonin and dopamine, your natural antistress, antidepressant internal medicines.

TEN STRESSBUSTERS EVERY PREGNANT MOTHER CAN LEARN

You have already learned some super stressbusters in the previous chapters. Grazing on good food stabilizes blood chemistry, which helps stabilize stress hormones. The same goes for exercise, one of the most time-tested mood mellowers. Stress management is a key tool throughout life, especially in those early years of childcare. Here are ten additional stressbusters you can use:

Stressbuster 1: You can't always control situations, but you can control your reactions to them. If you can't change it, don't worry about it. For example, say you lose your job. Come to grips with the fact that you're not going to get your job back. Try to accept it and move on. It's the feeling of loss of control that causes harmful stress. How your mind reacts to the stressor is now the only thing that is totally under your control. Try not to dwell on why you lost your job, because all that will do is rev up your stress. Address the financial situation. Look for what good will be coming from this. Volunteer your time or go back to school. Don't look back; the past is unchangeable history. You can only change the future. This is especially important if you are an overreactor, as many people are.

Stressbuster 2: Focus on solutions, not problems. Suppose you develop a medical complication during pregnancy. You can't change this fact. It is not under your control. What is under your control is what you can do about it — for example, how you can teach your body to muster up its own internal medicines ("happy hormones") for support. By immediately focusing on a solution, you regain your sense of control. As we said above, it's the feeling of helplessness that causes prolonged stress. By focusing on solutions rather than dwelling on the problem, you divert your energy from the problem to how to manage it. This is a stressbuster most men handle better than women, which in itself can cause a bit of marital anxiety. How often have you felt, "If only he would listen to me instead of just rushing in to fix it"? Do what you can to get him to listen, and then shift your mind to consider his solutions, too. He may come up with some you didn't think of.

Stressbuster 3: Focus on biggies, not smallies. You and your baby don't deserve the mental and physical fatigue caused by life's many annoyances. When a stressor arrives, immediately put it into perspective — downgrade it to a "smallie." Tell your body and mind not to react to it. Suppose you're late for a meeting because traffic is delayed from an accident. That's a smallie, an inconvenience. And you can't change it. The "biggie" would be if you were the one involved in the accident. Spend the rest of the drive being grateful that you have your health, your job, and your car. Send up a prayer for the person who had the accident.

Stressbuster 4: Enjoy a positive replay. One of the most powerful stressbusters is mood switching. As soon as a stressful,

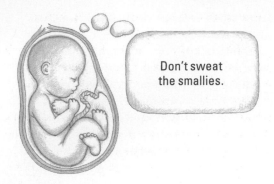

Don't sweat the smallies.

MISERY NEEDS HAPPY COMPANY

Especially during your pregnancy, surround yourself with positive people, preferably pregnant mothers who exude happy thoughts. Befriend those moms-to-be in your childbirth class who make you feel good just being with them.

depressing, or upsetting thought enters your mind, quickly program yourself to click into "don't go there!" mode. (Perversely, many of us "enjoy" dwelling on negative stuff.) Picture what happens in your brain when a stressor or upsetting thought or scene enters and you redirect negative thoughts to happy ones. As you're building a baby, build more pathways in the happy centers of your brain. When a negative thought arises, open up your mental library and replay serene scenes from your past. Dwell upon these joyful memories, such as your wedding day or the day you told your mate you were pregnant. As you fill your mind with these instant replays, the happy centers can take over.

Dr. BJ notes: *In your mama journal jot down a note to your baby to share a few happy thoughts. Writing to your baby allows you to center your thoughts on joy and focus on your unique journey, no matter what crops up. Notes to baby will be precious to both of you someday — and therapeutic right now.*

(See page 140 for some tips on journaling.)

Whenever I get stressed, I look at happy photos or listen to pleasant phone messages that I saved on my smart phone. As soon as I feel a negative thought coming on, I tap into my techy de-stressor.

Stressbuster 5: Relax and take a deep breath. Your body is composed of all kinds of biochemical up/down hormones and on/off switches. Some hormones rev you up. Some hormones calm you down. The rev-up mechanism is called your sympathetic nervous system (SNS). It shifts your body into high gear when you need it to be. When the SNS is hyperactive, it floods your body and brain with stress hormones needed to manage some crisis. Balancing this turn-up mechanism is the turn-down part, called the parasympathetic nervous system (PNS).

Taking a deep, relaxed breath turns up the PNS and turns down the SNS. Once every hour (or more!) take a breath break, a moment off from your busyness to take a deep breath. Here's how:

1. Breathe in slowly through your nose, relaxing your abdominal muscles to expand your belly, and let your pelvic muscles descend. Inhale to the count of four. As you are breathing in, imagine the cleansing air traveling deep into your lungs and delivering more oxygen to your baby.

2. Hold your breath for a count of two to four while you think about your baby.

Slowly exhale through your mouth for a count of six. Exhaling slowly through pursed lips improves oxygenation to your body, and possibly even to your baby. If you have a negative thought, imagine it leaving your body during exhalation.

3. Breathe with a mantra, a word or phrase that prevents your mind from getting sidetracked with anxious or negative thoughts. A mantra is a centering device that helps quiet the clutter of disturbing self-talk. Use a two-word mantra, one on breathing in and the other on breathing out, such as "Thank (inhalation)...God (exhalation)"; "Feel...Good"; "Love...Baby."

Stressbuster 6: Let music mellow your mind. Create your personal "mood medley," a playlist on your MP3 player or computer of music that helps you relax and de-stress. Treasure this medley because you're probably going to need it during the first few months (and years!) after birth. Music opens up the happy centers of the brain and releases happy hormones. It taps into the frontal lobe, the part of the brain that governs mood and emotion, enabling you to avoid thoughts that suck you into worry. Select music that helps you replay pleasant scenes, such as the music theme of your wedding or your favorite dance. The more you play your mood music, the more you imprint the association: "I feel stressed, I hear this, I feel calmer." You can program your mind to enjoy this music-mood connection, even during labor!

Stressbuster 7: Move to mellow your mind. You've heard the old sports advice, "Walk it off!" By increasing blood flow to the brain, vigorous exercise stimulates neurochemicals that have a natural calming effect. In addition, vigorous exercise lowers

the alarm hormone, called ACTH, which activates stress hormones.

What's one of the healthiest therapies you can use when pregnant and stressed? The swimming pool. "Swim it off" could be just what the stress therapist ordered. (See page 66 for more information on swimming while pregnant.) If swimming is not an option, take a walk while humming a happy tune to add music to movement.

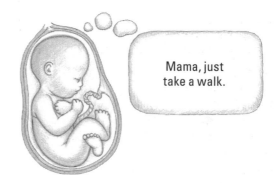

Mama, just take a walk.

Dr. BJ notes: Dance the stress away. The combination of music and movement is a great stressbuster. I advise mothers to plan a personal "happy hour" every day. In late afternoon or early evening, enjoy thirty minutes of dance or other exercise, twenty minutes of meditation, and ten minutes of healthy hydration and snacking.

Stressbuster 8: Meditate to self-medicate. Meditation mellows the mind by shifting your brain focus from the stress centers to the peaceful centers. It also turns down your SNS and turns up the PNS pathways in your brain.

You can meditate anytime and anywhere, but it helps to have a quiet meditation space in your home or at work where you can center your mind using your mantras or prayer phrases. Schedule a twenty-minute

SCIENCE SAYS: MEDITATE FOR A HEALTHIER PREGNANCY

Here's what science says about the healthful things that happen to your pregnant body while meditating:

Pregnancy Quirk	How Meditation Helps
High blood pressure	Lowers blood pressure
Weakened immune system	Boosts immune system
Rapid heart rate when stressed	Steadies heart rate
Restless sleep	Improves sleep
Anxiety and depression	Relieves anxiety and depression
High stress hormone levels	Lowers stress hormone levels

silence break into your day to practice your favorite form of meditation or prayer. Mellowing your mind through meditation will be a valuable stressbuster to continue once your cute little "stressor" starts throwing temper tantrums. Once you've learned the meditation practice, you can more easily create the moments of peace you'll need as a busy mom when you may not always have the luxury of twenty minutes of downtime.

Stressbuster 9: Laughter is your best pregnancy medicine. Laughter balances your immune system. It lowers the excess stress hormones epinephrine and cortisol, in addition to boosting your natural germ-fighting cells. Consider putting together your own humor library so you can read a joke or watch a short, funny video on your mobile phone. Store funny scenes or jokes in your mental file cabinet to replay and "laugh it off" when you feel a stressful thought or situation coming on.

LOVE AND LIGHTHEARTEDNESS

The relation between love and health has been known for centuries. Love strengthens your immune system and turns on the cerebral happy centers. Being able to turn your love inward to your baby is a unique stress-relieving perk of pregnancy.

Stressbuster 10: Have a happy home. Moms, this is a fine time to shift some of your stressors to others, such as dad. You've heard of the "honey-do" stage of older age. Start with daddy-do's now. Delegate to your mate as many tiring and mental energy–draining tasks as you can. Unlike mommy stress, daddy stress doesn't directly bother baby. Pregnancy is also a good time to work on your marriage relationship, so you bring your baby into a happy home.

7

How to Sleep Peacefully while Pregnant

As your pregnancy progresses and your little passenger starts taking up a lot more room, quality sleep becomes more of a challenge. You get more tired and need more sleep, but the changes of pregnancy can keep this from happening.

WHY YOU WAKE UP SO OFTEN

Early in pregnancy sleep simply overtakes you — you have no choice but to sleep a lot.

But later on, the very marvels that are taking place inside your body and in your growing baby conspire to keep you awake. This just goes with the territory. One way to cope is to understand this "territory."

Difficulty sleeping. Your body is working day and night to grow a baby, and your hormones never rest, so it's no wonder you have difficulty settling into a restful sleep. As your pregnancy progresses, your sleep patterns become similar to those of a newborn infant. The amount of deep (non-REM) sleep

---

WHY PREGNANT MOTHERS NEED MORE SLEEP

During sleep the following healthful things happen to you and baby:

- Tissues grow and heal.

- Heart rate goes down.

- Stress hormones diminish.

- Growth hormone increases.

    But those aren't the only reasons you need a good night's sleep:

- Your body's metabolism is working overtime, so it needs more rest.

- Sleep deprivation causes a decrease in leptin, the appetite-control hormone, resulting in overeating.

- Sleep deprivation can worsen depression.

- Sleep deprivation increases the risk for type II diabetes and/or gestational diabetes.

you get decreases, and REM sleep increases. REM stands for "rapid eye movement," the state of sleep in which you are more aware of your environment and arouse from sleep more easily. Though it's hard to imagine a physiological purpose for this change, it does prepare you for a realistic fact: motherhood is not a nine-to-five profession.

While sleep loss is one of the inevitable side effects of motherhood, night feedings and diaper changes have yet to begin. While you must accept the fact that a sleep-through-the-night pregnant woman is as rare as a sleep-through-the-night newborn, there are a few ways to help your mind and body enjoy a better night's sleep. (See also page 82 for our pregnancy sleep prescription.)

Heartburn. As we discussed earlier, the pressure from your growing baby pressing against your diaphragm can cause irritating stomach acids to be pushed up into your esophagus, causing gastroesophageal reflux. Sleeping on your left side in a semi-upright position helps gravity keep stomach acids down, whereas the horizontal position of sleep is a recipe for reflux.

Need to urinate. Downward pressure on your bladder, requiring frequent urination, happens in the first trimester, before the uterus is large enough to move up out of the pelvic cavity into the abdominal cavity and away from your bladder. In the third trimester your bladder will be squeezed for room again by your uterus, now full of baby, amniotic fluid, and placenta. Another cause of frequent urination is the high level of progesterone necessary in pregnancy.

If frequent treks to the bathroom disrupt your sleep, avoid beverages containing caffeine (coffee, tea, cola) after 3:00 p.m.

Also, use the triple-voiding technique to empty your bladder just before retiring. ("Grunt" three times before you get off the toilet to be sure your bladder is empty. This is a good time to exercise your pelvic muscles, too; see page 68.) If you wake up in the middle of the night feeling the need to urinate, just get up and go. The sooner you do it, the sooner you'll get back to sleep.

Baby kicking. Babies, whether born or unborn, often have their days and nights mixed up. If your enlarging uterus doesn't wake you up, its occupant will. Whereas your daytime motion lulls baby to sleep, when you rest, baby awakens, stretches, and wakes you with all the wonderful movements she's learning.

You've heard the phrase "sleep like a baby." Well, that's only partially true. While it's nice to enjoy that deep zoned-out sleep that babies periodically have, you may not realize that babies have longer periods of light (REM) sleep throughout the night. Pediatricians theorize that babies have more REM sleep to gift them with easier arousability so they can wake up more readily to signal a nighttime need.

Body aches and pains. Leg cramps, skin itching, and swelling breasts are nighttime nuisances that commonly keep pregnant mothers awake. Especially in the third trimester of pregnancy, leg cramps and "creepy, crawly" sensations in the legs can be particularly annoying. Flex your toes toward your head to ease a cramp — pointing your toes down usually aggravates cramps. Calcium and potassium deficiency can make cramps worse, so eat more fruits and vegetables and limit carbonated drinks, since the phosphoric acid can steal calcium.

Worry and stress. With all the changes going on inside your body and your home environment, it's easy to carry daytime worries — and the associated high level of stress hormones — into your precious sleep time. Reread chapter 6 for tips on keeping anxiety at bay so you can get the sleep you need.

Vivid dreams. Pregnancy dreams tend to be more intense, vivid, disturbing, and bizarre than your nonpregnant dreams. Women we have interviewed report that pregnancy dreams seem more real than regular dreams and that the usual "life worries" themes seem more grossly exaggerated. Pregnancy dreams also occur more frequently than nonpregnancy dreams, and are recalled more easily because a pregnant woman wakes up so frequently, often during a dream, when it's fresh in her mind.

I dream a lot anyway, but my pregnancy dreams were so realistic! I dreamed that I told my husband he could date his ex-girlfriend, and the dream went downhill from there. I dreamed he took her out to dinner on my birthday, and eventually ran off with her. I woke up drenched with sweat, shook my husband, and screamed, "How could you do that to me?"

You dream differently while pregnant because you sleep differently. As we've said, during pregnancy, especially during the last trimester, you spend a larger percentage of your nap and nighttime sleep in REM, the stage that encourages dreaming and easy awakening. However, pregnancy dreams cannot be blamed entirely on hormones, since many expectant fathers also report having more vivid, even scary, dreams. A baby on the way means big life changes for everyone in the household. Because of these changes, a pregnant woman's mind is ready for thought and introspection day and night.

I dreamed we left our two-year-old with my parents and forgot to pick her up. I think this dream means I'm scared I will neglect our older child when the new baby comes.

Pregnancy dreams often reflect a woman's pressing concerns, which change with the stages of pregnancy. Early in pregnancy, dreams seem to focus on fertility symbols: potted plants, fruit, seeds, water, ocean waves. Toward the middle of pregnancy, dream babies appear in your fantasies, and your dream life may be filled with images of your baby, babies in general, and even tiny animals, such as puppies or kittens. Some women dream that they aren't pregnant at all and wake up confused and horrified. Many women find the "builder" theme repeated in their dreams, reflecting the role of Baby Builder. Toward the end of pregnancy, the dreams may become nightmares: your baby is not healthy, you have a problem delivery, someone is stealing your baby. It's also normal toward the end of pregnancy for dreams on other topics to become more anxious — you might dream about career upsets or problems with your spouse. Most women report that their fearful dreams are baby-related, such as having empty breasts when baby wants to nurse, or doing something terrible as a mother. Dreams of dropping the baby are common.

I kept dreaming about deformed babies. My therapist says this is a common dream for pregnant women and perhaps symbolic of the real threat the baby poses to an established lifestyle and body image.

It is best not to overanalyze your dreams and become anxious about their content. Sleep, especially pregnant sleep, distorts and exaggerates realities anyway. If you dream you deliver a deformed baby, it just means that you have the normal, healthy fears a good mother has for her child. Many women find it helpful to write down a negative dream and then rewrite a happier ending.

While dreams do not foretell the future, pregnancy dreams, especially those that have a recurring theme, can reveal hidden anxieties and bring your attention to issues that need to be dealt with. It's helpful to record the recurring story lines of your dreams to see whether a pattern emerges that might reflect some hidden issue that needs to be addressed. While you don't need to attach a great deal of meaning or importance to your dreams, some women find that reflecting on them can actually alleviate a lot of their anxiety. Encourage your husband to talk about his dreams as well. He's making a big adjustment, too.

THE PREGNANCY SLEEP PRESCRIPTION

Now that you are aware of all the pregnancy quirks that may keep you awake, here are some time-honored ways to help you sleep.

Have a restful day. Try to keep emotional stress to a minimum — a day filled with emotional ups and downs is likely to carry over into a fitful night. Learn ways to stay peaceful and relaxed. Read about methods for relaxing or try a relaxation tape. If you've been to a childbirth class, use the relaxation skills you learned there to relax into sleep. (Review the stressbusters on page 75.)

Enjoy more exercise. The more you move during the day, the better you're likely to sleep at night. Revving up your body during the day through exercise is not only a good stress reducer, it also increases the percentage of time you're likely to spend in the deep and rejuvenating stages of sleep. The best time of day for exercise for the best sleep effect is morning and early afternoon, rather than within a couple of hours of bedtime: a racing heart and an invigorating surge of hormones do not help bring on sleep.

Enjoy a couple of catnaps during the afternoon. Try to sneak in one or two twenty- to thirty-minute naps during the day, preferably when your body prompts you to lie down. It's therapeutic for a pregnant working woman to retire into a quiet room and enjoy a couple of catnaps while at work. You need these more than coffee breaks.

Enjoy earlier to bed and earlier to rise. The human body is actually programmed to go to bed shortly after the sun sets and wake up with the sun, yet few of us have the luxury of doing this. While you may crave time for yourself after a hectic day, listen to your body and retire when you start craving sleep. Certainly, you're likely to need to retire at least an hour earlier than your usual bedtime. The age-old wisdom of "early to bed, early to rise" fits your natural hormone cycles. Your rev-up hormone (cortisol) is highest at 6:00 a.m. and starts to dip in the evening when your turn-down hormone (melatonin) clicks in.

Eat for sleep. Your sleep can be highly affected, for better or worse, by what you eat. During your pregnancy you will discover which foods are "sleepers" (those that help you sleep restfully) and "wakers" (those that stimulate neurochemicals that perk up your brain). "Sleepers" are foods that contain tryptophan, the nutrient that helps make serotonin and melatonin, which slow down nerve traffic in your brain and stimulate sleep. "Wakers" are high-carb foods or junk foods, especially chemical foods that contain artificial food additives (such as MSG and aspartame) that you may find you are more sensitive to.

Observe the wisdom, "don't dine after nine." Most pregnant mothers find that they enjoy a better night's sleep if they make their evening meal their lightest of the day, and then enjoy a 100- to 150-calorie bedtime snack, emphasizing the snooze foods (one or two eggs are a favorite). A carb-only bedtime snack is likely to be a waker if it's not partnered with protein, since after the carb wears off your blood sugar crashes, which triggers stress and night-waking hormones that perk up the blood sugar and are likely to keep you awake. Finally, don't go to bed hungry, as hunger can stimulate night-waking hormones.

Enjoy before-bed rituals. A bedtime ritual is similar to foreplay in the way that it sets up the mind and body for the pleasure of delicious sleep to follow. Put your mate to work to help you relax mind and body with a massage. This skin-to-skin bedtime ritual can be carried over into after-baby pampering. Massage, whether soft touch or deep tissue, helps relieve and prevent cramps and itchy skin, common nuisances that cause night waking.

SNOOZE FOODS

Snooze foods partner healthy carbohydrates with high tryptophan-containing proteins. This before-bed partnership is likely to help you sleep. High-calcium foods, such as dairy products, also help the brain use tryptophan to make melatonin. Here is a list of high tryptophan-containing foods to enjoy for your evening meal and before-bed snack:

- Beans
- Cheese
- Cottage cheese
- Eggs
- Hazelnuts and almonds
- Oatmeal
- Pumpkin seeds
- Salmon and tuna
- Sunflower seeds
- Tofu
- Turkey and chicken
- Yogurt

Don't worry, be sleepy. As cortisol decreases in the evening and melatonin increases, it's important not to counteract these natural sleep-inducing biorhythms by allowing stress to linger. You might try the following to help wind you down:

- Prayer
- Light reading
- Soft music
- A warm shower
- Aromatherapy from lavender oil

It's also a good idea to jot down "to do" thoughts that pop up so you can forget about them for now. Practice the relaxation techniques you are learning in childbirth class, such as mental imagery (see page 299). The images that tend to work best for pregnant mothers are those in which you imagine you are being lulled by floating in warm water or moving back and forth, cradle-like, on a swing. Breathe your way to sleep using the deep-breathing technique you learned on page 76. Reserve a special collection of sleep-inducing rituals for use only at bedtime.

Make the bedroom boring. Remember, bright lights and stimulating noises turn up your waking hormones. On the other hand, increasing darkness and mellow, soothing sounds turn down the rev-up hormones and turn up the sleep-inducing hormones. To set up your bedroom for sleep:

• Don't use the computer or watch TV within an hour of going to bed, as these artificial lights turn off melatonin. Light stimulates serotonin; darkness stimulates melatonin. It's as simple as that.

• As you are turning off the lights, turn on soothing music. Make a medley of your tried-and-true sleep inducers.

• Keep your bedroom cool, airy, and allergen-free. During the winter months, turn down the central heating in the bedroom and turn on one or two vaporizers. Hot steam humidifies the air and helps keep nasal passages open, in addition to providing a more breathing-friendly source of warmth in the bedroom.

Enjoy aromatherapy. Sniffing lavender oil has some support in science. Japanese researchers at the Meikai University School of Dentistry studied people after they sniffed lavender oil for five minutes and found that the levels of the stress hormone cortisol in their saliva decreased.

Wake up to your body's own alarm. The absolute worst way to wake up is from a mechanical alarm. You don't really want to "alarm" your brain and heart rate, do you? The most natural way to wake up is with gradually increasing light as the sun rises or soothing music with gradually increasing volume. On days when you can sleep in, try blackout curtains. This may help you steal an extra hour or two of slumber. (P.S. Keep those curtains for when your baby becomes an early-waking toddler.)

Position yourself comfortably for sleep. The most comfortable sleep position for most pregnant women is on your left side with a firm pillow between your knees and another one against your lower back. Sleeping on your left side lessens reflux because it allows gravity to keep the stomach contents down. It also keeps the pressure off your liver, which is on the right side. Besides taking stress off your lower back, sleeping on your side prevents against the narrowing of the airway that is often caused by back-sleeping and the resultant obstructive sleep apnea and snoring that can occur. If you're experiencing nighttime reflux, try a 30- to 45-degree wedge-shaped pillow to sleep more upright.

Once I got larger in my pregnancy I began to snore, which constantly woke me up. I found that sleeping semi-upright in a cushy recliner with my feet up not only relieved the pressure on my back and hips, but also lessened the snoring and gave me a better night's sleep.

Later in pregnancy, back-sleeping causes your uterus to compress the blood vessels between the uterus and spine. This can compromise circulation, lower blood pressure, and increase pressure on your back. It can also exacerbate leg swelling and hemorrhoids. Sleeping on your left side enables the best blood flow to baby. Your body will naturally tell you how to comfortably shift sleeping positions as you and your baby grow.

(See page 80 for information on restless leg syndrome, an uncomfortable sensation that some mothers describe as feeling "creepy crawlies" on their legs.)

Use care when getting out of bed. Roll onto your side and use your arms to slowly push yourself up into a sitting position. Then slowly put your legs over the side of the bed. Plant your feet firmly on the ground, then use your arms to push yourself up into a standing position. This precaution can save you back strain.

Enjoy white noise. Try sleep-inducing bedside sounds from a noise machine, such as a babbling brook, ocean sounds, rain, or monotonous low-pitched music. You may not realize it, but baby is probably enjoying — and sleeping to — the white noise inside the uterus, such as your heartbeat and the swooshing sounds of the blood flow through the uterine vessels. This prenatal programming may be why lullabies, gentle

SLEEPING COMFORTABLY

Firm pillows are a pregnant woman's sleep friend. You may find as your pregnancy progresses that you need as many as five pillows for comfortable support: two under your head, two supporting your top leg, one wedged between your back and the mattress, and a foam wedge between your abdomen and mattress. If you feel off-balance lying on your side, roll slightly onto your stomach, moving your top leg forward so that it is completely off your lower leg, and let your abdomen snuggle onto the pillow or the mattress. You might want to try some specially designed maternity pillows.

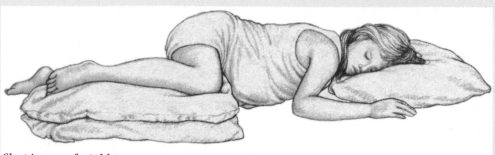

Sleeping comfortably.

"shushing," and white noise are so effective in lulling babies to sleep later on.

Cool it! Before pregnancy you may have needed a warmer bedroom than your mate — some couples experience blanket battles early on in marriage. During pregnancy, your bedmate may actually enjoy the fact that your body heats up more so you can enjoy a cooler bedroom and fewer blankets. Because a mother's pregnant body runs hotter, some couples find that they need separate blankets.

8

Go Green!

Many mothers naturally "go green" when they become pregnant. We don't mean morning-sickness green here, though there is the fact that pregnancy gives your body a heightened sensitivity to the food you put in your mouth and the air you breathe. Pregnant women can often smell smoke, gasoline, and other harmful fumes from twice the distance than before they were pregnant. We've often heard expectant mothers say, "That stuff never used to bother me, but now it does." Feeling and being protective comes with the profession of motherhood, and it begins at conception.

It's no coincidence that a pregnant mother is most sensitive to environmental smells and toxins at the time when her baby is most vulnerable to them — the first trimester. Developmental defects are most common in the early weeks when organs are forming the fastest. Statistics are on your side. Even though most babies are born "prepolluted," the good news is that almost all of these babies turn out to be just fine.

How pollutants bother baby. While the exact mechanism of how toxins increase the chance of birth defects is not entirely known, we do know what happens when a toxin gets into your baby's rapidly dividing cells. Each organ in your baby's body grows according to a genetic blueprint, a biochemical architect that directs cells how to divide and grow. Suppose the genes, due to a nutritional deficiency or exposure to a chemical toxin, fail to direct the organ to develop according to the right genetic blueprint. For example, let's look into a baby's heart. Genes direct the heart to divide into four chambers. But

GO GREENEST EARLIER IN YOUR PREGNANCY

Environmental toxins are most likely to interfere with the development of your baby's organs in the first trimester, a time when birth defects can develop. Later on in your pregnancy environmental toxins can interfere with baby's growth rather than the formation of her organs. The fetal "garbage disposal system" is too immature to handle these toxins, so they can build up in a baby's bloodstream in proportionately higher levels than in the mother's.

suppose some of these genes are turned off or changed by a chemical in baby's blood. The tissue dividing one chamber, such as the two ventricles, may not develop completely. This could result in a hole or opening between the two ventricles, called a ventricular septal defect. Similar problems in gene-directed "closure" may lead to cleft palate, spina bifida, and other birth defects.

Since not every mother may be able to go entirely green, there are degrees of green that you should consider.

THANK YOU FOR NOT SMOKING

Obstetricians, pediatricians, and every healthcare provider conclude: smoking while pregnant is child abuse in the womb. When Mommy smokes, baby smokes. Nearly everything you're about to read below also applies to breathing secondhand smoke, which means that even when Daddy smokes, baby smokes.

Suppose you are about to enter a room when you see a warning sign on the door that says, "This room contains the poisonous gases of approximately 4,000 chemicals, some of which could kill or injure your baby and increase your risk of miscarriage." Most mothers would insist, "There's no way I'd take that chance!" But that's exactly what happens when a pregnant woman smokes or when she inhales someone else's cigarette smoke.

Among the many poisonous gases in cigarette smoke are nicotine (an addictive drug known to narrow blood vessels), carbon monoxide (an oxygen robber), benzene (a potential carcinogen), ammonia, and formaldehyde. The harmful effects of cigarette smoke on you and your baby increase with each cigarette smoked each day. And new research shows that smoking causes more lung damage in women than in men, presumably because women's lungs are smaller.

Smoking robs babies of nourishment. Many studies have shown that infants of mothers who smoke have lower birth weights than infants of mothers who don't smoke. Nicotine passes from the smoke a mother inhales into her bloodstream. The poisonous nicotine narrows uterine blood vessels, thus reducing blood flow to the baby in the womb. Baby depends on this blood flow for healthy growth — less blood flow means less nourishment and, therefore, less growth. As a general rule, bigger babies are healthier and less likely to need special care in the days after birth.

New studies refute the theory that the placenta may act as a barrier, preventing the toxic cigarette chemicals in mother's bloodstream from reaching her baby. When researchers examined the cord blood of newborns whose mothers either smoked or were exposed to secondhand smoke during their pregnancy, they found the presence of cancer-causing chemicals. The newborns had received around 50 percent of the carcinogens that were in the mother's blood, and the greater the maternal exposure to smoke, the higher the levels of these poisons in the babies' blood.

Smoking robs baby of oxygen. Besides restricting blood flow to the womb, ingesting cigarette smoke decreases the amount of oxygen available to the baby from the blood. The level of carbon monoxide in the blood of pregnant women who smoke is 600 to 700 percent higher than in those who don't smoke. Carbon monoxide is an oxygen blocker; it prevents blood cells from carrying a full load of oxygen. Researchers equate carbon monoxide levels in cigarette smoke to those in automobile exhaust; in effect, smoking partially smothers the baby in the womb. Lack of oxygen can affect the development of every organ in the baby's body.

Smoking injures little brains. New studies suggest that the developing baby's brain is injured not only by lack of oxygen, but also by the chemicals in cigarette smoke, which may be directly poisonous to developing brain cells. Children of mothers who smoked during pregnancy, especially those of mothers who smoked more than one pack a day, have been found to have a smaller head circumference as infants, decreased mental performance scores at one year, reduced IQs, and diminished academic performance scores in school compared to the children of mothers who did not smoke.

Even passive smoke hurts babies. New research shows that when pregnant mothers are exposed to secondhand cigarette smoke, their babies are at risk of having lower birth weights and show an increased risk of sudden infant death syndrome (SIDS), just as the babies of smoking mothers do. If father and mother both smoke, the risk of SIDS is nearly double. The risk of SIDS if father smokes but mother doesn't is still greater than if no one in the family smokes. Insist that your husband, relatives, friends, and coworkers respect the life inside your womb and not smoke in the same room with you. If your job requires working in a smoke-contaminated environment, you have grounds for a reassignment; pregnant women have a legal right to work in a smoke-free environment.

What about public places frequented by smokers? "But we always sit in the no-smoking area," you rationalize. No-smoking areas in public places are a step in the right direction, but many still contain significant levels of airborne pollutants. Trying to create a no-smoking area within a room is like trying to chlorinate half a swimming pool. Pollutants travel through the air. To be safe, stay as far away from cigarette smoke as you can.

Kicking the Habit

The earlier you stop smoking, the healthier you and your baby are likely to be. The best decision is to quit smoking as you prepare to become pregnant. At the very least give it up by the fifteenth week of pregnancy. Smoking after the fifteenth week of pregnancy triples the risk of having a premature baby and doubles the chance of having a small-for-date baby — the old term being "growth retarded." While the harmful effects of smoking seem to be greatest in the first trimester of pregnancy, even babies of "late stoppers" seem to fare better than infants whose mothers continue to smoke throughout their pregnancies. While there are few hard-and-fast rules in this book, this is one of them: Quit smoking.

Of course, this is more easily said than done. Smoking is an addiction, and addictions are hard to kick. You are accustomed to feeling the strong physiological effects of smoking. Nearly every system in your body is affected by nicotine. You may also be psychologically addicted to the oral sensation of smoking. It may take a while for your body to get used to feeling right without that hit of nicotine. Quitting will be one of the hardest things you'll ever do. Here are some suggestions:

> ## ADVANCE WARNING: "BIRTH-DEFECT CONTROL"
>
> If you are planning to get pregnant or trying to get pregnant, it is best to avoid alcohol, nicotine, and other drugs *before* becoming pregnant, to give your baby the greenest start at a stage when it makes the most difference.

Try stopping cold turkey once you're pregnant. The best time to extinguish your last cigarette is the moment your pregnancy test turns positive, and some women do just that. Others find that sudden cigarette withdrawal makes them extremely anxious, and this is not good for baby either. A gradual weaning may make more sense. Some "lucky" women find that they develop a natural aversion to the smell of smoke when pregnant, and this forces the issue.

Try goal setting. If you can't quit on the first day you know you're pregnant, set a goal for tapering off by, say, the tenth day. Plan a reward for your efforts. You might calculate how much money you would save in a year of not smoking and spend it on something special for yourself or your baby.

Choose your poison more carefully. Switch brands while you taper off. Some brands are higher in nicotine and carbon monoxide than others.

Cut down on how much poison you inhale. As you attempt to stop the smoking addiction, try taking fewer puffs. Or, smoke only the first half of the cigarette. (More poisons are concentrated toward the end of the cigarette.) Better still, don't inhale. This can cut down your nicotine dose by half.

Make it inconvenient to smoke. Buy only one pack at a time. Leave the pack somewhere inconvenient — for example, in the garage.

Fill the void. Think about what led you to start smoking. Once you identify the psychological reasons that might have led to this addiction, it might be easier for you to stop, or at least to find a safer substitute habit.

Try healthier substitutes. If you need to hold something and keep your hands busy, try writing, drawing, knitting, or working crossword puzzles. If you need something in your mouth, try chewing on carrot or celery sticks, cinnamon sticks, or straws; or try sucking on ice, juice popsicles, or hard candy. Nibble on sunflower seeds or granola. Chew gum. If you smoked for relaxation, try listening to soothing music, reading, or paying for an occasional massage. Take a walk. Go swimming. If you smoked for pleasure, indulge yourself in fun at a nonsmoking place: go to a movie or a nonsmoking restaurant, go shopping, go visit a nonsmoking friend.

Create unpleasant associations. Addictions thrive when they are associated with pleasant thoughts or events. Try associating the desire to smoke or the act of smoking with an unpleasant image. When you get the urge to smoke, for instance, imagine your baby gasping for air inside your womb.

Try scare tactics. Compose your own antismoking warnings, such as "Each puff could cost my baby another thousand brain cells" or "Smoking could damage or kill my baby," and hang these reminders in places where you are most likely to want to smoke. Wrap these warnings around your cigarette packs, too.

Get a stop-smoking buddy. If your quitting needs company, enlist the help of a friend or your mate. When you feel the urge to light up, call this person or share in an activity that you both enjoy.

Give yourself credit. Rather than losing hope when you occasionally give in and smoke, pat yourself on the back for each puff you resist. Resolve to do better each day.

Get professional help. If after two weeks you have made no progress on your own, you might want to contact a local quit-smoking resource or seek professional help to resolve deeper issues. The cost of counseling may be covered by your health plan. Regardless, it will be money well spent.

Dr. Bill notes: One day I was in a hospital meeting with a group of pediatricians and obstetricians. The topic was mothers smoking during pregnancy. While we realized how addictive this habit is, we doctors were horrified that any pregnant or new mother would smoke, given the widespread knowledge of how smoking harms babies. The general consensus was that smoking while pregnant, or around babies, should be considered child abuse.

Mothers who smoke during pregnancy are likely to continue smoking after birth,

HOW SMOKING HARMS BABIES AND MOTHERS

The incidence of just about everything you don't want to happen to you and your baby goes up when you smoke:

- Prematurity

- "Growth-retarded" baby

- Sudden infant death syndrome (SIDS)

- Smaller head circumference

- Reduced IQ and mental retardation

- Poor academic performance

- Complications of pregnancy and delivery

- Miscarriage

further increasing the risk of health problems for their infants. Respiratory infections, ear infections, and SIDS are all more common in the children of smokers.

Furthermore, studies show that mothers who smoke have lower levels of prolactin, the hormone responsible for both milk production and calm "maternal" behavior. Mothers who smoke are likely to have more breastfeeding problems and to wean earlier (probably because of inadequate prolactin). Babies of breastfeeding mothers who smoke tend to have nicotine in their blood, suggesting that they receive tobacco chemicals through their mother's milk (although it is still better for a mother who smokes to breastfeed than to give her baby formula). Quitting now rewards your baby fourfold: first, because she is spared toxins in utero; second, because she will not be exposed to them as an infant and child; third, because she will not learn the harmful habit of smoking from you; and fourth, because she will have a healthier mother who isn't at increased risk of heart disease, stroke, emphysema, lung cancer, and many other disabilities.

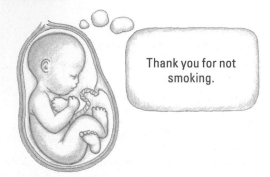

Thank you for not smoking.

THANK YOU FOR NOT TAKING ILLEGAL DRUGS

Heroin, cocaine, crack, meth, LSD, and PCP. When a mother uses any substance or drug, so does her baby. When she is addicted, so is her baby. After birth, the addicted baby suffers symptoms of drug withdrawal (extreme irritability and jitteriness). Infants of mothers who use addictive drugs during pregnancy are more difficult to care for after birth, and can show lifelong effects of their mother's drug use.

Drugs affect a baby throughout pregnancy but are most dangerous in the first trimester. Possible effects of illegal drugs on the developing baby include stillbirth, miscarriage, reduced birth weight, mental retardation, prematurity, and an increased risk of SIDS. In fact, the risk of SIDS may be increased as much as twenty times in infants of opiate-abusing mothers. Researchers believe that drugs such as opiates and cocaine also harm developing babies

indirectly by constricting blood vessels in the placenta and thus reducing the oxygen supply to the unborn baby — a suffocation effect similar to that caused by nicotine. Cocaine confuses baby's brain, contributing to hyperirritability.

Marijuana. Until recently, maternal marijuana use during pregnancy was not proven to be harmful to babies. Newer studies, however, suggest that marijuana can harm the fetus in all the ways mentioned above, thanks to its active ingredient, THC. In addition, marijuana smoke may contain carbon monoxide and hazardous chemicals found in cigarettes, only in doses that may be greater than those found in commercially available tobacco products.

Amphetamines (speed). These addictive drugs are also harmful to the developing baby and increase the chances of prematurity and intrauterine growth retardation. Newborns of speed-addicted mothers show typical speed withdrawal symptoms (rapid heart rates and breathing) immediately after birth.

If you are addicted to drugs, make an appointment with a professional counselor or enroll yourself in a drug withdrawal program the day you discover you are pregnant. It goes without saying that you should quit drugs the moment you make plans to become pregnant.

THANK YOU FOR NOT DRINKING ALCOHOL

While not as harmful as smoking, it's best to avoid drinking alcohol while pregnant, or at least greatly limit it. The relationship between fetal defects and alcohol excess was recognized in the early 1900s when obstetricians observed that there were more birth defects in babies born nine months after certain European drinking festivals. The same alcohol level you have in your blood reaches baby.

Obstetricians used to advise pregnant mothers to "limit alcohol during pregnancy," because it wasn't known how much alcohol could bother baby. It has long been known that heavy drinking during pregnancy can cause babies to be born with fetal alcohol syndrome (FAS), a disorder causing babies to be shorter and lighter, have smaller brains, and have unusual facial characteristics such as short noses, thin upper lips, and small eyes. FAS babies also have a higher incidence of other malformations, such as in the heart and limbs. Excessive alcohol consumption is most harmful in the first trimester, when it can contribute to miscarriage, low birth weight, and prematurity. Because alcohol is a "fat solvent," it seems to most bother baby's brain, one of the fattiest organs in the body.

In recent years more and more doctors have reasoned that if a lot of alcohol bothers a baby a lot, perhaps a little alcohol could bother baby a little, but not enough to be obvious. This has led the U.S. Surgeon General and the American Congress of Obstetricians and Gynecologists to recommend that mothers avoid alcohol entirely while pregnant. We second that advice.

Don't drink, but don't worry either. An occasional glass of wine sipped slowly with dinner is unlikely to bother baby. Yet you must avoid both binge drinking (five or more drinks on one occasion) and drinking an average of two drinks per day throughout pregnancy, as you risk harming your baby at those amounts. (One drink is 1 ounce of hard alcohol, one 5-ounce glass of wine, or one 12-ounce bottle of beer.) And remember, the fetal alcohol effect is riskiest in the first trimester, when your baby's organs are just developing.

FOOD CHEMICALS TO LIMIT

Most of the following chemicals fall into the "we're not sure" category. So, as much as possible, we recommend adding them to the "when in doubt, leave it out" list.

While we are fortunate to live in a country where foods are policed, special interest groups have tainted the trustworthiness of the FDA and other government agencies. Consider hydrogenated fats, or trans fats, which were known to be unhealthful in scientific and regulating circles for twenty years before the FDA finally "discouraged" (but didn't ban) them in 2006. Don't expect these agencies to protect your baby from chemical additives — *you* must do it. Here's why:

Never been proven safe. Most chemical additives are tested on experimental animals. If the rats pass the test, then they are tested on humans (usually adult volunteers) for a short period of time. If the rats survive and the humans don't get sick, these chemicals get the FDA stamp of approval. In the meantime, there is lots of lobbying going on since foods that are "preserved" (to sit on the shelf for a longer time) or "flavor enhanced" (to get you to eat more) enjoy economic advantages. Remember that the purpose of the USDA (United States Department of Agriculture) is primarily the economic development of the meat and agricultural industry, not the health of babies. Consumer advice about food additives should come from trusted medical authorities, such as the National Institutes of Health or the Institute of Medicine.

Scientists have long known that feeding certain chemical additives to baby animals increases the chances of their growing up to be sick adults. Dr. Russell Blaylock, author of *Excitotoxins: The Taste that Kills,* estimates that the developing brain of a baby is four times more vulnerable to the harmful effects of neurotoxins than the adult brain. This is because certain food additives cross the blood-brain barrier and can cause the developing nerve fibers to be miswired. One of the effects of this miswiring is called premature pruning. The baby's brain grows like a tended garden, pruning the connections that aren't needed, allowing more growth for the connections that are needed. Too many additives could lead to overpruning.

Blaylock singled out monosodium glutamate (MSG) and aspartame (a sugar substitute marketed as NutraSweet or Equal) for study. Since these substances are approved by the FDA, you may believe they are safe. This is not necessarily so. As of this writing, the FDA has received more health complaints about MSG and aspartame than any other chemical additives. Science says that:

- High doses of MSG fed to pregnant experimental animals can damage the brains of their babies.

- Young animals fed MSG showed changes in brain cell development and grew up to become obese and have autism-like symptoms.

When it comes to babies, there should not be any label loopholes.

THE DIRTIEST DOZEN

Here is a list of chemical additives that, according to science, may not be safe for growing babies:

Acesulfame
potassium

Artificial colors

Aspartame

BHA (butylated
hydroxyanisole)

BHT (butylated
hydroxytoluene)

Hydrolyzed
vegetable protein

MSG
(monosodium
glutamate)

Partially
hydrogenated
oils (trans
fats)

Potassium
bromate

Propyl gallate

Sodium
benzoate

Sodium nitrate/
sodium nitrite

Source: Environmental Working Group

Aspartame and sucralose—*not* for babies. Here are some reasons why, in our opinion, a steady diet of these two commonly used artificial sweeteners, aspartame (NutraSweet, Equal) and sucralose (Splenda), would not be healthy for you or your baby:

- **The science is suspect.** The science claiming the safety of these artificial sweeteners was funded by the manufacturers. It's noteworthy that research has discovered that, in general, company-funded studies are four times more likely to report favorable outcomes than those conducted by independent investigators. Add to this the fact that they've never been tested on babies and you have a double reason for leaving them out of your shopping cart.

- **Baby's body can't break them down.** Aspartame, for example, is broken down into chemical by-products, one of which is formaldehyde, the embalming chemical. Yet, aspartame supporters preach that this formaldehyde is rapidly metabolized into water and carbon dioxide and excreted from the body. This would demand a mature garbage disposal system, which, as you previously learned, a baby doesn't have. Another by-product is phenylalanine, a neurostimulant — just what a growing brain does not need.

So should you switch from aspartame to sucralose? Not so fast. The same problem exists: It has been tested mainly on animals, not on children, and certainly not on babies in the womb. Furthermore, sucralose doesn't behave in the body — especially not a baby's body — in the way that manufacturers claim; it is not "natural" just because it's made from sugar. The manufacturer also claims that the body does not digest and metabolize sucralose, leading you to conclude that it doesn't cross the placenta and get into baby. This has never been proven. While researching this topic, we had the opportunity to read the *Federal Register,* the official publication of the U.S. Food and Drug Administration, which revealed that 20 to 30 percent of the sucralose a person eats is metabolized, so it really does get into the body. And, even though only a small percentage of the sucralose that's in food may get into the mother's bloodstream, no one knows what it does once it gets there — or, more important, what it does inside baby's bloodstream.

High-fructose corn syrup (HFCS)—also not for babies. Now that you've crossed off aspartame and sucralose, here's why high-fructose corn syrup is not so sweet for the health of your baby:

- **Scientists question its safety.** A number of years ago when I (Dr. Bill) was on the TV show *The O'Reilly Factor,* after making the case that hydrogenated oils (trans fats) may turn out to be the worst FDA-approved fake food in the history of the food industry, Bill O'Reilly asked me what I thought the next food on the hit list might be. I responded, "high-fructose corn syrup." Needless to say, I got lots of calls from the Corn Refiners Association, which is commissioned for the "economic health" of the government-subsidized corn industry. They tried to convince me that it's been tested and found to be as safe as ordinary "natural" sugar.

As a confirmed show-me-the-science doctor, I have concluded, as have most other nutrition-savvy doctors, that HFCS is unfit for human consumption, especially for babies. Recent studies suggest that HFCS may increase excess body fat more quickly than table sugar and decrease insulin sensitivity — two top health problems that pregnant mothers need to avoid. The general consensus among nutritional researchers is that the high consumption of HFCS over the last thirty years has been a major contributor to the obesity epidemic and its health consequences of diabetes and cardiovascular disease.

• **HFCS has never been tested on babies.** We are not aware of any research on the effects of HFCS on a pregnant experimental animal and the developing baby.

• **HFCS keeps bad company.** Even if high-fructose corn syrup is eventually determined to be safe for babies, take a trip around your local supermarket and examine a collection of foods that contain HFCS. You're in for a shocking label lesson. Foods that contain high-fructose corn syrup are more likely to contain other suspect ingredients. Compare, for example, plain yogurt (or those sweetened only with fruit or honey) with yogurt sweetened with HFCS, and you'll notice that the artificially sweetened yogurt label reads like a chemistry test. That's because HFCS and other chemical additives are cheaper than real sugar and real fruit. You and your baby deserve not only the best foods but the safest foods.

Dr. Bill notes: In my office I tell kids to play "I spy with my little eyes. Look for the bad word on food labels: high-fructose corn syrup."

CAFFEINE CONCERNS

Drinking caffeinated beverages while pregnant falls into the category of "when in doubt, leave it out." While a couple of cups of coffee a day are probably safe for baby, scientists are not sure how much is safe and how much isn't. You'll commonly see 200 to 300 milligrams of caffeine given as a safe daily upper limit, but there really isn't a lot of

scientific basis for this recommendation. Consider these caffeine concerns:

• During pregnancy your body's ability to eliminate caffeine slows. Usually half of the caffeine you drink is eliminated within 3.5 hours. During pregnancy, especially in the last trimester, caffeine can linger in your system for as long as 18 hours.

• It's tough to set a safe upper limit because different coffee beans, processed in different ways, contain varying amounts of caffeine. So in reality a coffee drinker doesn't know how much caffeine she's getting per cup.

• Not only is caffeine metabolized more slowly in a pregnant mother, but it crosses the placenta and is metabolized even more slowly in a baby whose liver is not yet mature. Caffeine is a drug, and there have been infants born of heavy caffeine drinkers who actually showed caffeine-withdrawal symptoms shortly after birth.

• Keep in mind that "decaf" is often "low-caf" rather than "no-caf." Even if the caffeine content is less than 10 percent of an ordinary cup of coffee, don't fool yourself into thinking you are completely avoiding caffeine.

• Studies have shown that high doses of caffeine — 1,000 milligrams of caffeine (four or five cups of coffee a day) — can increase the risk of miscarriage. A 2008 study in the *American Journal of Obstetrics and Gynecology* reported that women who drink 200 milligrams or more of caffeine a day (about a 10-ounce cup of coffee) can as much as double their risk of miscarriage. Yet another study by the National Institutes of Health found no association between miscarriage and caffeine intake up to 300 milligrams a day. Since the research is not conclusive on how much caffeine is safe during pregnancy (and the caffeine effect may be different for many mother-baby pairs), we suggest most mothers limit their daily caffeine to no more than 200 milligrams per day.

• Consider that caffeine effects on mother — increased heart rate, increased blood pressure, increased stress hormone adrenaline (to name a few) — could also occur in baby, who doesn't have the metabolic reserve to handle these physiological changes.

• Caffeine can be a nutrient depleter by increasing the amount of calcium mothers excrete in their urine and interfering with the absorption of iron.

If you do habitually enjoy your daily caffeine buzz, try to withdraw from this habit before you're pregnant. Listen to your body. Remember, caffeine is a cardiovascular stimulant that increases your heart rate and blood pressure, and it can also act as a diuretic, causing you to urinate more and get dehydrated. Chances are if you drink enough to feel a caffeine buzz, it's probably not healthy for your baby.

Try these ways to decaffeinate your pregnancy:

• *Try herbal tea for two.* Herbal teas are caffeine-free. Enjoy! Sometimes just the habit of enjoying a hot beverage will suffice. Other alternatives are warm milk, lemon in hot water, and hot apple cider.

• *Low-caf your own tea.* If you use a caffeinated tea bag, dip the bag in a cup of hot water for twenty seconds, then discard that tea and reuse the tea bag. Since caffeine is water soluble, this process removes much, but not all, of the caffeine. If you must drink coffee, use water-processed decaffeinated coffee instead of the less safe chemically processed decaf.

• *Try half-caf.* Gradually dilute the caffeinated java with increasing amounts of decaffeinated coffee.

• *Check labels.* Caffeine lurks in soft drinks and some over-the-counter and prescription medications, so be sure to check labels.

• *Shorten your preparation time.* If you cut the percolating or steeping time in half, the resulting brew will have less caffeine.

If you must caffeinate yourself (and your baby), do so in the morning so that the caffeine effect wears off and doesn't interfere with your nightly sleep. On a sweet note, don't worry about the minimal caffeine effect of dark chocolate, which averages only 20 milligrams per ounce. A few squares of dark chocolate (60 to 80 percent cacao) a day is one of the most enjoyable — and healthy — treats.

ELEVEN MORE WAYS TO GO GREEN

There are three ways that toxins can get into your body: through your mouth, through your lungs, and through your skin. These are the avenues we're going to try to barricade. While your lungs, liver, kidneys, and placenta provide filters that these environmental chemicals have to go through to get to baby, some chemicals can get into the bloodstream that you and your baby share.

Here are simple ways to protect against toxins, now that you have a vulnerable little person inside.

1. Purify your drinking water. Install a water purifier on your kitchen faucet.

2. Detoxify your home. Remember that your baby lives here, too. As a general guide, if you're bothered by chemical odors, consider that it could also bother baby's development. First and foremost, ban smokers from your home, even if the smoker is your best friend or your father or mother. Consider hanging a sign on your door: "No smoking allowed. Baby inside."

You also need to be careful about cleaning products. Instead of chemical cleaning products, go greener by using a solution of vinegar, lemon juice, and baking soda. Never mix chlorine bleach with ammonia, vinegar, or other cleaners because a chemical reaction will occur and produce a toxic gas. Go as green as you can by avoiding highly pungent aerosol sprays that contain volatile organic compounds (VOCs) and other chemicals that form toxic gases in the air. Think twice before using furniture polish, spray disinfectants, carpet cleaners, room deodorizers, toilet bowl cleaners, flame retardants, paint thinners, antifreeze, and garden pesticides and herbicides. Skip odor-masking products, such as air fresheners, especially in your car. Not only do they often contain VOCs, but you don't want to desensitize your sense of smell. Use your supersniffer — if it smells toxic to you, it could be. Do an online search by typing in the name of each household cleaning product in question followed by the letters MSDS (Material Safety Data Sheet) for information on whether it contains VOCs and other chemicals. Another resource for environmental chemical safety is CosmeticsDatabase.com.

3. Use an air filter, especially in your bedroom. HEPA filters remove more than 99 percent of VOCs in the air. Be sure to change the filter according to the manufacturer directions.

4. Clean up your kitchen. Look for the "BPA-free" symbol on plastic bottles, plates, cups, and other containers. Recyclable plastics marked with the codes 1, 2, 4, 5, and 6 are unlikely to contain BPA (bisphenol A, a possible carcinogen); those marked 3 or 7 may contain BPA. Avoid canned foods that do not feature the "BPA-free" symbol, since many cans contain BPA as well. In one study, people who consumed canned vegetables at least once a day had 44 percent more BPA in their urine. Don't put any plastic containers in the microwave; choose glass or ceramic instead.

Think about what is important to you and how you want to honor this very special time in your life. Be a strong "mama bear" and focus on protecting yourself and your baby.

5. Better your bed. If you can afford it, buy a "green" mattress, one that is free of flame retardants classified as persistent organic pollutants (POPs).

CELL PHONE SAFETY WHILE PREGNANT

Scientific research has not yet determined whether cell phone radiation is harmful to mother or baby. A 2011 study by researchers at Yale University Department of Obstetrics, Gynecology and Reproductive Sciences revealed that newborn mice that were exposed to cellphone radiation while in the womb were more likely to show neurodevelopmental problems. Don't wait for the science to be "conclusive," because it may never be — there is too much financial interest in protecting the status quo. So play it safe. Certainly don't sit around with your tablet or your cell phone propped up on your belly. All that radiation hovering around rapidly dividing baby cells can't be good for them. As we discussed earlier, these cells, especially those in baby's brain, absorb more radiation than do adult tissues. Follow these precautions:

- Use a landline when you can.

- Use a cell phone with the lowest radio frequency.

- Try to wear or carry your cell phone as far away from your belly as possible, although that may be difficult in later pregnancy. Even stashing your cell phone in your purse may be too close.

See ewg.org for more information.

6. Be careful with candles. When possible, use natural beeswax candles, which have a safe fragrance. Be sure the candle and the wick are certified "toxic-chemical free."

7. Find a greener dry cleaner. Studies reveal that fumes from dry-cleaned clothing can become toxic, especially in small, unventilated areas like closets or dressing rooms. While pregnant, try to avoid dry cleaning entirely or look for a green dry cleaner.

8. Don't change cat-litter boxes. They can contain infectious germs, such as listeria and toxoplasma.

9. Say no to nail and hair salons. Go back to your natural nails while pregnant and skip the acrylics, which contain some of the most toxic solvents. If you do frequent a salon, find one that is well ventilated; book the first appointment of the day, before the fumes increase; and go when there are no perms, pedicures, or manicures being done. When applying nail polish at home, do it next to an open window or, better yet, outside. If possible, avoid hair salons while pregnant, especially during the first trimester. Hair color chemicals have never been proven safe. If you must color your hair, temporary or semipermanent dyes contain fewer toxic chemicals than permanent ones and are therefore likely to be safer. Try to avoid getting chemicals on your scalp, as some could be absorbed through the skin. Better yet, try natural vegetable dyes. If you must use a hairspray, use a pump instead of an aerosol, which may contain phthalates, and be sure to use it in a well-ventilated room. Not yet scared out of smelly salons? Consider the 2009 study in the journal *Environmental*

Health Perspectives, revealing that women who work in beauty salons are twice as likely to have babies with birth defects, probably because of the toxins they inhale daily.

10. Drive green. Whenever possible, avoid driving behind high-exhaust vehicles, such as trucks and buses, and during rush hour. Keep your windows closed while driving in heavy traffic. Certainly, don't let your car idle in the garage. If possible, delegate filling the gas tank to someone else. Drive less during smog alerts, if applicable where you live. If you live in a smoggy area or near busy traffic interchanges, and you are considering a move anyway, now would be the time. Studies show that women living in heavily polluted and smoggy areas have a higher incidence of babies with heart defects, preterm birth, and miscarriages compared with pregnant mothers who live in areas with cleaner air.

11. Get a greener job. If possible, change jobs if your present one exposes you and baby to harmful chemicals. A study in *Reproductive Toxicology* revealed that mothers who were exposed to BPA in their industrial job had babies with a lower birth weight than babies of nonexposed mothers.

SCIENCE SAYS: WATCH WHERE YOU WORK

Animal studies have clearly shown that a variety of fat-soluble, chemical solvents readily cross the placenta and that maternal inhalation of these compounds results in nerve and neurodevelopmental deficits in newborn animals. A study reported in the *Journal of the American Medical Association* showed a thirteenfold higher risk of major malformations, as well as increased risk for miscarriages, in women who work with chemical solvents during pregnancy. The greater their exposure, the higher the risk of malformations.

In a 2004 study in the journal *Archives of Pediatrics and Adolescent Medicine,* thirty-two pregnant women in occupations in which they were exposed to chemical solvents were followed for several years after giving birth. Compared to a matched unexposed control group, the children exposed in the womb to chemical solvents tested lower on language, motor, intellectual, and behavioral functioning. While heavy metals, such as lead and mercury, deservedly get a lot of bad press, in this study there was no difference from controls in exposure to lead and mercury. Our concern is that the "modern" placenta has not perfectly adapted to filter these "modern" chemicals. So, for baby's safety sake, when in doubt, leave them out.

MAKE YOUR PERSONAL CARE PRODUCTS SAFE FOR BABY

All that stretching of the skin and the hormonal happenings beneath it cause the feel, color, and texture of your skin to change during pregnancy. (See page 181 for information on what changes you may experience, and why.) Yet, it's important for the health of your skin and the overall health of your baby to be careful what you put on your skin since everything is absorbed through it. Go green with all those lotions and potions you put on while pregnant:

- Go organic! Just as you should eat organic food (see page 41), you should use organic body care products. Look for products that display the seal "USDA organic."

- Avoid plastic containers with the recycling code 3 or 7, which may indicate the presence of BPA.

- Beware of the term "fragrance" or "scented," which may mean that the product contains phthalates, substances shown to be hormone disrupters.

- Avoid nail polish, deodorant, shampoo, lotion, and cosmetics containing the phthalates DBP and DEP.

- Avoid products containing retinols, vitamin A, or salicylic acid, all known to cause birth defects. Lotions that contain glycerin, hyaluronic acid, cocoa butter, coconut butter, or shea butter are safe.

- Avoid insect repellents containing DEET, which has never been proven safe, especially for pregnant women.

- Sunblocks are generally safe because only a very little of the chemical gets through the skin into your body.

- Try natural skin softeners such as an oatmeal and milk bath, coconut milk, and aloe oil or lotion.

The Environmental Working Group's Skin Deep Cosmetics Database (ewg.org/skindeep) provides health and safety information as well as lists of ingredients for all kinds of cosmetic products, including makeup, skin care, hair care, nail care, sunscreen, fragrance, and more.

For more tips on caring for your skin during pregnancy, see page 183.

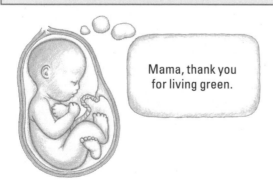

Mama, thank you for living green.

9

Practice the Pills-and-Skills Model of Self-Care

That pill-sensitive little person inside may be just the motivator you need to lower your dependence on prescription medicines. Recently the mother of one of our patients came to our office for a consultation. She was taking several medications for different conditions: an anti-inflammatory, an antihypertensive, and an antidepressant. Because she was planning to get pregnant again, she was rightly worried about the effects of this drug cocktail on her baby. I (Dr. Bill) surprised her with this question: "How would you like to learn how to help your body make its own internal medicines?" She was overjoyed, as if I had in some way "delivered" her from reliance on doctor-prescribed medicines. Our consultation continued as I taught her the pills-skills model of healthcare, better called self-care. Here are the steps to go through to shift from pills to safer self-help skills while pregnant.

Develop a pills-skills mindset. Next time you have an ailment, instead of thinking or asking your doctor, "What can I *take?*" ask yourself and the doctor "What can I *do?*" This also prompts your doctor to shift from a medical mindset into more of a self-help mindset, from what the doctor *prescribes* to what the doctor *advises.* Remember, the word *doctor* means "teacher." We have noticed that pregnancy is often a time when mothers finally get the pills-skills concept. Because they are afraid to continue taking pills, they are more motivated to muster their own preventive-medicine skills.

We have discovered in our practices that the pills-skills model is actually what most people want, especially during pregnancy. Now that you've made up your mind to take charge of your health and are willing to devote more time to self-help skills and less reliance on pills, consult your healthcare provider. Some medications require a gradual weaning; others you may be able to stop abruptly. Your provider may prescribe a lower-dose or safer medication. Doctor/ midwife consultation is especially important if you are taking medication for a chronic illness, such as diabetes or another hormonal or metabolic disorder. It is not safe for you or your baby to mess with your medications without consultation and ongoing supervision.

SELF-HELP SKILLS FOR COMMON PREGNANCY ILLS

Here's a list of the most common ailments mothers experience while pregnant and the most useful skills you can try to reduce your need for pills:

Common Pregnancy Ills

- Blood clots
- Gestational diabetes
- Heartburn or reflux
- High blood pressure
- High blood sugar
- Immune system dysfunction
- Inflammation or "itis" illnesses
- Mood disorders

Skills

- Increase daily exercise. (See page 59.)
- Graze according to the rule of twos. (See page 21.)
- Follow the 5-S diet. (See page 44.)
- Try the sipping solution. (See page 22.)
- Eat more seafood and less meat. (See page 29.)
- Eat a real-food diet. (See page 54.)
- Relax and use stressbusters. (See page 75.)

Open your personal pharmacy. You learned on page 59 how your body can make its own medicines. The nine health tips in Part I, especially the big three — following the Healthy Pregnancy Diet, grazing, and moving — are the best ways to keep your personal pharmacy open. Review those pages for details.

The keys to opening your personal pharmacy are sort of like the wise advice your mother gave you to keep you healthy as a child: "Eat more fruits, vegetables, and seafood, and go outside and play." Your mother would be pleased to know that you plan to use these self-medicating tools to help yourself have a healthier pregnancy. For an in-depth discussion of how you can teach your body to make its own internal medicines by practicing the pills-skills model, consult *Primetime Health: A Scientifically Proven Plan for Feeling Young and Living Longer* (William Sears and Martha Sears).

POPULAR PILLS WHILE PREGNANT: BE CAUTIOUS

Besides increasing the skills to reduce or avoid pills during pregnancy, there are popular pills you need·to be extra cautious about:

Antidepressants and anti-anxiety medicines. While recent research links the use of mood mellowers, such as selective serotonin reuptake inhibitors (SSRIs), during pregnancy with increased rates of birth defects, the science is a bit conflicting. There seems to be a slight correlation between SSRI use in mothers and heart defects in babies, though it's very low: 0.9 percent in women who took an SSRI compared with 0.5 percent of women who didn't. It was also found that newborns who are exposed to SSRIs while in the womb may experience a temporary withdrawal-like effect, including low blood sugar, unstable body temperature, and irritability.

These medications belong in the "when in doubt, leave them out" category, unless you have tried all alternatives and your fragile mental health jeopardizes your healthy pregnancy and healthy baby. Be sure to consult with your healthcare practitioner. (See the stressbusters on page 75 for natural ways to mellow your mood.)

Cholesterol-lowering drugs. Your baby's growing body and brain — as well as yours — need extra cholesterol. Cholesterol is one of the top brain fats in growing your little "fathead," and you need additional cholesterol to make the pregnancy-maintaining hormones progesterone and estrogen. The good news is that except in the case of a rare genetic quirk called familial hypercholesterolemia, the skills of diet and exercise we present here will usually work as well as and much more safely than the pills to keep your cholesterol at a healthy level.

Botox. This drug has not been proven safe. Don't use it while pregnant.

Over-the-counter pain and fever reducers. While a few occasional doses of ibuprofen (Motrin, Advil, Nuprin) or aspirin are unlikely to harm your baby, prolonged use requires medical supervision. Both ibuprofen and aspirin can interfere with prostaglandins, the natural labor-inducing hormones. Also, because of its prostaglandin-lowering effect, prolonged use of ibuprofen could theoretically interfere with normal blood flow in the baby's blood vessels. (Prostaglandins regulate widening and narrowing of blood vessels.) Aspirin is an anticoagulant and theoretically can cause bleeding. Acetaminophen (Tylenol) is considered the safest analgesic. If taken in the standard dose for only two to three consecutive days, it gets the green light.

RESOURCES FOR MEDICATION USE DURING PREGNANCY

- Thomas Hale, *Medications and Mothers' Milk 2012*. Also see Dr. Hale's website: InfantRisk.com.

- Gerald Briggs, Roger Freeman, and Sumner Yaffe, *Drugs in Pregnancy and Lactation* (Lippincott Williams & Wilkins, 2011).

II

Your Pregnancy: Month by Month

For the next nine months the big theme of your life will be trans-formation. *Your body will change right before your eyes. Your perspective and views on life will broaden and evolve. Most significant, your life will be altered forever because you now have the most magnificent privilege of growing, then parenting, a human being. In each of the following eleven chapters we will show you what most expectant mothers experience most of the time. More important, we will help you channel the many aspects of this transformation into becoming (and staying!) a radiantly healthy mother growing a healthy and happy baby. Whether this is your first child or your fourth, get ready for a glorious adventure.*

If you're already pregnant, you probably can't wait to start reading about the month-by-month changes. After you read about the month of pregnancy you are in now, be sure to go back and read (and follow!) the healthy pregnancy guidelines in Part I.

FIRST-MONTH VISIT TO YOUR HEALTHCARE PROVIDER*
(1–4 WEEKS)

On your first visit to your healthcare provider, expect to have:

- Confirmation of pregnancy

- A general medical history taken, plus a previous obstetrical history, if you have one

- A general physical exam, including a vaginal exam

- Blood tests: hemoglobin and hematocrit for anemia, blood typing, rubella titer, hepatitis B screen (optional: HIV screen, sexually transmitted disease screen, and sickle cell screen)

- Possible cultures for vaginal infections

- A Pap smear for the detection of cervical cancer

- A blood test for genetic diseases, if your history warrants it

- Urinalysis to test for infection, sugar, and protein

- A weight and blood pressure check

- Counseling on proper nutrition and on avoiding environmental hazards

- An opportunity to discuss your feelings and concerns

* This month-by-month schedule of visits to your healthcare provider is recommended by the American Congress of Obstetricians and Gynecologists.

10

First Month: Newly Pregnant

What? Really? Impossible! Oh, thank God! I knew it! Whatever your initial thoughts may have been, congratulations! You are now a mother. Ahead of you lies one of the most exhilarating experiences of your life, one that leads to unprecedented change and growth. There's much to think about, adjust to, and prepare for as you anticipate the birth of your baby. It might seem overwhelming at first; but by taking it one day at a time, arming yourself with information, and relying on the abundant wisdom within you, you will navigate this momentous time of your life with confidence.

Even though you are pregnant, you may not feel it yet. Perhaps your pregnant "feelings" are so far only emotional. You may have eagerly awaited pregnancy and now you are happily anticipating any signals (beyond a missed period) your body might give you that "this is it." Or, you may be feeling slightly nauseated already. Maybe you were caught a bit off-guard by the knowledge that you are pregnant. You may initially have thought you had the flu until your body or your doctor told you otherwise. Perhaps you simply "knew" when you became pregnant, even before you experienced any symptoms.

Whatever your physical symptoms, the early part of your pregnancy is likely to be an adjustment. You may find yourself feeling elated, scared, nervous, relieved, unbelieving, confused, or all of the above. Of course, your initial reaction will depend greatly on whether your pregnancy comes as a shock or as welcome news after months of planning and hoping. Don't be surprised if you have to let the news sink in a bit before you act on the fact that you are pregnant. Every woman who discovers she's "with child" goes through this. As you ponder and prepare, here is an overview of what lies ahead.

HOW YOUR BABY IS GROWING, 1–4 WEEKS*

Even before you emotionally or physically "feel pregnant" or "look pregnant," a lot is

---

* Throughout this book, the number of "weeks" refers to fetal age, or the age of baby beginning at conception, not menstrual age, the age from mother's last menstrual period (which average two weeks longer than the fetal age). These growth figures are

107

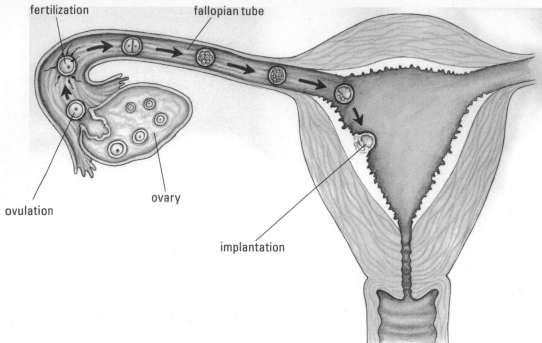

Week one: from fertilization to implantation

going on inside you. A wonderful new little person is busy growing and developing. Let's follow this little person along from conception to those beginning buds.

Week 1: Fertilization

Sperm meets egg, and together they start growing a baby. The twenty-three chromosomes in your egg couple with the twenty-three chromosomes of your mate, and lifelong traits are determined instantly: gender, skin color, body type, and so on. If two sperm fertilize two eggs (or more multiples), you are growing fraternal twins, genetically similar but not identical. They are

averages and may vary from baby to baby. (See page 125 for an explanation of baby's age.)

simply siblings who happen to occupy the uterus at the same time. A single fertilized egg can also split into two, and this creates genetically identical twins.

Now that sperm and egg get along and decide to stay together and multiply, this two-, then four-, then eight-, then sixteen-cell little bundle of baby rolls down the 4-inch fallopian tube in a several-day trip toward baby's first cradle, the uterus.

Week 2: Implantation

As if hunting for food and protection, baby finds a comfortable nest in the plush lining of your uterus. Meanwhile, that lining is growing a web of blood-rich vessels to envelop, nourish, and protect this precious person. Baby burrows into this blood-rich nest in search of a secure home for nine months. (A small amount of vaginal bleeding may occur during implantation.)

At this point your uterine lining is like a vascular sponge; these vessels envelop baby and start to deliver nourishment directly while disposing of any metabolic waste products from the life-supporting process taking place. Around the end of the second week this web of blood vessels forms a primitive placenta, a spongy pancake that delivers nutrients to baby.

This little person is obviously more than just a mass of cells. By a marvelous protective biochemical plan, baby, now called a blastocyst (literally, "sprout pouch"), signals mother's biochemical sensors and immune system to accept his presence. Baby's biochemical language says to his mother's immune system: "Don't reject me, I belong here. Exception alert! It's OK — I'm depending on you. I will need your immune system to protect me until I can make my own."

Week 3: Placenta and Baby Grow Together

All this growth requires both nutrients and biochemical direction. Enter hormones, the biochemical architects that direct baby's growth — and mother's as well. One of these early hormones is human chorionic gonadotropin (HCG), whose main function is to grow the placenta. HCG prompts the ovaries to make more of the baby-growing hormones estrogen and progesterone. These hormones signal your ovaries to suspend ovulation, and they signal your master gland, the pituitary, to not menstruate naturally. You "miss your period" because the uterine lining you would have lost is now retained to nourish and protect the baby.

By the end of the third week, this little person who began life as the union of two cells has now multiplied to millions of cells, all of which are biochemically guided into the organs they will soon form.

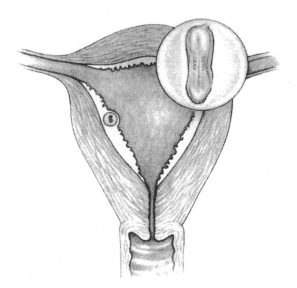

Embryo at 3 weeks.

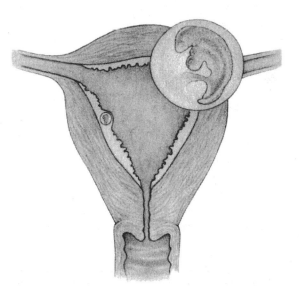

Embryo at 4 weeks.

Week 4: Baby's Body Takes Shape

Toward the end of your baby's third week of development, the cellular components inside your baby are ready to become the organs they are programmed to be. First, they huddle into three teams of cells, each with a predetermined destination in baby's body. One group of cells will combine to form baby's nervous system, hair, and skin. Another group will team up to form the digestive system and lungs. The third group will combine to form baby's cardiovascular system, kidneys, muscles, and bones. The blood vessels also team up to form the umbilical cord vessels. With baby now about the size of a curved grain of rice, the rudimentary organs begin to bud:

- The heart, until now just a tube, circulates baby's blood and begins to beat. By the end of the fourth week it becomes a ball and starts dividing into four chambers that pump blood into bigger vessels, but you can't yet hear the heartbeat.

- Tiny bones stack up to begin the backbone.

- Barely visible arms and legs bud out from the tiny torso.

- What looked like another tiny tube, called the neural tube, now bulges out and curves as the head bump reveals the rapidly growing brain.

By the end of the first month, you might still be wondering why your period is late, but most of your baby's major organs, though tiny, are already in place.

HOW YOU MAY FEEL

Joyful. The news that you are pregnant may leave you feeling over-the-moon ecstatic, especially if you have been trying to get pregnant for a long time. You may feel complete and fulfilled, and have an overall sense of well-being.

Knowing there is a little person growing inside me who is so dependent on me for love and life is not only an awesome responsibility but also a great blessing. It is the most fulfilling experience in my life.

Confused. While you may think the words mother/mom/mama/mommy have a nice ring to them, you may also feel overwhelmed anticipating the life changes that come with the job. It's incredibly common to have mixed feelings about being pregnant, especially if your news comes as a surprise. It's normal to be happy about the prospect of becoming a mother, yet also feel sad or worried about what you'll have to go through or give up to get the title. Many women find it comforting to consider pregnancy a developmental stage, like adolescence. Pregnancy is one of life's most incredible transitions, and a natural way to prepare for the next stage, when baby arrives. You can think of it as somewhat of an identity crisis. The realization "I'm going to be somebody's mother!" leads to the question "What will happen to the 'me' I am now?" It is normal to feel unsure about surrendering your life to such a major change. Even when a pregnancy is planned and longed for, a woman may wonder if she's as ready or as capable as she thought she was. Change can be intimidating and seem overwhelming, even when it is positive.

You may also feel like a dual-career woman even in the first month of pregnancy. There may be days when you are so excited (or anxious) about the pregnancy that you can't focus on anything else. You might fear that if you don't come down to earth soon, you could lose your job. You may be worried about leaving your job, whether for maternity leave or permanently, and about taking on the responsibilities of motherhood. Other days you may be so engrossed in your current life you almost forget you're pregnant (and then feel guilty for forgetting). Just remember that it's normal to have difficulty staying enthusiastic about your job while pregnant. For some women biology takes over and they come to the realization that they can't work to their full capacity, physically or mentally. Most women, however, soon settle into the pregnancy, embracing a "new normal" daily routine.

My mother told me about her first pregnancy, "I got up, threw up, made breakfast, and then your dad and I went to school to teach."

How you feel about your body may also have its ups and downs. You may experience pride in your femininity and fertility, and such delight in nourishing another life within your own body that you can't wait to show or tell about it. You may be glowing. On the other hand, you may not enjoy relinquishing your comfortable, familiar body to the widening and bulging of pregnancy. Maybe you have heard from friends that they looked and felt awful when they were pregnant. Many women worry about becoming less attractive to their husbands.

Some women, expecting to feel ecstatic when they discover they are pregnant, are surprised that those feelings aren't there yet. Don't be alarmed if you don't immediately experience those warm and tender feelings of bonding with your baby. It's not unhealthy or abnormal in the early weeks or months to feel more like an incubator than a mom. Many women don't feel motherly until they feel the first kick or see the ultrasound picture of their moving baby. Getting connected with your baby is a long process that works differently for different mothers and babies.

Dr. Linda notes: Women who have had difficulties with miscarriage, infertility, or other pregnancy uncertainties often have more problems feeling connected to the growing fetus. This is normal.

Anxious. It's normal to feel anxious about the unknown. If you have been settled in a childless, adult lifestyle for more than a few years, the prospect of diapers, middle-of-the-night feedings, and a tiny person controlling your life may leave you feeling more than a little freaked out. When you close one chapter in your life to open another, expect to have some misgivings. When you announce to your friends that you are pregnant, you also invite an army of veterans to share their birth and pregnancy stories. Some tales from the front can be interesting, some overwhelming. Learn to take these stories with a grain of salt. Your experience will most assuredly be uniquely yours. You can also take comfort in knowing that women have been birthing babies for millennia; have faith in nature's process and the wisdom of your body.

Dr. BJ notes: Surfing-the-Internet syndrome can produce anxiety.

Additionally, trepidation about the discomfort of pregnancy and the pain of childbirth produces its own anxiety. Worries about miscarriage are also common early in pregnancy, though the odds against having one are in your favor. The longer your pregnancy progresses, the less you need to worry about a miscarriage. A certain amount of worrying is normal during pregnancy. The heightened awareness of being an "overprotective mother" begins. It's healthy, yet it may not make you happy. If you already are prone to anxiety and your "awareness" dial is already set on high, pregnancy may push it to overload. If you find your concerns escalating as your pregnancy progresses, or if anxiety prevents you from living your life as usual, consider seeking professional help.

Dr. BJ notes: Several times a day close your eyes and envision your healthy growing baby, and take a deep breath to reduce stress.

Moody. A completely blissful pregnancy is as rare as a perfect parent. In other words, it's not going to happen. As the initial elation of discovering you're pregnant subsides and the reality of impending parenthood sinks in, it's common to have great days and then not-so-great days. There are several reasons for these mood swings. One is the normal letdown that naturally occurs after an intensely emotional experience; in human emotions, lows usually follow highs. Another reason is purely physiological: it's those hormones. The pregnancy hormones that are surging through your body also account for the volatility of your emotions. Of course,

feeling depressed may catch you by surprise, especially if this is a long-anticipated pregnancy. This is supposed to be the happiest time ever, right? And, of course, feeling bad or guilty that you don't always feel joyous just makes it worse. Add in the nausea and fatigue of early pregnancy, and it's no wonder that most mothers go from glad to sad and back again several times a day. When hormone levels are changing dramatically in the first three months (and final weeks) of pregnancy, mood changes, even dramatic ones, are to be expected. After all, these are the times when anticipation increases and fatigue sets in. Try to recognize and embrace all of your emotions, even the ones that aren't so happy.

Fatigued. Most likely, you are tired. Sometimes *very* tired. That little energy-draining creature growing inside you will naturally sap your strength, as if mommy's bed and breakfast is working overtime to accommodate her special guest. Of course, you are also dealing with the emotional upheaval caused by those darned hormones, so your exhaustion is both physical and mental.

Being very tired was always the first sign for me that I was pregnant. I would fall asleep on the couch at 8:00 every evening. My husband called it "sleeping for two." It's funny, but it's true.

The overwhelming tiredness that many newly pregnant women experience is also your body — and your brain — forcing you to rest. Pregnancy fatigue is the first of many biological signals that flash in your mind and body urging you to tune in and nurture yourself and your baby. It's also the earliest pregnancy prompt that prepares you for one of the most essential mothering lessons: *Baby needs a happy, rested mother.* Take good care of yourself so you can take better care of your baby. This holds especially true once baby arrives! In fact, all of this is excellent preparation for the adventure that lies ahead.

Dr. BJ notes: *With my first pregnancy the fatigue was profound and I did not expect that. My routine was impacted as I was asleep by early evening. I realized early on that the fatigue was actually a blessing because it stopped me in my tracks and made me recognize how important it was to honor the process that my body was managing and to surrender to it.*

While your "three-month exhaustion" will lessen somewhat in the middle trimester, don't expect your energy level to return to its pre-pregnant peak. Your body has been reset to what's best for you both.

I found it helpful to make a list of all the tasks I had to do and divide them into three sets. The first set was things I absolutely had to get done and could only do myself; the second set was tasks that I could delegate — and I really had to delegate these; the third set was tasks that could be ignored, and I crossed them out with a big, red pencil. Whenever I started feeling overwhelmed, I simply asked myself, "What are the consequences of not getting something done?" I discovered that 90 percent of the time, life went on if I simply ignored the tasks.

Me first. Now that you're a mother, and a tired one, you can no longer be all things to all people. Set priorities. Your first priority is to be a healthy mommy growing a healthy baby. It is OK to multitask less and say "no" more. You may need a day or two of "sick leave" now and then throughout your pregnancy, and if you have a demanding job, you may also need to negotiate flexible or even reduced working hours. Learn to delegate tasks to others and focus on doing what no one else can do but you. Don't feel guilty; remember that you are doing the most important job in the world: growing a human being.

When I first found out I was pregnant, we called a family meeting. My husband announced that mommy had a new job description. The older kids would have to do more themselves. Mom would be partially going off call. The kids got it. I'm so glad my husband did this for me.

Let them know. It may be difficult for your husband and child(ren) to fully understand the life-altering and fatigue-causing changes of early pregnancy. Since you need cooperation from your family, it is important not to wait too long to share the news. After all, your kids need to understand why mommy drifts off to sleep in the middle of that bedtime story and is a bit crankier than usual. They might as well start adjusting to their roles as big siblings. Impress upon your family all the energy this new little person demands. You may be surprised by how well they understand and how compassionate they can be when you aren't feeling well.

Dr. Bill notes: *In my office when an expectant mother comes in with older kids, I have the kids repeat after me: "Mommy needs more rest."*

Sleep like a baby. Babies have the luxury of listening to their bodies and sleeping when they need to. While few moms have such a pregnancy perk, you should still try to sleep when you are tired. Enjoy a mid-morning and afternoon catnap when you can. Few pregnant mothers can keep going from sunrise to sunset without turning off at least briefly. Try going to bed earlier and waking up naturally instead of to the sound of the alarm. While "early to bed and early to rise" is healthier for your body's natural sleep rhythms, that may not be possible every day. Use blackout curtains, white noise, and/or earplugs to extend your sleep a couple of hours whenever you can.

Guilty. Many women who are surprised to find themselves expecting are immediately consumed by guilt. They think of that big margarita they had, the cigarettes they snuck in, the sleeping pill they took, and guilt and panic set in.

Dr. Linda advises: *Relax! While in the best of worlds all women of childbearing age would be living perfectly healthy lives, we all live in the real world:*

- Half of all pregnancies in the United States are unplanned.

- Most of the things that we wouldn't do if we knew we were pregnant don't actually damage the baby in those first few weeks. Heavy exposure to things like alcohol, cigarettes, and certain drugs can cause birth or developmental defects in babies, but the small exposures that might have already taken place probably won't.

- Today is a new day — if you are doing things that are bad for your baby, stop now. If you find that you can't stop, get professional help.

- Contact an obstetrician or prescribing physician quickly if you are on prescription drugs and don't know what you should do in early pregnancy. While some drugs should be stopped immediately, it can be dangerous to stop certain medications suddenly. Sometimes the medical problem the drug is treating is much more dangerous to your baby than the drug itself.

- Be honest with your caregiver about exposures and concerns — if you have an addiction you can't stop, your doctor or midwife can probably help. The more your caregiver knows about exposure to drugs, sexually transmitted infections, and so on, the more she can help.

EARLY SIGNS OF PREGNANCY	
What You May Experience	*Comment*
Missed menstrual period	There are also some non-pregnancy-related reasons for menstrual irregularity, such as stress.

Fatigue	You no longer have the stamina for usual activities, such as walking quickly up a hill or staying awake after supper.
Nausea and vomiting (morning sickness)	Morning sickness may be confused with the flu or feeling like you're "coming down with something." And it may not be confined to the morning.
Aversion to odors, alcohol, and smoke	Baby-protective mechanisms click in.
Food cravings	Surprisingly, you may crave foods that you seldom ate before or previously found distasteful.
Slight staining or spotting	Bleeding or spotting at the time of implantation can be mistaken for menstruation.
Breast changes	Nipples tingle, breasts feel tender and fuller, the areola begins to darken, and tiny glands on the areola enlarge. Changes may be similar to premenstrual feelings in your breasts, only more dramatic.
Abdominal discomfort, bloating	Feeling gassy and crampy may be confused for GI upset.
Crampy pelvic discomfort	You may feel generalized discomfort throughout the lower abdomen and pelvis; however, *sharp one-sided pain is not normal and should be reported to your doctor.*
Frequent urination	Early on, you will urinate more often due to pregnancy hormones. Later on, this will be caused by pressure of the enlarging uterus on the bladder.

Keep a peaceful home. The pregnant mind needs rest just as the pregnant body does. Try to maximize the factors in your home and work environment that give you peace and minimize those that don't. Arrange for childcare for a few hours during the week to give you a break from your other children. Try classical or relaxation music, or a warm soak in the tub. Now is a good time for your partner to learn and implement the fine art of massage. Do not feel guilty about the time you spend relaxing; you and your baby need it.

Let nature nurture you. A change of scenery is good for a tired mind and body. Call it green therapy. During times when your body is willing, treat yourself to exercise: a long walk in the park or along a nature trail, or a relaxing swim.

Eat when you need to! Not eating enough can lower your energy and aggravate fatigue. Choose nutritious food and nibble frequently throughout the day. (Reread chapter 2 for guidelines on healthy eating during pregnancy.)

Notice that the suggestions outlined above incorporate the mainstays of everyone's well-being and self-care: eating right, sleeping enough, relaxing, and exercising. While pregnant you need an extra dose of these energy-replenishing practices.

NAUSEA AND MORNING SICKNESS

Yes, that feeling that you've been hearing about and dreading may have started by now. The term "morning sickness" is misleading, as this queasiness can occur in the morning, afternoon, evening, or middle of the night. Instead of calling it morning sickness, in our practices we refer to it as pregnancy-induced nausea (PIN). The intensity and duration of PIN is as individual as a mother's weight gain. For most women, it seems to peak at four to seven weeks.

Some research shows that the severity of PIN increases proportionally with the increase in thyroid hormones, and also human chorionic gonadotropin (HCG), the main growth hormone of pregnancy. For most women, PIN ends when the thyroid hormone returns to normal, usually around twelve to sixteen weeks. Women vary in their sensitivity to rising HCG, just as they do to seasickness.

The two primary miseries of PIN are hypersensitivity to odors and aversion to certain foods. This heightened sensitivity is believed to be a genetic carryover from the days when the pregnant woman foraged for food: her gut spoke loudly, prompting her to avoid foods potentially harmful to baby. Certain smells may "go right to your stomach," triggering nausea and queasiness. The usual odors that women find most offensive are garlic, peanut butter, alcohol, coffee, traffic and fuel fumes, and cigarette smoke. Some pregnant women complain that typical household odors that didn't bother them before become intensely unpleasant. The family dog may smell more "doggy." Some women find the normal masculine odors of their beloved man repulsive. A lovely perfume may send a woman running outside to retch. Even favorite foods may now be inedible because the smell triggers a gag response.

It is biologically correct to blame your mood swings and your morning sickness on "those hormones." It might help to think of pregnancy hormones as a miracle drug necessary for maintaining the well-being of you and your baby. Yet those hormones, like most drugs, have a few unpleasant side effects, namely, intestinal upsets. HCG supports your pregnancy, but also unsettles your stomach. The hormone cholecystokinin, which increases in pregnant women, increases the efficiency of digestion by making better metabolic use of food within the mother's system. But while increasing the body's ability to store energy, this hormone also contributes to low blood sugar, nausea, dizziness, delayed emptying of the stomach, and the after-meal sleepiness that many pregnant women experience. Rising estrogen and progesterone levels also contribute to nausea by their direct influence on intestinal hormones.

You are likely to feel the worst when hormonal changes are the greatest — in the first trimester. By the end of the third month, when blood levels of some of these hormones level off or start to decline, so (usually) do the intestinal maladies. Expect to have more than your fair share of morning sickness if you are carrying twins; you are producing more hormones, so your nausea may be more intense.

This hormonal havoc also slows the action of your intestines, causing accumulation of stomach acids, indigestion, and heartburn. The slowing of your intestines and the decreasing amount of space for them (because of your expanding uterus) may leave you feeling constipated. All of these factors contribute to morning sickness.

We believe that PIN is a treatable, or at least partially treatable, side effect of pregnancy. Lemon, ginger, and peppermint are time-tested tummy relievers because the taste and the aroma of these foods distract the nausea receptors in the brain.

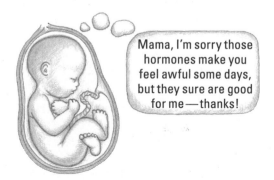

Mama, I'm sorry those hormones make you feel awful some days, but they sure are good for me — thanks!

Questions You May Have about Morning Sickness

I know I'm supposed to gain weight, but I'm afraid I'll lose weight since I feel so sick. Will all my nausea and vomiting hurt my baby?

Don't worry about losing weight during periods of sickness. In fact, most women continue to gain weight quite well, even during these weeks or months, probably because in order to feel better, they are eating frequent small meals. Even those women who do lose weight make up for it by gaining weight quickly once the sickness subsides. When there aren't enough nutrients for two, baby will get what she needs from nutrients stored in mother's body. This nutrient balance will be restored once mom feels better and is eating normally and healthily again.

Fewer than 1 percent of pregnant women suffer a severe form of persistent vomiting called *hyperemesis gravidarum* (Latin for "excessive vomiting in pregnancy"). In this condition, the body is unable to compensate for the relentless vomiting. You lose body fluids and valuable body salts called electrolytes; in other words, the mother becomes dehydrated. If unrecognized and untreated, this severe vomiting can make you very sick, which can, in turn, compromise your baby. With treatment, even babies of mothers with severe hyperemesis stay remarkably healthy.

Here are signs that you are becoming dehydrated and should call your doctor:

- You're urinating less and your urine appears darker in color.

- Your mouth, eyes, and skin feel dry.

- Your mental acuity seems compromised.

- You feel increasingly weak and faint.

- You haven't been able to keep down any food or drink for twenty-four hours.

In addition to preventing dehydration, you need to prevent a condition called *starvation ketosis.* When your body is starved for nutrition, especially carbohydrates, your tissues begin to break down, and an excess of ketones (an organic compound) is produced in your blood, which aggravates nausea. To keep this from happening, try sipping salty fluids, such as chicken broth, oral electrolyte solutions, and coconut water (see the recipe for our pregnancy supersmoothie on page 24).

My obstetrician told me that morning sickness could be a sign of a healthy baby, but I suspect she said this just to make me feel better.

It may help to know that the high levels of pregnancy hormones that contribute to nausea also suggest a well-implanted embryo. In fact, statistics show that the more nausea a mother has, the more likely she is to deliver a healthy baby. This does not mean, though, that if you don't feel sick, you won't deliver a healthy baby. Many mothers coast through pregnancy with a minimum of morning sickness and are blessed with healthy babies.

My unsympathetic husband thinks it's all in my head when I feel sick.

How frustrating! Sometimes when men (or anyone for that matter) can't understand or experience exactly what you are going through, they react by being critical. They often feel helpless, then frustrated that they can't fix what's wrong. It's hard for your husband to stand by and see the person he loves suffering. Start by explaining your queasy feelings by telling him to imagine feeling seasick or carsick all day while having the flu, or however else you might describe your own personal experience. You can ask him for his support in specific ways.

HOW HUSBANDS CAN HELP

Attention, Dads! Support and TLC are the name of the game when it comes to taking care of your wife during her first trimester. Many of these gestures will also help support her throughout the entire pregnancy:

- Find out which chores most upset mom-to-be and do them yourself — for example, walking the dog, changing the cat's litter box (a must anyway; see page 99), and even feeding the little ones while she sleeps in. Your newly pregnant wife deserves to wake up to a clean-smelling kitchen and settled kids.

- Do the shopping and run errands. Some pregnant women find supermarket aromas intolerable, especially in the early months of pregnancy.

- Brainstorm with your wife a list of all the de-stressors that will help her feel better and keep things in the house running smoothly. Support her in taking care of as many things as you can.

• Use the power of touch! A massage, or even just a foot rub, can help mom get her mind off her queasy tummy.

• Since your wife's senses are heightened, you may need to change your clothes more often, brush your teeth more often, and go easy on foods like garlic, onions, and hot peppers.

• Be the cook. If she is hypersensitive to the usual kitchen odors or to handling raw meat, you and your family can do the cooking and call mom in when the food is ready. And don't forget to open the windows to air out the kitchen!

As your expectant wife is learning to cope with these discomforts, part of your training is to become sensitive to her needs and learn ways to make her life easier now and when your baby arrives.

Dr. Bill notes: *Martha had a pregnancy craving for zucchini, and I would often make midnight treks to the supermarket to satisfy her cravings for before-bed zucchini pancakes. Late one night as I was going through the checkout counter with a foot-long zucchini, the clerk concluded, "Your wife must be pregnant."*

How long will these miserable feelings last?

Many mothers are rewarded with "well windows" — hours of the day or even whole days when they feel well enough to function normally. As your pregnancy progresses, keep your perspective positive. The good days will get better, and there will be fewer and less intense bad days. Sooner or later, the morning sickness will pass.

Dr. Linda notes: *I could identify no rhyme or reason to my own morning sickness. I had very little with my first pregnancy, a boy, and almost none with my third, a girl, but was violently sick practically all of the first few months with the middle pregnancy,* *also a girl. This was completely unrelated to my stress level, which was consistently high during all three pregnancies.*

Fifteen Stomach-Friendly Tips

Here are some easily digested tips on managing morning sickness:

1. Begin the day in a stomach-friendly way. If you start the morning off sick and don't take the appropriate measures, you are likely to stay sick all day. Instead, give your stomach a friendly start by eating something before you go to bed so it won't be empty when you wake up. You can also stash an assortment of easy-to-digest favorites at your bedside. (The classic favorite is salty crackers.) When you trek to the bathroom in the middle of the night, treat your stomach to a nibble. A good rule is to put food into your mouth before your feet touch the floor. Once you are awake in the morning, give your gut a good breakfast and continue to munch all morning, carrying your nibble pack around with you if necessary.

Sudden transitions often trigger nausea. And what could be more unsettling than being abruptly awakened by an inconsiderate alarm? Ease into your day. Try awakening to soothing music from a clock radio or a noiseless alarm light, which gradually increases brightness at a preset time. If you don't have to awaken at a set time, don't. If your partner gets up early, get him his own noiseless alarm, then let him wake you in a gentle way when it's time for you to get up.

2. Track the trigger. Keep a list of which foods cause you the most discomfort. While this may change throughout your pregnancy, here are the usual suspects:

- Cabbage

- Caffeine-containing beverages, such as coffee and colas

- Cauliflower

- Foods containing monosodium glutamate (MSG)

- Fried foods

- Greasy foods

- High-fat foods (read labels)

- Onions

- Sauerkraut

- Spicy foods

Besides keeping tabs on your trigger foods, note your favorite comfort foods as well. Many women keep their personal "desired dozen" comfort foods handy to nibble on during the days when they feel the worst.

3. Graze on stomach-friendly foods. Some foods are just naturally harder on the stomach than others. High-fat, spicy, and some high-fiber foods are hard to digest. Try to follow these easy-on-the-stomach tips:

- Consume foods with nutrients that are easily digestible and pass through the stomach quickly, such as liquids, smoothies, yogurts, and low-fat, high-carbohydrate foods. Avoid hard-to-digest fatty foods and greasy fried foods, such as French fries, fried chicken, and sausage.

- Eat nutrient-dense foods such as avocados, kidney beans, cheese, fish, nut butter, whole-grain pasta, brown rice, tofu, and turkey. If peanut butter doesn't appeal to you, try a milder-tasting nut butter, such as almond or cashew butter. Spread it thinly on crackers, bread, apple slices, or celery sticks; a large glob of it may be slow to digest due to its high fat content.

- If your prenatal vitamins trigger nausea, try taking them midday, with a meal.

- Foods with a high water content are not only easy on your intestines but also prevent the dehydration and constipation that aggravate nausea. Try melon, grapes, frozen fruit bars, lettuce, apples, pears, celery, and rhubarb.

4. Grazing is the way to go! Follow the rule of twos that you learned on page 21. Low blood sugar, which can trigger nausea, can occur upon awakening or anytime you go many hours without food. The traditional eating pattern of three square meals a day is not meant for pregnant women. A more digestible pattern is six smaller meals, which can be especially helpful when your stomach thinks it doesn't want anything at all. Grazing on nutritious snacks throughout the day keeps your stomach satisfied and your blood sugar steady. You may find that this is a biologically ideal way to nourish yourself even when you aren't pregnant.

I felt like I was always hungry, always thinking about my next meal. As my stomach got empty, I would get sick, so I had to keep my stomach not just partially full, but full all the time. Right after breakfast I would think, "What am I going to eat for lunch?" My days revolved around food and what I was going to eat next.

5. Select the sipping solution. Sipping on blended food throughout the day provides easy-in/easy-out "good gut" feelings. Blended food is more easily digested, and sipping throughout the day also helps ensure you get enough fluids. Dehydration aggravates nausea, which makes you not want to eat or drink, which makes you more dehydrated, and the cycle intensifies. (See the recipe for our pregnancy supersmoothie on page 24.)

Try lemon anything: lemonade, lemon drops, sucking on lemons. My husband gagged when he saw me eating a lemon, but it wasn't even sour to me. It really took the bite out of my nausea.

6. When it's good to suck. Sucking keeps saliva flowing, and if queasy stomachs could talk, they would ask for a steady supply of saliva, which is like health juice for your stomach and intestinal lining. Saliva buffers the acid and coats the esophagus, preventing and relieving the pain of heartburn. Besides, digestion begins in the mouth — the more saliva mixes with food, the better it is predigested. But avoid letting saliva hit an empty stomach, or nausea will soon follow. Most women produce an excess of saliva while pregnant, and even thinking about food can stimulate you to salivate. Lining your stomach with milk or yogurt before eating a saliva-stimulating food (such as salty or dry foods, like crackers) may keep

STOMACH-SOOTHING FAVORITES

- Applesauce
- Bananas
- Candied ginger or ginger tea
- Celery sticks
- Chamomile and peppermint tea
- Chewing gum
- Fruit juice popsicles
- Grapes
- Hardboiled eggs
- Lemon drops, lemonade, sniffing cut lemons

- Licorice
- Pudding
- Rice cakes
- Salty sunflower seeds
- Sorbet
- Toast
- Yogurt
- Zucchini

saliva-induced nausea from striking. Many pregnant women claim that peppermint candy or gum helps nausea, but it's best not to use either on an empty stomach, as these foods increase saliva production but put no bulk in the stomach. Experiment with various all-day suckers, such as lemon drops. Choose what works best for you and tote around a pocketful.

I learned to stay away from anything that could cause heartburn. For me, heartburn and morning sickness were a drastic duo I didn't want.

7. Eat out. Not necessarily at a restaurant, but in the great outdoors. There will be days when it's a chore just to get moving and you'd rather be a couch potato. But it can be well worth the effort, physically and mentally, to get up and go. One of the keys to overcoming nausea and other pregnancy discomforts is to get your mind off them. Your gut is called the second brain for a reason: it is richly supplied with nerves and neurohormones that trigger emotions. Getting outside and enjoying the sights and sounds of nature helps your head brain overcome your gut brain. If you work in an office and normally eat lunch at your desk, for example, go out and nibble while you walk.

Dr. Linda notes: Even when I felt like staying home from work, I was actually better off at work. At least while I was working I had less time to think about how awful I felt.

8. Sniff ahead. If you know what aromas trigger your nausea, it makes sense to arrange for detours around those things. If cooking odors bother you, consider precooking and

freezing foods on days when you feel well. Or you might lower your standards temporarily and buy more convenience foods. If you are invited to another home for dinner, offer to bring a dish you know you'll be able to eat. When you're at work or running errands, be sure to carry your reliable edibles with you; when a hunger surge hits, the nausea is sure to follow if you don't have a tried-and-true snack handy.

9. De-stress. Your brain and stomach share nerves, so when you are upset, your stomach can be, too. Many mothers get stuck in a stress-nausea cycle. The worse they feel, the more stressed they become, and then they feel worse.

Because you and your baby are so hormonally connected, you want to spare your baby a steady barrage of stress hormones. If your job is giving you lots of stress and little satisfaction, you may need to negotiate some changes in hours or responsibilities. Spouse and kids excluded, rid your home of unnecessary stressors. Learning to reduce stress now is good practice for maintaining serenity as a new mother. Remind yourself that what your baby needs most is a happy, rested mother, both before and after birth.

Pregnancy for me was a chance to retire from the rat race. It was a time for me to get out of the high-pressure stockbroker profession. I started looking for opportunities to work from home.

10. Dress comfortably. There is absolutely no reason to continue wearing clothing with zippers, buttons, or snaps that make you feel tight, constricted, or uncomfortable. Just because it still fits, doesn't mean you have to wear it. Instead, go for comfort as soon as you desire! Many pregnant women find that anything pressing on their abdomen, waist, or neck is irritating and nausea-triggering.

Martha notes: A few days after a positive pregnancy test, in anticipation of soon losing my waistline, I cinched my belt in a notch as a way of "holding on." I regretted it immediately when a wave of nausea reminded me who's boss.

11. Sleep it off. It's fortunate that the increased need for sleep coincides with the morning sickness phase. At least you can count on sleep to bring some blessed relief. Martha remembers craving sleep for this reason alone — to escape nausea. So precious is this rest that you will want to ensure that sleep goes on for as long as possible. For some women, though, bed rest doesn't help. They need to do something mind absorbing to get their focus anywhere but on their queasy stomach. If you have a toddler running around, you will not have the luxury of staying in bed or sleeping in.

If you go to bed stressed, you are more likely to awaken in the same state. A sleepless night is likely to be followed by a day of vomiting and nausea. To avoid entering sleep with unsettling thoughts on your mind, read or do something relaxing before going to bed. Avoid watching television because it can be overstimulating, especially the news or other potentially disturbing programs. Many couples enjoy using this time instead to talk about the joys of upcoming parenthood or to talk to their growing baby. Pregnant women report that this is a very relaxing practice that helps carry them into sleep.

Dr. BJ notes: Enjoy a warm bath in the evening with a cool cloth over your eyes while you meditate on your baby floating inside.

12. Try acupressure. Both Eastern and Western medical practitioners describe a pressure point on the forearm about 2 inches above the crease, on the inner aspect of the wrist, that, if stimulated, may relieve nausea and vomiting associated with pregnancy and other conditions (such as seasickness). Acupressure bands, available without prescription at pharmacies and marine stores, are meant to be worn around one or both wrists. Each band contains a button that presses on the nausea-sensitive pressure point. A study published in the journal *Obstetrics and Gynecology* compared the incidence of morning sickness in pregnant women who wore the real band with that of women who wore a placebo band, one on which the button had been blunted so as not to exert pressure on the adjacent point. Around 60 percent of women felt better during the three days they wore the actual acupressure bands, while only 30 percent in the placebo group felt better. The physicians who organized the study concluded that this method of acupressure was both safe and effective. Acupressure and Sea-Bands work by stimulating the pressure points that dampen the hypersensitivity of the nausea center in the brain.

13. Keep your eye on the prize. Surround yourself with encouraging and supportive people and try to emphasize the positive parts of pregnancy to your children. When you're having a day when you can't keep anything down, remember, this too shall pass.

I felt fine in the morning because I had a good night's sleep, but I felt miserable in the afternoon when the kids came home from school. They would see me only tired, grumpy, and needy. The poor kids didn't get too many decent meals either. One time our fourteen-year-old heard me complaining and groaning and asked, "Mom, are you sorry you're having a baby?" That made me stop and realize that I had better soft-pedal my complaining a bit and try to present a more positive attitude around the children. I didn't want to model all that negativity to my daughters. Our new daughter was worth every moment of morning sickness!

14. Position yourself for comfort. As if nausea and vomiting were not enough, many women experience heartburn as part of the morning sickness package. This burning feeling, which is caused by reflux of stomach acids into the lower esophagus, occurs more frequently during pregnancy than at other times. This is one more ailment attributed to those pregnancy hormones, which relax the stomach walls. For heartburn, gravity will be your best remedy. Keep upright after eating. Sleep on your left side to keep the inlet of your stomach higher than the outlet, allowing gravity to lessen reflux. You may need to sleep propped up 30 degrees on a wedge; see more about sleeping positions on page 84.

15. Monitor treats that relieve nausea. Stress can cause nausea, and eating sweets can trigger the brain to release stress mellowers, such as serotonin. So, many mothers will occasionally be tempted to ignore the nutritional label on the food and just eat what stops the nausea. Keep a log of stomach-friendly sweet treats that are not too junky and not eaten too often. (See our list of snacks on page 22.)

I decided that "three squares a day" meant chocolate, not meals.

FOOD CRAVINGS

Often the best way to handle food cravings, especially during periods of morning sickness, is to give in to them. Treating your stomach to what it's asking for may make the difference between a queasy day and a comfortable one. Cravings during pregnancy may in fact reflect the wisdom of the body: many nutritionists who study food cravings conclude that several common cravings actually serve vital nutritional needs during pregnancy. Consider two common cravings: pickles and potato chips. These foods are high in salt, which your body needs, and they stimulate thirst, so you drink more water. Perhaps your body knows that it will need a lot of extra fluid to fill up baby's amniotic sac. Some women even yearn for foods they never liked before, perhaps because their changing bodies have nutritional needs they didn't have before. Most women find that their cravings change throughout pregnancy, perhaps in keeping with their changing nutritional needs.

If you feel your cravings are getting out of hand, take a closer look. Make a list of them, noting the amounts you eat, and the frequency with which you eat them. Consult your healthcare provider or nutritionist for help in determining whether these cravings are in your and your baby's best interest. As a general rule, when it comes to food cravings during pregnancy, what you *want* to eat is likely to be what you *need* to eat, unless the food you are craving is clearly unhealthy.

Of course, there may be those gut-wrenching days when the only thing that makes you feel better is to give in to your food cravings, but then you worry that you're not eating a balanced diet. When you are feeling sick, the last thing you think about is the nutritional content of what you are eating. Remember, any food (except foods known to be incredibly unhealthy or unsafe) that helps mother feel better by staying down and giving her energy will be good for baby. There may be days when you seem to overdose on carbohydrates, other days when you consume megadoses of protein, and days when you simply eat or drink anything that will stay down. You may be surprised to find that the variety of food cravings you experience over a month leads you to a diet that is not so unbalanced after all. When nausea is at its worst, forget about a balanced day's nutrition and aim for a balanced week instead.

A treat a day may actually keep food cravings at bay. Enjoy a nutritious treat each day, such as a couple of squares of dark chocolate or a homemade healthful cookie. As you reshape your tastes to nutrient-dense snacks to satisfy your cravings, even though it may not be what you initially "want," eventually you will train your cravings to be satisfied with what's good for you and your baby.

Dr. Linda notes: *There is a time and place for medical treatment. Sometimes all efforts at diet and lifestyle management for hyperemesis (extreme vomiting) fail. Simple treatments, such as IV fluids — which might include salt, potassium, and* *glucose — can treat dehydration, low blood sugar, and electrolyte imbalances. There are also safe and effective medications to treat extreme cases of nausea.*

CONCERNS YOU MAY HAVE

As your baby grows, here are some of the concerns you might have.

Due Date

"When are you due?" is a question you will continually get. Here are some do-it-yourself methods to calculate your due date as well as the ones your healthcare provider uses to make the best guess.

Conception dating. If you know when you conceived, your healthcare provider will calculate your date as 266 days (thirty-eight weeks) after you conceived.

Menstrual dating. You can use an online due-date calculator or a due-date calculating wheel that simply plots out the weeks on a calendar. Or, you could do the math: Take the first day of your last normal menstrual period (LNMP), add 280 days (forty weeks), and that becomes your due date, or in medical jargon your estimated date of delivery (EDD). This calculation is accurate only if you have regular twenty-eight-day cycles and assumes ovulation approximately fourteen days after the first day of your period; it can be corrected for long or short cycles. This initial guesstimate is later refined by measurements of leg bone length on ultrasound images, as well as when the heartbeat can be heard.

Ultrasound dating. If you are not sure of the date of your LNMP, or if your periods are often irregular, many obstetrical caregivers establish a due date from the first ultrasound, which is helpful, but not infallible.

Dr. Linda notes: The earlier in pregnancy an ultrasound is performed, the more accurate it will be for dating. After twenty weeks, ultrasound becomes less useful for delivery dating, since natural variations in the size of babies will affect ultrasound measurements.

Ultrasound also helps obstetricians establish an accurate date for challenging deliveries, such as multiples or babies who require a surgical or induced delivery. While an accurate due date is convenient for you and your baby, don't fret if your doctor or midwife hedges a bit about giving you an actual date.

A SIMPLE DO-IT-YOURSELF METHOD:

- Note the first day of your LNMP (e.g., January 1, 2013).

- Add 1 year: January 1, 2014.

- Subtract 3 months: October 1, 2013.

- Add 7 days. Your EDD is October 8, 2013.

How accurate are due date predictions? While these numbers are nice to put on your calendar and tell your friends, only about 5 percent of babies arrive on their predicted due date. Most mothers give birth within two weeks before or after that date.

You may notice that your own "guess date" differs by a few days from the one given to you by your healthcare provider. That's because your healthcare provider may use a chart that calculates gestation in terms of days, yet you use a calendar, and not all months have the same number of days.

"PENCIL ME IN"

To avoid due date anxiety, pencil in your expected date of delivery on your calendar, as you'll likely need to erase it and pencil in an update.

Dr. Linda notes: While there may be a few days' discrepancy between menstrual dating, conceptual dating, and early ultrasound dating, for many pregnancies this is inconsequential. However, since obstetricians need to time certain tests according to how far along you are, it is important to establish a reasonably accurate due date early in pregnancy. It is routine to use the menstrual dating, or corrected menstrual dating, if it is within a few days of ultrasound dating. If menstrual dating differs too much from ultrasound dating, then ultrasound will be more accurate.

To relieve due date anxiety, some mothers move the EDD out one week on their calendar to avoid the "I can't stand being pregnant any longer" feelings as the calendar date arrives but your baby doesn't. This will also help you avoid those "Are you still pregnant?" phone calls from your family and friends that start as soon as the elusive due date has come and gone.

PREGNANCY TESTS

Urine test. Instead of making the long trip to your doctor or midwife's office, you can make the short trip to your own bathroom and get your answer from a couple of drops of urine. Here's how those telltale signs in your urine develop: When implantation occurs by the end of the first week after conception, the budding placenta begins to produce the pregnancy growth hormone human chorionic gonadotropin (HCG). This hormone will be present in your urine six to twelve days after conception, just around the time that your menstrual period is due. Because you need a high enough level of HCG in your urine to reflect a positive test, if the test is done too early, there may not be a high enough concentration to register.

So if you get a negative test at six days, repeat at twelve or fourteen days. During the first week after a missed period (two to three weeks after conception), these tests are 97 percent accurate, as long as you follow the directions.

Blood test. This is performed in your practitioner's office or a laboratory. It measures the level of HCG in a blood sample. The blood level of HCG may be detectable as early as a week after conception.

If the tests are negative or HCG levels are low yet you still think you are pregnant, notify your doctor or midwife, because problem pregnancies are often associated with lower than normal levels of HCG.

Early Spotting

As baby nestles into the blood-rich lining of your uterus, a small amount of bleeding or "spotting" can occur. You may mistake this for menstruation because the timing of implantation and the expected date of your period can be within a few days of each other. Usually this normal "implantation bleeding" is lighter in color and amount than menstruation, but it can be confusing. If you are concerned, check with your doctor or midwife. (See the related section on bleeding later during pregnancy, pages 154 and 384.)

"We're Pregnant!"—Sharing the News

You will most likely be aching to tell your friends and family right away, before you show. Or, you may choose to wait before telling your loved ones. No matter whom you tell and when, this is a very special announcement! Using the phrase "*We're pregnant!*" lets your mate know right from the start that the two of you are in this together. However, don't be offended if he does not initially share your excitement, especially if the news comes as a surprise. You have already had a little time to experience your feelings, and it may take him a while to adjust. He may need to work through his concerns: "Is the timing right?" "Can we afford a baby?" "How's this new person going to affect our marriage?" Some new dads-to-be need a bit of time before the reality sinks in and they can get excited about becoming a father.

Dr. Bill notes: *Twenty-eight years later, I still remember the setting in which Martha told me she was pregnant with our sixth* *child, Matthew. On Christmas Day she gave me a gift-wrapped box that contained the results from a pregnancy test. I remember opening the package and seeing the purple ring, revealing a positive test. I especially enjoyed reading her attached love note.*

Telling kids. Once you tell your children, expect everyone else to know, too. Different kids at different ages need different approaches. Most little ones like picture books about pregnant mommies and new baby siblings, such as *Baby on the Way* (William Sears, Martha Sears, and Christie Watts Kelly). You can introduce the subject to older children by showing them the how-baby-is-growing pictures in this book. Even fairly young children will sense that something is different, so you do need to talk to them, especially if they're hearing pieces of adult conversation about the pregnancy. They'll be proud to be among the first to know. Just realize that they have no concept of "nine months."

It is also important that they understand that you are going to need more rest, more help, and more understanding. Explain to them why you may have grouchy days and sick days, but also reassure them that you will be fine and that, of course, you will continue to love and take care of them. This may be the first time in their young lives that your children get the message that someone else's needs are as important as theirs. Use age-appropriate explanations, such as "Baby uses a lot of mommy's energy to grow, so mommy is feeling tired and needs a lot of rest. Mommy needs you to be as quiet as a mouse so she can rest and the new baby can rest."

Telling your larger community. You both can decide together when to tell others. You may choose to wait before telling friends and

family. If you feel you aren't yet ready for a barrage of questions and advice about pregnancy and baby care, you may elect to tell only a chosen few. If you are private types, you may wish to keep this delicious secret to yourselves at first. Whenever you do go public with your news, be prepared for increased attention as people may want to shower you with help, advice (solicited or not), gifts, and support.

Telling employers. When to break the news to your employer may be an exercise in career strategy more than anything else, especially if you are concerned about how your pregnancy may affect your job description or job security. Legally, you can't be discriminated against because you're pregnant, but you may want to think carefully about your plans for returning to work after the baby is born before you tell your supervisor about your pregnancy. (See the related section, Working while Pregnant, on page 185.)

I knew my company would start mommy-tracking me as soon as I told, so I waited. Sure enough, they gave me a huge raise when, unbeknownst to them, I was two months along, and then they were shocked when I announced, at four months, that I was going to have a baby.

When to go public with your news is a personal decision. Even if you say nothing, sooner or later your body will give your secret away.

Assembling Your Birth Team

With the privilege of pregnancy — and parenting — comes the responsibility of making the best possible decisions for you and your baby. One of the first issues you must tackle is selecting your birth attendant. Whom will you trust to help you have the healthiest pregnancy and safest birth possible?

Interview yourself. Before you interview birth attendants, it is helpful to do a little soul-searching: What is truly important to you to create the birth you want? Finding a healthcare provider who shares your birth philosophy requires you to first develop one of your own. But if this is your first pregnancy, you may not yet know what type of birth you want or what "philosophy" to have.

For most women, a birthing philosophy evolves throughout pregnancy, often with the input of her healthcare provider. As your pregnancy progresses, so will your knowledge of birthing alternatives and the needs of your particular pregnancy. Nevertheless, you need to pick a caregiver now, one who will work with you as your pregnancy evolves. If this is your first baby or your first major relationship with the medical system, you may find caregiver-choosing somewhat unsettling. How can you know ahead of time what you'll want at delivery? You want to have a healthy pregnancy and give birth to a healthy baby; but you also want to cope with pain in appropriate ways, take advantage of relaxation techniques, and enjoy an emotionally satisfying beginning to your parenting career.

Even if this is not your first pregnancy, you might still be looking for the right caregiver. Perhaps you were unsatisfied with your previous birth experience or birth attendants and want to do it differently this time. Perhaps your first practitioner retired or you

moved away. You now know the questions to ask and may have resolved to be more assertive about your birth vision. You may also be more willing to be flexible and listen to the wisdom of your advisers.

In determining what you want from a healthcare provider, it may help to ask yourself the following questions:

- Do I have a specific vision of what I want for the birth? Can I articulate it to others?

- Do I want/need a professional labor coach? (See page 260.)

- What are my fears?

- What do I want from my office visits? Will I have time to ask questions?

- How comfortable am I with hospital procedures?

- How will I react if I have to have a cesarean?

- Do I care whether my practitioner is male or female?

- How involved does my husband want to be in the pregnancy and birth? What do I expect of him?

- Will my husband be a good advocate for me if things don't seem to be going as planned?

Interview friends. Talk to your friends about their birth experiences to get an idea of what giving birth is really like. Ask like-minded friends what they were happy with and what they would do differently next time. Read all you can on birthing alternatives. Be aware that friends and family with good intentions may not be comfortable with alternatives and may try to persuade you to do it their way. Have a good sense of what you want before you visit your healthcare provider. Hearing lots of "birth stories" may open your eyes and mind to what birth can be like. However, try not to be scared by others' experiences. Each birth is unique.

Interview birth attendants. After interviewing yourself and your friends, you are ready to interview birth attendants, the people who will care for your health during your pregnancy and be with you during delivery. If you have your heart set on being both the leading lady and director of your birth, most practitioners are happy to take on the role of consultant, provided you have studied your part. Midwives are very comfortable with facilitating your birth experience rather than trying to direct or control it. If, on the other hand, you want to keep the starring role but have your birth attendant direct, you may feel best in the hands of an authority-figure type, usually an obstetrician rather than a midwife.

Good communication from the start helps you avoid the "my way versus the doctor's way" clash that can arise at crucial moments during your pregnancy and delivery. Even at this early stage, remember that as you grow in knowledge and experience, roles might change along the way.

CHOOSING DR. RIGHT

Ask friends and healthcare professionals for doctor recommendations. Obstetric nurses are excellent resources, having seen many local obstetricians in action. Narrow the list down to several candidates and call to make an appointment to interview these physicians. Be sure to ask whether the prospective doctor accepts your insurance plan. (If your insurance plan limits your choice of obstetrician, you can still interview several birth attendants from the pool of choices.) Tell the receptionist that your visit is for an interview only. If the receptionist has time, you may even want to run your most important concerns by her or one of the nurses before you make an appointment. Ideally, visit the doctor at a time when both you and your husband can attend. Don't be offended if the doctor does prenatal interviews only once a week or if on interview day you are bumped because the doctor is at the hospital attending a delivery. His first priority is to the patients — something you'll appreciate if you become one of them.

Interviewing the office. Arrive early and browse around the office a bit. Introduce yourself to the office personnel. Are they friendly? Accommodating? You'll be spending a lot of time on the phone with these people if you choose this practice. Sometimes, unpleasant exchanges with receptionists or nurses can ruin your experience, even if you love your physician, so be discerning as you observe the office in action.

You can learn many of the important facts that you need to know from the office staff before even meeting the doctor: the doctor's call schedule, vacation plans (in case it is during your due month), how many doctors are in the practice, accepted insurance plans, fees, hospital affiliations, and, if the doctor is in solo practice, who covers for her. If you ask the office personnel these questions rather than the doctor, the doctor will appreciate your respect for her time, and you'll be able to concentrate during your interview on the specifics of the doctor's philosophy of birth and care of your pregnancy and birth. If you can, chat with other clients in the waiting room. "Interviewing" other expectant moms can give you a sense of the doctor's birthing philosophy and how women feel about this practitioner. But remember, the qualities one mother absolutely feels she must have in a birth attendant may be just the ones you don't want.

Questions to Ask the Doctor

Make a list of important questions you must have answered. Keep your list with you at all times and jot down concerns as they occur to you. It might be helpful to keep notes on your cell phone to stay better organized and avoid forgetting or misplacing a paper list. While you won't get the answers to all these questions on your interview visit, you will need to ask them at some point during your pregnancy. Bring them up as your birth philosophy and your relationship with your practitioner evolve.

• What hospital(s) is this doctor affiliated with? The doctor and the birth place often come as a combined package, but some doctors deliver at more than one hospital. After working out your birth wishes, which birth place would this doctor suggest? Some hospitals are high-tech, others are high-touch, and some are both. Find out which one is right for you.

• Ask about the doctor's call schedule. Who covers for this doctor, how often, and what are these physicians' birthing philosophies? If the doctor is part of a group practice, will you meet each of her colleagues during your prenatal visits?

• What exercises are safe to do during pregnancy? How often should you do them? Should you stop doing them as your abdomen gets heavier?

• What prenatal screening tests does the doctor advise and why? If she suggests routine tests, ask her to be more specific, since you don't consider your pregnancy to be "routine."

• What childbirth classes does this doctor advise you to take?

• Would this doctor support you if you chose to employ a labor coach or doula for your birth, and does the office provide referrals?

• What is the doctor's recommended schedule of prenatal visits?

• What are this doctor's views concerning walking and changing positions during labor? Will he help you improvise labor and birthing positions, such as standing, squatting, and side-lying? You'll want to have a good idea of whether the doctor uses the force of gravity during labor or if his birthing philosophy is stuck in the horizontal position.

• What about pain management? What are this doctor's views on the epidural, pain relief by injection, use of labor tubs, and how to find a balance between natural and medical pain relievers during birth?

• What alternatives to episiotomy does he suggest and use at delivery?

• If you have had a previous cesarean section and wish to try a VBAC (vaginal birth after cesarean), what is this doctor's VBAC success rate, and what specific measures will he offer to increase your chances? Does she believe you can have a VBAC?

• What are this doctor's views on electronic fetal monitoring: continuous, intermittent, or only if a complication is suspected?

Conducting the interview. Your main goal in the initial interview with the doctor is to determine whether she can deliver the birth experience you want. If this is your first baby and your first interview, you may not know yet what you want. You are still learning what your birthing options are. Share where you are in your homework stage with this prospective doctor. Perhaps this practitioner can discuss your options with you, guide you through some of the decision-making process, and help you make informed choices. The doctor's ability and willingness to have a give-and-take discussion will tell you whether you can comfortably work with this person through your pregnancy and labor.

A few notes on interview etiquette: Negative openers do not make good first impressions, so don't begin with a barrage of "I don't wants" ("I don't want an IV, electronic monitoring, stirrups," and so on). Ease into your interview with positive statements about the birth experience you want. You don't want to come across as a wet-behind-the-ears recent graduate of the school of birthing books that unfairly portray all doctors as adversaries. Even if your mind is made up as you enter the doctor's office, you owe it to yourself and your baby to be open to viewpoints you may not have considered. This doctor has had the benefit of perhaps thousands of birth experiences.

You want to come away from this interview with two pieces of information: how this doctor *approaches* birth and how this doctor *manages* birth. You should also get a feel for the doctor's communication style and willingness to address any concerns with helpful discussion. The doctor's answers to your questions will give you a clue to the mindset she will bring to your delivery. One of the best indicators of a doctor's birthing philosophy is whether she views you as a *participant* or a *patient* during birth. Another is whether this doctor realizes the value of a woman's laboring in different positions at different stages of birth to alleviate pain and enhance progress.

A perceptive doctor knows by experience that birth does not always go "according to plan," so once you have let the doctor know your wishes for birth, be prepared to receive an answer like this: "I respect your desires completely but I must, in the best medical interest of you and your baby, reserve the right to intervene medically should the need arise, and I ask you to trust my judgment." The doctor is asking of you the same respect and flexibility that you are asking of him.

Dr. Linda notes: *One of the problems I often note during interviews is mother rigidity. A rigid woman comes in with inflexible expectations for a "good" birth, and this may set her up for a bad experience. Good birthing experiences may require flexibility and a little bit of a "go with the flow" attitude.*

One first-time mother empowered herself with all the tools she could find to increase her chances of a satisfying birth experience. She told us how her partnership with her birth attendant worked:

I wanted to be in complete control of my faculties — no drugs or intervention unless there was a need. But I also wanted the security of a doctor's knowledge. And I wanted to know from the nurses and doctors what was going on at all times and why. I didn't want to be left out of the decisions, but at the same time I didn't want the sole responsibility for making them.

This mother took the best of herself and the best of her birth attendants and had a satisfying birth experience.

How to Get the Most out of Your First Prenatal Checkup

Once you've selected your birth attendant, you will schedule your first appointment. Here's how you can get the most out of that visit.

Do your homework. Before your visit, ask yourself, "What do I want to get out of my checkup?" and make a list of questions and concerns you have. Prioritize your list to make sure you cover what is most important on your first visit. What may happen in six to nine months can be held for a future visit. For instance, you'll want to know what prenatal supplement your doctor recommends. (See our recommendations on page 23.)

Play doctor. Put yourself behind the eyes of your healthcare provider and ask yourself, "If I were the doctor, what would I want to know about this new patient?" This exercise may help you come up with some details about you and your pregnancy that you hadn't thought your doctor needed to know.

Inspect your insurance. Want to make first-visit points with the office staff? Do your insurance homework. Before your visit, call your insurance provider and get the answers to the following questions:

• Is my doctor's medical practice on my insurance plan?

• Which obstetrical services are covered by my policy, and which aren't?

• What is my deductible and have I met it this year? If my pregnancy covers two separate calendar years, will I have to meet my deductible twice?

• What's my copay?

If you really want to make points, call the office first and ask what they need to know, and ask your insurance company to fax this information directly to their office. The less paperwork the staff and the doctor have to do, the more time they have for you.

Arrive early. As soon as you arrive, formally greet the staff (you're going to get to know them — and need them). Hand them your insurance information and ask if there is any information they need from you before you see the doctor. Some practices will have a form for you to fill out.

Write all about it. Bring along your journal so you can make notes about your visit, namely, answers to your questions and advice your healthcare provider gives.

What may happen at your first prenatal visit. While each visit will be a bit different as your pregnancy body and your education develop, here is what you might expect to happen at your first visit:

Fill out a medical history form. The following information may be requested: allergies; medications you are taking (prescription, over-the-counter, nutritional supplements, vitamins, and so on); family medical history; genetic disorders; your past gynecological history (pregnancies, births, miscarriages, surgeries, etc.); exercise habits; nutritional habits; use of alcohol, cigarettes, or illegal drugs; pertinent medical history of the father; and any other pertinent history your doctor should know.

Confirm that you are pregnant. You may simply show or tell the results of your home pregnancy test or your healthcare provider may repeat the urine test or do a blood test for confirmation.

Set the due date. You will be asked for the date of your LNMP (last normal menstrual period). Your healthcare provider will then use charts and mathematical calculations, and possibly an ultrasound to increase accuracy, in order to arrive at an educated guess as to when baby is most likely to arrive.

Perform an ultrasound. Some obstetricians routinely recommend early ultrasound to establish a due date and the location of the pregnancy in the uterus, and also to get an early heads-up on multiple pregnancies. Other obstetricians recommend early

ultrasounds only if there is some specific problem, such as bleeding, unusual pain, or a dating issue.

Do a complete examination. Your healthcare provider and/or physician's assistant will examine you from head to toe, including possibly an internal exam of your vagina and cervix, similar to a routine gynecological exam. A vaginal exam may be deferred until after your first trimester as benign spotting can commonly result.

Perform tests. Routine tests may be done in the office or at an outside laboratory. Many of these tests are recommended by professional organizations and/or mandated by law for public health, specifically maternal and infant health. A urinalysis will be performed to check for infection, protein, and sugar, and you may have a Pap smear, although some doctors delay this test until the next trimester. In addition, you will have blood drawn for a variety of reasons:

- Determine complete blood count, blood type, and Rh factor, and check for blood-type antibodies.

- Check the level of HCG and other hormones, such as progesterone.

- Check for antibodies to infectious diseases such as rubella (German measles).

- Perform a blood chemistry profile, including liver function, kidney function, and electrolytes.

- Check blood sugar, if indicated.

- Conduct genetic tests (see page 401).

Obstetrician or Midwife? Consider Both!

Since we began writing about parenting and birth, we have envisioned the ideal birth team that would give the mother and the baby the best chance of the healthiest and most satisfying birth. During the course of prenatal visits you would see both an obstetrician and a midwife. Depending on your individual obstetrical needs, you would see one more often than the other. This would give you the best of both worlds: If your pregnancy is progressing healthfully with no complications, most of your prenatal visits would be attended primarily by the midwife, as would your birth. The obstetrician remains "on standby" should medical complications arise, for example, if a mother and baby require a surgical birth. (The word *obstetrician* comes from the Latin *obstare,* meaning to "observe" and be on standby in case a medical problem develops.)

Choosing a Midwife

We strongly believe that this obstetrician-midwife partnership will play an increasingly important role in the future of obstetrical practice. Dr. BJ shares her perspective about some historical information about the rise and fall, and rise again, of midwifery:

In the 1970s, outcome in the care of women during pregnancy and childbirth in the United States was similar to outcome in Europe. The cesarean section rate was about 7 percent on both sides of the Atlantic. Then technology began to rule obstetrical care, and in the thirty-five years that have followed, the U.S. cesarean rate has exploded

to 33 percent nationwide, and in many areas the rate is over 40 percent.

Some years ago, when medical authorities in Great Britain recognized that the increase in technologically augmented birth created a significant rise in delivery costs, a review of practices ensued and positive changes were made. Midwifery was reintroduced, ultimately resulting in improved outcomes and decreased costs. As midwife-attended births contribute to a decrease in the cesarean section rate, the overall economic and personal cost is lower (since vaginal birth without anesthesia is less costly, in both the short and long terms). In the UK, most women are seen initially by a midwife and are triaged to physician care only if needed, following an assessment and review of risk factors.

Why and how birthing practices have changed. In general, the midwifery-based model used in Britain and many other developed countries is associated with lower intervention rates and lower healthcare costs. The reasons for increased technological interventions and costs in the United States are complicated. In addition to the rise in electronic fetal monitoring, there is a widespread belief that epidural anesthesia should be universally offered as an option for women in labor. Additionally, professional organizations such as the American Congress of Obstetricians and Gynecologists have made safety-based recommendations that have increased technological interventions, which in turn have increased costs. Examples include the recommendations that breech (bottom- or feet-first) babies be delivered by cesarean section and that women who have had prior cesareans should be offered trial of labor and vaginal birth only in hospitals that have immediate 24/7 emergency cesarean capabilities.

In addition, modern obstetrical care has enabled women who would not have been able to carry babies to term in the past to deliver healthy babies, but these pregnancies require intense monitoring. Modern infertility treatments, particularly among older women, have resulted in more multiple births, which can also carry greater risks. More Americans are overweight and obese than ever before, resulting in more complications during both pregnancy and birth. And finally, many women in the United States don't have economic and geographic access to a comprehensive maternal health program, so problems that might have been addressed early in pregnancy might not even be detected until labor and delivery. All these factors have combined to increase the use of technological interventions during birth — and their associated higher price tags.

Fortunately, most of the readers of this book will have adequate prenatal care and understand that technology can be a two-edged sword. When you need it, modern technology can be lifesaving for mother and baby. When you don't need it, technology can add to costs, discomfort, and unnecessary interventions.

Midwives in the twenty-first century are very different from the practitioners of the past. They must complete a rigorous nationally accredited education program and be certified through the American College of Nurse-Midwives. Midwifery is recognized in all fifty states and all U.S. territories. Midwives are specialists in normal pregnancy and natural birth; they can provide all prenatal care, including laboratory and diagnostic tests that any healthcare provider would recommend.

A hallmark of midwifery practice is the advocacy for informed choices and shared decision-making. Midwives specialize in discussing care and outlining options and opportunities, and they recognize the importance of joint decision-making. These principles apply from the initial visit through all of the prenatal care and during the birth itself. A midwife honors a mother's deep sense that pregnancy and birth are sacred experiences.

Yet, one of our birth *fears* (if we can use the "bad word" appropriately) is that hospital midwives will be forced, for economic and perhaps legal motives, to behave like obstetricians and increase their use of pharmacology and technology. We also fear they will be forced to work like all other medical professions to adapt to the new healthcare reform — dubbed *volume-oriented medicine:* push more mothers through labor in shorter times. We hope that the profession of midwives is professional enough not to let this happen.

Why choose a midwife? Many women report satisfaction with the medical model of birth, especially when they had or were at risk of having a complication during pregnancy or delivery. Some women also welcome the medical pain relief a physician can provide and feel safe in the hospital birthing scene. Other women, however, want a less medically managed birth. Midwives generally spend more time with women during prenatal visits and have a more holistic approach to aspects of care, focusing especially on nutrition, exercise, stress management, and preparation for birth and early parenting.

The most appealing aspect of a midwife-attended birth is that, ideally, a midwife provides hands-on-labor support from early contractions through the final push. An obstetrician, on the other hand, will check you periodically during labor, but will probably not stay with you until your delivery is imminent. A midwife patiently blends into the birth scene, sometimes simply watching and waiting and other times giving hands-on support to ease the discomfort or accelerate the progress of labor.

With a midwife, the mother is the star and director of the show, and events proceed at her pace. The midwife assumes that the birth will go well, because most of the time and with the right support it does. However, she is also trained to look for complications and work with a physician, if necessary, to ensure the safety of the mother and baby. The midwife understands that fear is one of the primary inhibitors for the laboring woman because it increases the pain and slows the progress of labor. An experienced midwife is a valuable person to have around an otherwise anxious birth scene for her knowledgeable, compassionate, and calming presence.

If the obstetrical system in your community is not set up for midwife-attended births, you can still enjoy this "best of both worlds" approach by having an obstetrician-attended birth and employing a professional labor coach or doula. (For information on how these professionals work, see page 260.)

Are you a candidate for a midwife-attended birth? Because most women are healthy and do not have medical conditions that would complicate pregnancy, a midwife is a valid option. Before you consider interviewing a midwife to care for you during pregnancy and birth, ask yourself these questions:

• Are you currently in good health, and is your pregnancy uncomplicated? Or do you already have a medical condition that requires attention, such as diabetes or high blood pressure? Depending on the practice, your health care issues may not preclude midwifery care, since there are collaborative practices in which physicians and midwives work closely together.

• Do you have any reason to anticipate special medical needs at the time of delivery, such as a preterm labor?

• Is the medical system in your community set up for midwife-attended births? Not only should your midwife be professionally trained and licensed, but she should also have a regular working relationship with qualified doctors who will act as her backup should an unforeseen emergency arise.

DOES YOUR INSURANCE COVER MIDWIFERY SERVICES?

Midwifery care is mandated by all federally supported insurance, such as Medicaid, Federal Employees Health Benefits, and insurance for members of the military and veterans. In addition, many other insurance plans offer midwifery as a benefit, but if you do not ask, they are under no obligation to tell you. If midwives are a benefit of your plan and there are no referrals on the list, you can search in your area for certified midwives and work with your insurance to cover their care in the same fashion that they would cover a physician's care.

Selecting a midwife who's right for you.
If you decide to interview midwives as part of your healthcare provider selection process, ask them the same questions you would ask a doctor (see page 131), along with these:

- Where did you receive your education in midwifery? Are you also a nurse? Are you certified and licensed — by whom?

- How long have you practiced? Approximately how many births have you attended?

- Do you have an arrangement with a hospital that allows you to attend or co-manage my birth in the hospital?

- If I am found to be "high-risk," can you and a specialist co-manage my care?

- Who is your backup doctor and hospital? What percentage of the time is the backup doctor called in? How long will it take the doctor to get to me? At what point is the backup doctor generally called in? Will I have a say in the decision? Will I have a chance to meet the backup doctor ahead of time? Who covers for the doctor if he is busy with another delivery? Is the doctor's fee included in the fee I pay you? Are you allowed to stay with me during delivery, even if we have to call the doctor? (Call the backup doctors to confirm their relationship with your prospective midwife.)

- Will you stay with me during my whole labor if I want you to?

- Who covers for you if you are on vacation or occupied with another mother in labor? Are your backup midwives also certified and licensed, and what is their experience?

- Do you carry a pager or cell phone?

- Do you provide childbirth education or work with someone who does?

- Do you work with doulas, and can you suggest some?

- What arrangements do you make to transfer a home-birthing mother or baby to the hospital if needed?

- Are you certified in newborn resuscitation? What resuscitation equipment do you have?

- Are you experienced in giving medication to numb and repair a tear if I have one? Do you perform perineal massage? Episiotomy?

- What are your fees? (Some states mandate insurance coverage of certified/licensed midwives, but be sure to check with your insurance provider about whether your chosen midwife is covered.)

- Do you offer postpartum care? What postpartum services do you provide?

Dr. BJ notes: Many women who come for an interview or consultation recognize that midwives are comfortable with joint decision-making and keeping women informed. Many routine procedures, such as IVs, continuous fetal monitoring, and episiotomy are not required with midwifery care. When the provider is with the woman during labor rather than on episodic visits, the use of extra technology is rarely necessary. Lastly, midwives are very comfortable with Bradley childbirth preparation (see page 237) because it empowers women and decreases fear.

(see page 237)

MIDWIFERY SERVICES

To find the midwife who may be right for you, consult the following resources:

The American College of Nurse-Midwives (ACNM): midwife.org

American Midwifery Certification Board: www.amcbmidwife.org

Midwives Alliance of North America (MANA): mana.org

International Cesarean Awareness Network (ICAN): childbirth.org/section/ICAN.html

North American Registry of Midwives (NARM): NARM.org

Midwives can also be found through each state's certification body — generally the Board of Nursing has a listing for certified nurse-midwives. In a few states midwives are identified through a Board of Midwifery.

A growing number of pregnant women are choosing to deliver their babies with the help of midwives. The National Center for Health Statistics revealed that in 2006, 7.4 percent of all U.S. births and 11.6 percent of all vaginal births were attended by midwives. The largest percentage of births by certified nurse midwives, 96.7 percent, occurred in hospitals; 2 percent occurred in birth centers and 1.3 percent in homes.

Whether you choose an obstetrician, midwife, or both, you owe it to your baby and yourself to do your homework to help you make an informed choice.

Choosing Where to Birth Your Baby

While the majority of women probably start with the birth attendant and accept whatever facility their established doctor or midwife uses to deliver babies, there are times it makes more sense to start with a delivery site and work backward. Important issues to consider may include:

- *Philosophical.* If you want a birthing center or a home birth, you may want to contact the center of your choosing or find a local network of home delivery resources.

- *Geographic.* Take into account roads and climate. If you have a mid-January due date in upstate New York, for example, you want to be sure the facility is accessible in a blizzard.

- *Medical.* If you have an illness that could compromise your or your baby's health, you need to find out whether the facility is equipped to deal with high-risk pregnancies. Is there an intensive-care nursery that can care for premature or sick newborns?

- *Cost.* Is the facility covered by your insurance? If you will be paying for it yourself, is there a fixed price? How will your costs be calculated?

- *Birth options.* Have you had a previous cesarean section? Does the facility support vaginal birth after cesarean

(VBAC)? Many facilities either are not equipped for or decline to offer this option (for more on VBACs, see page 276).

- *Anesthesia.* Does the facility offer twenty-four-hour anesthesia epidural coverage?

Dr. Linda notes: We are a good team of authors in part because we have different perspectives on the birth process. There will be women reading this book who have chosen home births with "direct-entry" midwives, birthing center births with certified nurse-midwives, or hospital births with obstetricians. There are pros and cons to each of these choices.

As the obstetrician on the writing team, I do feel that I need to present the official stance of the American Congress of Obstetricians and Gynecologists (ACOG). The bottom line is that the vast majority of American births take place in hospitals and are attended by either obstetricians or family practice physicians, sometimes working in collaboration with certified nurse-midwives. Most of the time, these individuals follow standard practices as recommended by our various professional organizations. I will share my personal thoughts and philosophy throughout this book, but also try to present obstetrical practice as it is likely to be experienced by those of you who will deliver in mainstream settings.

JOURNAL YOUR BABY'S WOMB LIFE

Journaling is a time-honored home remedy for all types of stressful situations — ditto that for pregnancy. Martha enjoyed writing journals during "our" pregnancies, and now our children treasure reading them during their own pregnancies. You may find, as we have, that your personal pregnancy journal becomes one of your most prized family possessions.

Why write. Writing about your baby and about yourself helps you connect with your baby and can have tremendous therapeutic value. When you are struggling with difficult emotions, putting them into words helps you define and understand what you are feeling. Oftentimes, expressing your problems in writing helps you come up with solutions. And imagine this: one day

while reading your journal, you look up to see your rambunctious son run across the room. You realize, "There goes that little person whom we used to know only as 'Thumper.'" When you reread it in years to come, your journal will also help you replay one of the highlights of your life, and it will fascinate your child when she is ready to have babies.

Get it down. Don't let these precious moments go undocumented. What you write and how you write it is up to you. You might write a very simple chronicle of what you're doing and how you are feeling. Try writing letters as if you were talking directly to your baby; this is an especially meaningful way of connecting with your little one before her arrival. Record how you are feeling that day — your joys, your worries, especially what you did to help yourself feel better. The important point is to get it down; don't get hung up on how you say it. You may want to highlight special occasions, such as discovering you were pregnant, feeling the first kick, making the first baby-item purchase, and experiencing the first twinge of labor. Tell your baby how you felt at these moments.

Recording tips. You can collect your thoughts in an elaborate fill-in pregnancy journal or a simple blank notebook. Some moms have enjoyed keeping an online blog that they share with close family and friends. You can also "vlog" using a video camera or the camera on your phone. In fact, cell phones can be wonderful tools to allow you to record many aspects of your pregnancy. You can blog, take down notes, make voice recordings, and record videos. From first kicks to ultrasounds to messages from daddy, you can choose one or all

recording options to document your unique experience. Once you get hooked on recording your baby's story while he grows in the womb, you will want to continue this exercise during infancy and childhood.

At the end of the chapter for each month in this book, you will find a couple of pages to help you create your own pregnancy diary. After your baby's birth, you can photocopy these pages and collate them into a diary that will be treasured by you and your baby forever.

Post your pregnancy. If you enjoy social networking, post your pregnancy progress on Facebook, Twitter, or whatever social network you most enjoy. Share funny and not-so-funny experiences and invite your friends to comment. Then sit back and enjoy the likes and "can you top this" replies. Don't forget to proudly display your newborn's picture to your eagerly awaiting friends.

First hints I might be pregnant (e.g., breast changes, morning sickness, tiredness):

_____

_____

_____

_____

_____

My first thoughts:

_____

_____

_____

_____

_____

Memories of conception:

_____

_____

_____

_____

_____

My last menstrual period began on:

_____

_____

_____

_____

_____

MY PREGNANCY JOURNAL: FIRST MONTH

My most likely date of conception:

_____

_____

_____

_____

_____

Date of positive pregnancy test:

_____

_____

_____

_____

_____

Likely due date:

_____

_____

_____

_____

_____

My reactions:

_____

_____

_____

_____

_____

Dad's reactions:

_____

_____

_____

Others' reactions:

_____

_____

_____

My top concerns:

_____

_____

_____

_____

My best joys:

_____

_____

_____

_____

Lifestyle changes, habits to break:

_____

_____

_____

_____

SECOND-MONTH VISIT TO YOUR HEALTHCARE PROVIDER
(5–8 WEEKS)

During this month's visit to your healthcare provider, expect to have:

- An examination of your abdomen

- An examination of the size and height of your uterus

- A hemoglobin and hematocrit check for anemia

- Nutritional counseling

- A weight and blood-pressure check

- Urinalysis to test for infection, sugar, and protein

- An opportunity to discuss your feelings and concerns

Second Month: Feeling More Pregnant

During the second month this little life inside you really makes his presence felt. By now the hormone levels necessary for growing your uterus and your baby are causing emotional and physical changes. Your food may come up shortly after it goes down, your queasy tummy may nag with nausea, and those day and night treks to the bathroom will be a path frequently traveled. Embrace these feelings, even when they are challenging. You are entitled to feel proud, special, and part of a miracle. When you consider that you are creating another life in just nine short months, the inconvenience and discomfort become rather secondary.

HOW YOUR BABY IS GROWING, 5–8 WEEKS

Week 5. By the end of the fourth week after conception, baby is about the size of an apple seed. Even at this tiny age the tissue that forms baby's brain is the largest area. The heart divides into right and left chambers and starts beating. Pits that will become the eyes, ears, nose, and mouth begin to show. The arms and legs protrude from the body like tiny buds, and the paddle-like hands begin to show finger buds. Breathing passages begin to appear.

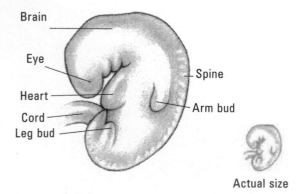

Brain
Eye
Heart
Cord
Leg bud
Spine
Arm bud

Actual size

Baby at 5 weeks.

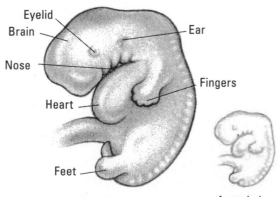

Eyelid
Brain
Nose
Heart
Ear
Fingers
Feet

Actual size

Baby at 6 weeks.

Week 6. Baby grows to around the size of a pomegranate seed. You may be able to see and hear the first sounds of life on a special ultrasound, although typically you'll have to wait until ten or twelve weeks to experience this. More than a million new cells are added to your baby's growing body each minute! Baby's heart beats faster, around 140 to 150 beats per minute, which is twice as fast as yours. Prepare yourself to be moved and inspired when you first hear those beautiful "whoosh-whoosh" baby heartbeats a month from now; there is absolutely nothing like it.

Arms lengthen, an elbow joint appears, and fingers become distinct. Feet are now separate from the leg buds, and tiny toe notches appear. The humped-over head looks as large as the rest of the body. Eyelid folds begin to form, and tiny eyes the size of a period already contain a lens, iris, cornea, and retina. The tip of the nose begins to show. Baby's beginning backbone looks like a stack of minuscule blocks.

Week 7. Baby is now about the size of a blueberry. A few first pees occur, put out by those tiny kidneys. Elbow, wrist, and knee joints are obvious; toes have formed; the fingers have lengthened. Eyelids are evident. Early facial features of eyes, ears, nose, and mouth are formed. An ultrasound can now

> ### SCIENCE SAYS: BABIES HAVE EARLY HEARTBEATS
>
> Through technology we now know that some organs mature earlier than once thought. Intravaginal ultrasounds have shown that at around six or seven weeks of gestation the heart is already pumping systolic and diastolic waveforms; and primitive valves, though somewhat leaky, are present.

show baby's body and limbs moving, though you won't feel them with your hand for a couple more months. Nerve cells in the brain branch out and touch one another, forming primitive nerve pathways. The lobes of the cerebellum begin to be seen through the transparent skull. Researchers estimate that one hundred thousand new nerve cells are created every minute.

Week 8. Baby is 1 inch long and weighs around ½ ounce — about the size of an olive. The previously hunched-over head and curved body are now more erect. All the internal organs that will be present in the fully grown infant have now formed.

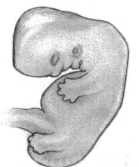
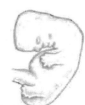

Baby at 7 weeks.   Actual size

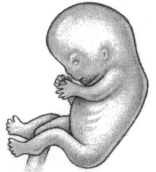
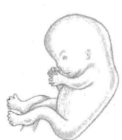

Baby at 8 weeks.   Actual size

The heart is now divided into four chambers. Hands, feet, fingers, and toes are fully formed. Major joints — shoulder, elbow, wrist, knee, and ankle — are evident. Mouth, nose, nostrils, and lips are more formed; earlobes show, and all the structures of the eyes are found. External genitalia may begin to show, but whether baby is male or female cannot yet be determined by ultrasound. Increased body and limb movements can be seen.

BABY TALK: WHAT TO CALL ME

Technically, the baby is an "embryo" up until eight weeks gestation, when the organ systems are formed; then it becomes a "fetus" (meaning "young one") and remains a fetus until birth. However, once conception has occurred, to most expectant parents "it" is known as "baby."

HOW YOU MAY FEEL

Wow! Many of the up-and-down emotions you felt in the first month intensify during the second month. Your mind may continue to be as unsettled as your stomach. Remember that it is normal to feel both happy about growing a baby and not so happy about the toll early pregnancy takes on your mind, body, and lifestyle.

Emotionally I'm feeling at odds with myself. One day I feel excited to be pregnant, the next day I almost forget I'm pregnant. One day I'm happy looking at the new maternity fashions, the next day I feel melancholy about losing my figure.

Aware of breast changes. Your breasts will declare that you are pregnant long before your belly does. The pregnancy hormones that are growing your baby also start enlarging your breasts. The earliest sensations of feeling slightly sore and swollen are similar to those you may be used to feeling in the second half of your menstrual cycle, only stronger. Breasts typically increase one cup size during the first trimester and another cup size during the rest of the pregnancy. Breast changes alone typically account for 2 pounds of your weight gain during pregnancy. Small-breasted women will notice these changes more, and first-time pregnant women may notice them more than they do in subsequent pregnancies.

Your breast changes are caused by a surge of hormones that stimulate the growth of milk glands. As the hormones are doing their work, you may notice throbbing sensations throughout your breasts. They may feel tingly, sore, warm, fuller, and more sensitive to touch. You may experience occasional shooting pains in your breasts that occur off and on for five minutes. You'll probably notice that your areolas (the darker areas around the nipples) enlarge and darken, and that the tiny glands on the areola that secrete lubricating, antibacterial oil become more noticeable, resulting in a bumpier look. The veins on your breasts may also become more noticeable, like rivers with tributaries branching out over your breasts to deliver increased blood supply.

Dr. BJ notes: I confirmed my pregnancy by the prominence of blood vessels in my breasts.

Although the rest of your body will eventually return to normal after pregnancy, your breasts will acquire a different shape. It's impossible to predict what your breasts will look like a year from now; a bit of your voluptuousness from pregnancy will linger while you are breastfeeding. Bear in mind that the changes your breasts undergo are due to pregnancy, heredity, and gravity, and will occur whether or not you breastfeed. Be kind to your breasts during pregnancy and enjoy the comfort of frequent, warm showers and a very gentle breast massage if that helps. If you are concerned about sagging, you can help the skin and muscles around your breast tissue by wearing a supportive bra throughout your pregnancy, even at night if you need it (see "Getting the Support You Need: Choosing a Bra," page 162).

Beyond tired. The occasional bouts of tiredness you experienced in your first month may now give way to total exhaustion. Last month you wanted to rest, now it's nonnegotiable! Many women describe their tiredness as "bone-deep." This feeling is nature's way of compelling a busy woman to slow down and direct her energy where it is needed, for growing her baby. You may find that you have to walk more slowly and that you get out of breath more easily, even during normal walking. Don't fight this fatigue. For your own sake and your baby's, listen to your body's message and rest as much as you can. If you have a demanding job or a demanding toddler, you may not have the luxury of staying in bed or sleeping in, but there will be days when your body simply forces you to get the rest it needs. If the time is not spent sleeping, at least get off your feet. If possible, leave work early or plug in your toddler's favorite video, sack out on the couch, and treat yourself to some much-needed rest.

I found it helpful to stock up on easy-to-prepare meals my husband could cook. For
the first few weeks, I wasn't sure what my name was let alone what was going to be for dinner.

Nauseated. The morning sickness that probably began last month often peaks in the second month. Hang in there! As you're wondering why you ever got yourself into this, a friend or your doctor offers the cheery dismissal, "Oh, that's just your hormones. Nausea is a sign that your baby is healthy." True enough, perhaps, but not much comfort when you feel seasick around the clock. (See page 119 for strategies to control nausea.)

Heart beating faster. As your body is making more blood to nourish that little person inside, you may notice that your heart beats faster, especially during workouts. The heart is one of the most adaptable organs in the body; it is as if baby is giving your heart the message, "You need to work harder and step it up a bit for me!"

Mouth watering. Most moms don't think they will have to deal with drooling until baby arrives, but around the second month the amount of saliva they produce can increase quite a bit. The taste can change, too, even becoming somewhat metallic. Yuck, right? The cause of this phenomenon is not understood, but it does no harm. Some mothers find that excess saliva can alleviate the irritations of heartburn by acting as a buffer against excess acids and a coating for the lining of the sensitive esophagus. On the other hand, excess saliva can trigger nausea. In any event, it usually lessens by the end of the first trimester. Try sucking on a mint or a lemon drop, or brushing your teeth with a minty toothpaste if the taste bothers you.

Urinating more frequently. Naturally, as you are making more blood to grow a baby, the necessary blood volume going through your kidneys results in more frequent urination. In addition, your growing uterus resides right behind your bladder and definitely makes its presence felt on a regular basis. Though you will continue to urinate more frequently throughout your pregnancy, the increased "urge to pee" is typically most noticeable during the first three months. In fact, if you're not urinating more frequently in the first trimester, take it as a sign that you may need to drink more fluids. Empty your bladder as thoroughly as possible when you urinate (bear down three times — review the Kegel exercises on page 68 — and lean forward as you do).

If you are concerned about your frequent urge to urinate, have your doctor rule out a bladder infection. Other signs of a bladder infection (cystitis) are burning when you urinate and/or low-grade fever.

Thirsty. Thirst is your body's normal signal that you and your baby need more fluids. And if you don't listen to your thirst signals you may become dehydrated, which only aggravates nausea and fatigue. Your body needs more fluid because your blood volume increases by 40 percent, and think of all that extra water needed to fill your baby's enlarging amniotic swimming pool. Drinking extra water helps flush the extra waste you now have from your kidneys. Since thirst is not an accurate guide of how much water you need, drink until you are no longer thirsty, then add an extra couple of glasses for good measure. Above all, don't drink less just so you will pee less; that's not good for you or baby. Remember, sipping your extra fluids slowly is more stomach-friendly than gulping it down. Also, drinking big glasses of water is not the only way you can get extra fluids. Try sucking on ice chips or homemade popsicles, drinking coconut water, and eating foods with a high water content, such as melons. The sipping solution (see page 22) might be just what the doctor ordered. Don't forget, too, that drinking more fluids helps ease constipation. We generally discourage sports drinks while pregnant. Although they do give you extra fluids, most are full of antinutrients (sweeteners and chemical additives) that neither you nor your baby need.

Dr. Linda notes: Fluids with some electrolytes keep you metabolically balanced; but natural nutrients, such as homemade soups, are healthier than chemically engineered bottled drinks.

Constipated. As we've discussed, early pregnancy hormones slow the movement of food through your intestines. The slower passage of food and fluid allows more water to be absorbed (perhaps another one of nature's ways of ensuring you get the extra

THE CHOCOLATE COMPROMISE

Having a sweet craving? Enjoy two or three squares of dark chocolate a day. Dark chocolate is good for you because it's high in antioxidants called flavonoids. The more growth that takes place in the body, the more oxidants (also known as free radicals, or "wear and tear chemicals") are produced. So pregnancy logic has it that you need to eat very high levels of antioxidants, since your body is going through the greatest growth spurt it will ever experience in your adult life.

Here are some sweet tips for enjoying the health benefits of chocolate:

- Choose dark chocolate, which has more flavonoids, less sugar, and less unhealthy fat than milk chocolate. Look at the cacao content — the higher the better, or in choco-speak: "The more bitter, the more better." To shape your tastes toward enjoying slightly bitter dark chocolate, begin with 60 percent cacao, then 70 percent, and gradually increase to 80 percent.

- Don't sour yourself on chocolate because it's high in saturated fats. The type of fat in cocoa butter — stearic acid — doesn't raise the blood level of cholesterol the way other saturated fats do.

- Unsweetened cocoa powder is the healthiest form of chocolate. A 2005 study in the journal *Food Science and Technology International* showed that cocoa powder has the highest concentration of flavonoids, around three times as much as dark chocolate. Milk chocolate, chocolate drinks, and chocolate syrup have the lowest concentration. Enjoy hot chocolate with all its rich antioxidants, the protein from organic low-fat milk, and the sensory appeal from the aroma and pleasant look of the foam. Sweeten with a bit of honey.

- Study the sweet facts on the label. Cocoa or cocoa beans should be the first ingredient, not sugar.

- Skip white chocolate, which has too much sugar and artificial flavoring and very little cocoa.

- Don't worry about the tiny bit of caffeine in three squares of dark chocolate.

fluids into your system). The combination of slower movement and increased absorption of fluids leads to harder stools. To better your bowel habits as your pregnancy progresses, continue your stomach-friendly habits: graze, eat more high-fiber foods, drink more fluids, exercise, and take probiotics.

Bloated and gassy. The bloated feeling may be similar to how you feel just before you begin your period, causing your lower belly to feel pregnant even when you don't yet look pregnant. As your gut and growing baby are learning to get along, the same intestinal upsets that cause constipation also give you gas. Besides the home remedies listed on page 119, try eating less of the common gassy foods, such as broccoli, cabbage, cauliflower, Brussels sprouts, beans, and carbonated beverages. Avoid greasy and fried foods, since foods with a high fat content take longer to empty from your stomach and intestines. A bloated feeling may cause you to feel as though your waistline is steadily expanding. In fact, this may prompt you to make your first wardrobe adjustment as you opt for more comfortable pants that don't irritate this highly sensitive area.

While drinking a carbonated beverage, I felt and heard every bubble until it came out the other end.

Heartburn. Shortly after eating, and sometimes even between meals, many pregnant women belch and burp and experience a burning, irritating sensation just below their breastbone. Oh joy, right? Once again, it's physiologically correct to blame heartburn on hormones. Pregnancy hormones (specifically, progesterone) cause an overall slowdown of the intestines, relax the stomach muscles, and delay the time it takes for food and gastric acids to be passed from the stomach. Thus, food and acids sit in your stomach longer than they do when you're not pregnant. Pregnancy hormones also relax the protective muscles at the entrance of the stomach, so it's easier for food and acids to travel back into the lower end of the esophagus when the stomach contracts. The medical name for this condition is gastroesophageal reflux (GER). GER also produces the uncomfortable sensation commonly referred to as indigestion. Later on, as your uterus grows and begins pressing upward, the pressure on your intestines and stomach may make your heartburn even more irritating.

Stomach acid is your intestinal track's natural antibiotic, warding off germs at the upper end before they have a chance to reach the lower end. For this reason, try to heal your heartburn without prescription or over-the-counter antacids, unless recommended by your doctor. The stomach lining naturally secretes a thick mucus that acts like a protective coating to keep the acid from digesting the stomach tissue, but the top area of the stomach and the lining of the esophagus don't share this protective sealant. Remember those three gut-friendly words: graze, sip, and chew.

Cramps. Many women feel cramps in their lower pelvis. Actually, these are generally "growing pains" and are a symptom of the ligaments that stabilize the uterus stretching. You may find that these subside after the uterus begins to grow up over the pubic bone but can return every now and then, especially if you overdo it — another way your body tells you to slow down.

If you suffer from leg cramps in the middle of the night, you might have a potassium deficiency. Eat a banana or drink a glass of OJ before bed. Works like a charm!

Listening to Your Hormonal Symphony Orchestra

To appreciate the marvelous music your pregnant body plays, we like to think of the hormones in your body as instruments in a symphony orchestra. When all the instruments play in harmony, beautiful music, or health, results. When they're out of tune, disharmony, or illness, results. Your brain (especially the hypothalamus) is the director of your hormonal symphony orchestra, which has more than a hundred players.

Your baby is "listening" to the music you are playing and feeling the effects, and so are you. During pregnancy, progesterone increases around one hundred times and estrogen levels skyrocket to fifteen times your pre-pregnant level. It's no wonder your body and mind are transformed. Estrogen rises daily throughout pregnancy and enhances baby's brain development.

When you conceive, you open your internal pharmacy, pushing out internal medicines you and your baby need to thrive. Yet, these medicines often have annoying side effects. (Dads, take note of this.) It's interesting how the hormones balance one another. Estrogen stimulates a heightened awareness and sensitivity, a sort of "upper." Progesterone, on the other hand, has more of a sedative effect, a sort of "downer." It's like having high doses of both stimulants and sedatives working for you, and when they're in balance they work well.

Here are the effects these two hormones have on baby and mother:

Good for Baby:

- Keep your uterus from untimely contractions.

- Promote growth of blood vessels in your uterus and placenta.

- Increase brain-tissue growth, facilitate nerve connections, and increase blood flow to developing organs.

- Promote growth of breast and milk-making tissues.

- Provide antioxidant protection to rapidly growing cells.

- Regulate insulin and other metabolic hormones.

- Help stimulate your metabolism to make more energy for two.

- Slow down your digestive system.

- Relax birthing muscles and ligaments.

Annoying for Mothers:

- Muscle fatigue

- Sedative effects

- Forgetfulness

- Heightened awareness of taste and smell

- Generally enhanced sensitivity

- Moodiness

- Food cravings — some healthy, some unhealthy

You put up with the annoyances of pregnancy because you keep your eyes on the prize. (See page 324 for an engaging performance of the hormonal symphony of birth.)

CONCERNS YOU MAY HAVE

Touchy and Hypersensitive

I get upset easily, and little things that didn't previously bother me now set me off. Why?

Your hormones are working overtime, and for good reason. Your hypersensitivity to sound, such as a dog barking or a doorbell ringing, is just part of the hyperalert state of being a new mom. Little nuisances may get big reactions. Typical toddler irritations may now drive you up the wall. And the normal hassles of daily living are magnified. Sometimes it feels as though *everything* is annoying. These are normal emotional fluctuations. Take this touchiness as a sign that you need to create an environment to allow as much rest as much as possible and conserve the energy you need to grow your baby.

Impatient with Husband

My husband is used to me having lots of energy, but now I'm sick and tired and need lots of rest. He doesn't understand why I don't want to do housework or even make love. How can I make him understand?

While the pregnancy is very real to you, for your mate it may take a while to sink in. He may not understand that you no longer have the energy to do what you did a couple of months ago. It's hard to feel sexy when you're tired and nauseated and preoccupied with your changing body. He needs to understand that certain quirks in his personality may be less tolerable for a while; it's not personal. You can tactfully remind him that you are pregnant, pumped full of crazy hormones, and then ask him to read the section on what dads can do to help (see page 118). Reassure him that you're likely to be feeling better, and definitely sexier, in another month or two.

Feeling Dependent

I've been so tired that my mother flew in to help me care for my other children for a few weeks. I feel so guilty; I am used to being independent at work and at home. Are these feelings normal?

You bet they are! Prior to being pregnant you were used to caring for everybody else's needs, and now you are the one needing the most care. Your body is so hard at work that it's time to let others pamper you. Try to give up feelings of guilt since you and your energy-requiring baby deserve to be taken care of and indulged.

Itchy Skin

My skin is getting dry and itchy, especially on the palms of my hands and soles of my feet. What can I do?

While dry, itchy skin is more of a problem later in pregnancy, it can start now. Supersensitive skin goes with pregnancy; sensitivity of just about every part of your body increases at least a little bit. (See the section on healthy skin care on page 183.)

Difficulty Sleeping

I used to sleep so soundly but now, although I'm going to bed earlier, I'm waking up more often. Help!

Since sleep challenges are a quirk during every month of pregnancy, we have devoted chapter 7 to helping you sleep more peacefully — reread it now for some helpful strategies.

BLEEDING AND SPOTTING

While vaginal bleeding of any sort can be scary, it does not necessarily mean that something is wrong with your pregnancy.

When not to worry:

- Implantation bleeding occurs between two and four weeks after conception, as your little baby burrows into the blood-rich lining of the uterus. This is usually of no significance, but may merit an ultrasound to be sure implantation is taking place in the uterus and not elsewhere (known as an ectopic pregnancy).

- Spotting after intercourse commonly occurs, but is harmless.

- You may have a tiny bit of red or pinkish blood, with no tissue fragments. Any time you have growing uterine tissue with lots of blood vessels, a few of those tiny blood vessels are going to break, so you may notice some occasional spotting or just a little bleeding.

When to worry:

- You have crampy abdominal pain occurring with the bleeding.

- There is a heavier amount of dark-brownish or clotted blood, possibly with clumps of tissue.

- The bleeding is heavy enough to begin to soak a sanitary pad.

- You feel faint or dizzy.

- The bleeding is getting increasingly heavy.

Basically, if you have any persistent bleeding and/or clumps of tissue, you should call your healthcare provider right away. How you describe the bleeding (amount, consistency, color), how persistent it is, and what other symptoms you have along with the bleeding will help your healthcare provider determine whether a problem is developing.

Genetic Screening: If, When, and How Much?

My doctor offered to do a bunch of screening tests for genetic abnormalities. I have mixed feelings about getting these done.

It's considered standard medical practice for your healthcare provider to make you aware of your options. While many of these tests are routinely done in the third month, obstetricians and midwives often discuss them during the second month to give you time to think about them. These tests are designed to detect birth defects, such as spina bifida, and chromosomal abnormalities, such as Down syndrome. Many pregnant women and their mates are not comfortable with the concept of testing and the implicit assumption that they would consider terminating the pregnancy if they discovered a problem with their baby. Still, some couples want to be tested in order to better prepare themselves and their families for the birth of a child with special needs. Fortunately, the vast majority of couples will get comforting results and have one less set of issues to worry about during their pregnancy. Which genetic tests to get and when to get them are decisions made by you and your doctor together, but here are some questions to consider:

- Is there a family history of any genetic or developmental condition?

- Does your age put you at a higher risk for having a baby with a birth defect?

- Are you in an ethnic group that has a higher risk of carrying a genetic abnormality?

- Are you worried about your baby having a particular genetic problem?

- How will you use the information you get? Will you worry more, or less?

- If the screening test comes back positive, will you follow up with an amniocentesis?

- Are the tests 100 percent accurate? Or, do some have a high incidence of "false positives" that will unnecessarily worry you?

Remember, as the name implies, "screening" tests for genetic and birth defects are not absolutely diagnostic. Some tests are accurate, others notoriously inaccurate. Understanding why they're done, what they reveal, and what problems may be associated with these tests will help you decide which ones you should consider. For more information on how to decide which genetic tests are right for you, see page 401.

ULTRASOUND: FOR MEDICAL PURPOSES ONLY

For safety's sake, ultrasound should be used as a valuable diagnostic aid, not as a pregnancy toy.

Dr. Linda notes: Ultrasound is a noninvasive technology for imaging based on bouncing sound waves from a transducer off fluid and solid surfaces, such as amniotic fluid, uterine walls, placenta, and fetal tissues. Ultrasound is used almost universally in modern obstetrical care. Standard indications for ultrasound include:

1. *Establishing the location and viability of an early pregnancy*

2. *Accurate dating of pregnancy if done in the first 20 weeks*

3. *Evaluation for birth defects, commonly done as part of chromosomal screening at approximately 13 weeks, broader structural screening at approximately 20 weeks, or evaluating for specific structural abnormalities later in pregnancy*

4. *Evaluation for bleeding during any stage of pregnancy*

5. *Monitoring the growth of the baby*

6. *As an aid for invasive procedures such as amniocentesis or chorionic villus sampling*

While ultrasound is generally regarded as safe for medical use during pregnancy, professional groups including ACOG and the American Institute of Ultrasound in Medicine (AIUM) have raised concerns about the boutiques that have offered "keepsake" pictures of fetuses without the benefit of facility accreditation or involvement of healthcare professionals in ordering and evaluation of the images. Ultrasound is a helpful obstetrical tool, but it should be recommended by your caregivers for specific reasons and performed at an accredited facility by qualified ultrasonographers.

For more information on diagnostic ultrasound, see www.aium.org.

MY PREGNANCY JOURNAL: SECOND MONTH

How I feel:

_____

_____

_____

_____

_____

My thoughts about you:

_____

_____

_____

_____

_____

What I'm eating:

_____

_____

_____

_____

_____

Most stomach-friendly foods:

_____

_____

_____

_____

_____

My food cravings:

_____

_____

_____

_____

_____

My top concerns:

_____

_____

_____

_____

_____

My best joys:

_____

_____

_____

_____

_____

THIRD-MONTH VISIT TO YOUR HEALTHCARE PROVIDER
(9–12 WEEKS)

During this month's visit you may have:

- An examination of your abdomen to feel the top of the uterus

- An examination of the size and height of the uterus

- Blood tests: hemoglobin and hematocrit

- Urinalysis to test for infection, sugar, and protein

- A weight and blood pressure check

- An opportunity to hear baby's heartbeat with a Doppler ultrasound device

- Discussion of tests if advised: ultrasound, chorionic villus sampling, amniocentesis, AFP, and prenatal screening for genetic problems

- An examination for swelling of hands and legs or fluid retention

- An opportunity to discuss your feelings and concerns

Third Month: Almost Showing

The highlights of this month are likely to more than offset the physical and emotional demands that have been so dominant for the past couple of months. You will likely find that the discomforts of the first trimester start to ease up now and that your energy level increases. Your emotional roller coaster may settle down as you can now connect with your baby through the delightful images and sounds you enjoy through ultrasound.

HOW YOUR BABY IS GROWING, 9–12 WEEKS

Now your baby really looks like a baby — from head to toe. As in previous months, baby's brain growth outpaces the other organs, occupying around half of baby's total size. Just imagine this budding baby brain working overtime to manufacture 250,000 new brain cells every minute. Baby is now 3 inches long and weighs nearly 1 ounce. Baby's little face really looks like a face. Twenty little tooth buds begin to form underneath the gums. Toenails, fingernails, and fine hair appear. Because heart valves are now in place, between ten and

twelve weeks you can begin to hear the fast fluttering heartbeat during a visit to your healthcare provider. Baby's endocrine system is now functioning, including the pancreas, which begins to produce insulin. A more mature urinary system allows baby to literally "pee in the (amniotic) pool." Toward the end of this month the external genitalia show either a penis or no penis, so that ultrasound can finally reveal whether baby is a boy or a girl. Boy babies may start producing testosterone this early.

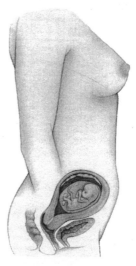

Baby at 9–12 weeks.

PREVENTING PREMATURITY

Once upon a time it was thought that premature births "just happened." New insights reveal that a mother can affect baby's maturity by:

- Getting diligent prenatal care

- Eating more omega-3s in supplements or seafood

- Eating green-light foods (Review the tips for good grazing on page 20 and the list of green-light pregnancy foods on page 45.)

- Having good dental hygiene (Why? See page 178.)

- Exercising regularly

- Not smoking

- Managing stress

Baby's mouth can open. He can move his tongue and swallow amniotic fluid. He can now open and close his fists. Even though baby is moving his hands and feet, you're unlikely to feel those little punches and kicks for another month.

HEARING BABY'S HEARTBEAT

Between ten and twelve weeks, you should be able to celebrate hearing baby's heartbeat via a Doptone, a wand-like Doppler ultrasound device that amplifies the sound through some gel applied to your abdomen. Baby's heartbeat is about twice as fast as yours (between 120 and 140 beats per minute) and will get even faster later in your pregnancy (140 to 160 beats per minute). It sounds like a rapid-fire "boom-boom," unlike the lub-dub of your own heartbeat, and is a sound you'll never tire of hearing.

Dr. BJ notes: When children attend prenatal visits with their mothers, which we encourage, they often say that the heartbeat sounds like a "galloping horse" or "Thomas the Tank Engine." We encourage the recording of the baby's heartbeat, especially when the father cannot be present. We got this idea from mothers whose husbands are deployed overseas. It makes such a special "singing message."

If you don't hear the heartbeat at this time, don't worry. Some babies won't dazzle parents with those marvelous musical sounds until fourteen weeks, especially if the due date calculations are a bit off or if baby's position or the amount of tissue between baby and the Doptone interfere.

(continued)

I was unprepared for how deeply I would be affected by the sound of my baby's heartbeat. The first time I heard that boom, boom, boom, it took my breath away. Much later in pregnancy I took my mother-in-law to an appointment with me. I had forgotten that this technology wasn't available when she was pregnant, and I neglected to prepare her. When she heard her grandchild's heartbeat, her eyes got very wide and she burst into tears of joy. It was a great moment!

HOW YOU MAY FEEL

You are in for at least a few more changes this month; that is, after all, the great theme of your life right now. As your baby grows, so do you!

Breasts go through a growth spurt. As your breasts gear up to feed your baby, they will grow as baby grows. Nipples get still larger, as does the areola. (Darkening of the nipple makes it an easier "target" for baby to latch onto when the time comes.) You're likely to experience some tenderness as your breasts get fuller and heavier. Since more breast tissue needs more blood supply, you may notice a more prominent spiderweb-like network of veins just beneath the skin. Tiny glands beneath the surface of your areola become more prominent, too, appearing like little bumps the size of pinheads.

Clothing doesn't fit. Around the third month you may be just between clothing sizes. Many women find this the most frustrating time in terms of fashion choices. Your old pants feel much too tight, yet the next size up still feels a bit loose. You're not physically, nor perhaps emotionally, ready to go crazy with the maternity clothes. A good compromise is to purchase (or borrow) some comfortable nonmaternity skirts and pants one size up with elastic waistbands. You'll probably outgrow these in another month or two, but you'll be able to wear them for a while again after baby is born, which makes them a worthwhile investment.

GETTING THE SUPPORT YOU NEED: CHOOSING A BRA

As your belly grows, so will your breasts. Looking ahead, by the fourth month of pregnancy, most women feel more comfortable wearing a maternity bra. Here's what to look for in choosing the right bra:

- **Fit.** Think comfort above all. Be sure the straps and closure system are adjustable to accommodate your expanding breast size. The cup should fit smoothly without puckering and the front of the bra should lie against your chest without any gaps. Even though most women find that their prenatal cup size peaks by the sixth month of pregnancy, continued expansion of your rib cage will require easing the band. When you purchase the bra, be sure it fits comfortably at the tightest hook closure. This will allow room for rib cage expansion.

- **Construction.** Choose cotton, which is comfortable and breathes. An underwire bra is a no-no for many moms during pregnancy and nursing because it can compress expanding, sensitive breast tissue. If you do buy an underwire nursing bra, be sure that it's not too tight. If it pinches as you grow, put it away until two to three months postpartum.

- **Band.** Feel how the band rests on your rib cage. In the back, it should fit comfortably below your shoulder blades. It should be loose enough not to bind your breasts, yet snug enough not to ride up when you raise your arms or shrug your shoulders.

- **Straps.** They should be wide so they don't dig into your shoulders as the weight of your breasts increases.

- **Nightwear.** Some women find that wearing a lightweight supportive bra at night gives extra support and eases discomfort.

- **Nursing bras.** The best time to buy your nursing bra is during the last few weeks of pregnancy. You want cups that open for baby's easy access. If you plan to use bras bought during pregnancy for nursing, buy them on the roomy side to allow for the rapid expansion of your breasts when your milk comes in. (Breast size can increase by two full cup sizes in the days after birth, but then settle down a bit after a couple of weeks.) Buy only two nursing bras to start out so you can reevaluate the fit later. Eventually, you will want three bras — one in use, one in the wash, and one on standby. Many mothers stick to maternity bras throughout their pregnancy and switch to nursing bras after their milk comes in. You will find a full range of maternity and nursing bras in maternity shops and catalogs, and online guides on how to get the best fit.

Pelvic discomforts even before you start to show. You may begin to sense a fullness between your pelvic bone and belly button. As your growing uterus stretches its supporting ligaments, you may notice twitches of pain on both sides of your belly. When tissue stretches, it's going to let you know. These pelvic discomforts will change as you and your baby grow.

DON'T WORRY, BE HAPPY

Worry tends to be an unproductive cycle: you read what you should worry about, then you wonder why you're not feeling all those things, and then you worry that you're worrying too much. Worry aggravates the tension-related discomforts

(continued)

you are already experiencing and releases more stress hormones. The last thing you need is another hormone challenge on top of the ones you're already dealing with.

Review the stressbusters on page 75, mainly the tips on mood switching. As soon as you find yourself worrying, resolve to relish the joys of pregnancy rather than focus on the problems. Ponder the miracle that's going on inside you to balance out the daily stress coming at you. The advice "don't sweat the small stuff" especially applies to pregnant mothers. Why waste energy on things you can't change when your growing body and baby need that energy? Remember, each year millions of women go through healthy pregnancies and go on to deliver healthy babies — and many choose to do it again and again.

Dr. Linda notes: Before being pregnant myself, as an obstetrician I had always been a bit annoyed by my patients' constant worrying. Once I became pregnant, I got it! If I didn't watch myself, I would worry incessantly. While as an obstetrician I had fewer worries about common complaints I knew were normal, I had entire textbooks of obscure, rare problems to worry about. I dealt with this by reminding myself to "get over it" and trying to channel worries into constructive activities of preparation and planning for our new lives.

CONCERNS YOU MAY HAVE

Enjoying Sex while Pregnant

Pregnancy can change your appetite for many of life's simple pleasures, from making dinner to making love. Once again you have those hormones to blame. Hormones will turn you on — and turn you off. Your feelings may go from "Please don't touch me..." to "I want you *now*..." and back again. Regardless, we can give you one guarantee: while pregnant you will feel differently about sex. How pregnant women experience sex varies greatly. Here is how you can use the hormone and sex-organ changes that occur while you are pregnant to enhance your sexual pleasure:

Expect mixed feelings. The changes in sex organs can lead to one woman's pleasure and another woman's discomfort. The same hormones that prepare your body for birth and nourish your baby also change the way your body experiences sex. As we've already said, your breasts become increasingly full and your nipples larger and more sensitive. During lovemaking, blood flow to your breasts increases even more. While your more voluptuous look can turn on your mate, the heightened breast sensitivity can be either irritating or stimulating for you. As their pregnant wives get curvier, many men find them sexier than ever and view these extra curves and softness as just "more to hold and love." But, there are weeks when a woman in bloom simply does not feel sexy.

As your breasts go through changes, so does your vaginal canal. Obviously, there is a lot going on there to ready this birth channel for baby passage. The increased blood flow to the muscles and lining of your vagina can boost sexual pleasure for some women or make things totally uncomfortable for others.

One perk, especially for women who previously experienced dryness during intercourse, is that vaginal secretions increase the lubrication of sensitive areas. However, you may experience an unwelcome change of odor to these secretions. While you both may appreciate the increased snugness and lubrication of the vagina, some couples find that the vascular congestion makes the vagina feel too snug.

Enjoy go-for-it days. Admittedly, in the third month, these days will likely be few and far between. The hormonal upheaval and the sick and tired feelings during the early months are more likely to press your turn-off switch. The good news is that during the second trimester, dubbed pregnancy's honeymoon, hormonal surges level off, and fatigue and morning sickness will lessen. Many couples discover that when these long-awaited-for, feel-good days occur, they want to spend a lot of time together, especially thinking ahead to that final month. These couples have that "enjoy it while we can" attitude, realizing that there will be a time when that ballooning abdomen literally comes between man and woman, and your focus starts to shift to becoming mom and dad.

***Dr. Linda notes:** Sexual activity is considered medically safe and healthy during most normal pregnancies. Obviously, you want to get your caregiver's recommendations as to whether there are any specific concerns. Caution, and even abstinence, may be recommended in the following circumstances:*

- *If the placenta is in a vulnerable location. "Placenta previa" occurs when the afterbirth is covering, or partially covering, the birth canal and can cause bleeding problems. Women with placenta previa are commonly advised to avoid intercourse.*

- *If you are bleeding, which can be a sign of placental problems or early thinning of the cervix.*

- *If you have risk factors for premature labor.*

Enjoy pillow talk. The language of lovemaking changes during pregnancy. Show and tell your man what produces pleasure and what produces discomfort. To increase your pleasure and help you avoid discomfort, tell him what feels good and what doesn't. There may be times when the increased sensitivity of your breasts and vagina gives you immense pleasure during foreplay; at other times, the ultrasensitivity makes breast-fondling and clitoral stimulation off-limits. When you enjoy being touched in those areas, welcome it; if not, nudge those caressing hands toward less sensitive areas.

Have a sex talk. Each of you should explain your feelings. Be sure that your partner does not interpret your lack of interest in sex as lack of interest in him, for example, and don't interpret his confusion over how to touch you now to mean that he's not interested. Tell your man about the way pregnancy is affecting your feelings about sex, and ask him to tell you how he feels about your new look. Talk to each other about your desires and try to find a way to satisfy the both of you.

Appreciate your changing body. Be proud of your body's new femininity: your darkened nipples, the emerging tummy bulge. Focus on what is new and exciting that you will both enjoy only during pregnancy. Your fuller breasts will be "all his" for the rest of the pregnancy — what a turn-on! In a month or so, you will enjoy lying down together, watching and feeling the baby move. One fun project can be taking "as you grow" photos: month-by-month photos showing your changing pregnant shape. Some women might not like the idea of a photo shoot, but they can all enjoy a new kind of intimacy with their partner during pregnancy. However you approach sex, be sure to appreciate each other during this uniquely fleeting time.

My husband took a video of me in the nude every month so we could document the exciting and beautiful changes my body went through. Now that I have my former body back and can hardly remember what being pregnant felt like, it's a wonderful reminder of a very special time in our lives.

Fling for fun! Plan to enjoy romantic weekend "dates" before your little traveling companion arrives. Future getaways may be harder with baby — if they happen at all — so the best time for romantic retreats is in the middle three months of pregnancy; make the most of this time to schedule some getaway weekends. If you already have one or more children, try to get away at least once before your family grows again. This is an important opportunity to share quality time as a couple, even if just for one night, now and then.

CHIROPRACTIC CARE DURING PREGNANCY

Diligent chiropractic care during pregnancy makes good sense. Women have found it especially helpful in relieving and preventing back pain. Your growing uterus exerts a downward and forward pull on the lower spine that, when combined with the gradually increasing changes in your gait and center of gravity, can set you up for back and neck pain. In addition, the ligament-loosening hormones of pregnancy can further aggravate pelvic and spine pains. Add to this the extra strain on your back of increasing breast size and weight. Pelvic adjustments help proper alignment and keep pelvic structures flexible. For further information on chiropractic care during pregnancy, see the website for the International Chiropractic Pediatric Association at ICPA4kids.org.

Fear of Miscarriage

Some women wonder whether having sex while pregnant could cause miscarriage. Science is on your side: there is no proven link between sexual intercourse/orgasm and miscarriage. However, doctors may advise women who have had several miscarriages to avoid intercourse while pregnant. The reason for this concern is that orgasm stimulates mild uterine contractions (orgasm *is* the uterus contracting). Timing is also on your side: when your risk of miscarriage is the highest, in the first trimester, your interest in intercourse is likely to be at its lowest. Your desire for intercourse usually increases after the first few months, while your chances of miscarrying decrease dramatically. (See page 259 for more about enjoying sex during the later stages of pregnancy and the risk of preterm labor after twenty weeks.)

If for medical reasons your healthcare provider advises you to abstain from intercourse, the warning of "no sex" need not mean "no closeness." If your physician recommends restrictions, it's important to understand the reasons. These restrictions might prompt you to invent ways of enjoying each other's affection, bringing you to a new level of intimacy. Communication is the key. Snuggling is, after all, highly underrated.

The Myth of the Deprived Man

Dr. Bill notes: As a man, I find this myth very guilt producing for women. The truth is that when a man puts his own needs aside temporarily, puts his wife's first, and doesn't make her feel guilty, they learn the nature of love: to will the good of the other. Women have long memories, and they don't forget. A healthy marriage can make it through this and come out stronger on the other end because the man was self-sacrificing. Guys, I have been there, felt that, and I know many men who have worked hard to blend their never-changing sexual appetite with their pregnant wife's ever-changing libido. You can do it, too.

Here are some turn-on tips for expectant dads:

Redefine "sex." True or false: a pregnant woman's desire for sex (translation:

intercourse) lessens during certain months? True! But a real fact of pregnant life is that a woman's need for sex (translation: security and affection) increases while pregnant. This may be the first time in your married life that sex does not have to equate with orgasm. It's a good idea to accept this definition upgrade now, as you're going to need to remember it during those tired months of early parenting.

"You first, me second!" It took me, Dr. Bill, forty years to fully appreciate this key to a happy marriage. It is especially difficult for men to learn this when they're in their career-building years. When you imagine the head-to-toe physical, emotional, and biochemical changes that are going on in your wife's pregnant body, just to deliver your baby, she deserves, and needs, a change in your priorities.

When we were pregnant, on one of Martha's grouchy days I was in a snit as I thought about how uncomfortable she was making me feel. That's when I realized I needed to practice what I preach by clicking into the mindset "don't go there!" Instead of selfishly thinking about my own discomfort, I filled my mind with what feelings I thought Martha must be having, and how uncomfortable she was. I told myself: "After all, it's half of my genes that are contributing to her discomfort. She is doing the most important job in the world: growing a human being." Every time I let myself fall into the me-first mindset, it really helped to focus on Martha's feelings, instead of mine.

Compliment her curves. The best way to turn on a pregnant woman is to help her realize that her body is sexier and more appealing to you, not less. If she feels you get excited about her changing shape, you're likely to be gifted with a livelier-than-ever sex life. Try these turn-ons:

- "I love the glow and feel of your skin."

- "I love how your breasts and belly are getting curvier."

- "Your body is amazing — I can't believe how sexy you look."

Lovingly acknowledge her beauty; this will help create intimacy and enhance your sex life as a couple.

Don't worry, enjoy intercourse. While certain conditions may preclude you from engaging in intercourse (see page 165), for most couples it can be mutually enjoyed right up until delivery.

Humor helps turn her on. It might be tempting to joke lightheartedly about her new shape, but that is risky. The joke may not be funny to a supersensitive, hormonal woman. Humor is good, but not at her expense. How about putting on a funny movie and watching it together to get her mind off her changing body, instead of focusing on it? A relaxed evening can ease even the tensest female. A freely given hug can lead to an honest cuddle, as long as she does not sense an agenda.

Empathize. While empathy means imagining how your wife feels, there is no way on earth you'll ever be able to really understand what she's experiencing and feel what she's feeling. That's why the cliché "I know how you feel" is a likely turnoff, because she's probably thinking "If he really knew how I felt, which he never will, he'd go to the kitchen and get me some cookies and milk instead of wanting to make love."

Evolve from lover to father. Some men start feeling more paternal than sexual as pregnancy progresses. As your mate is going through a body change, you may go through a mindset change and start to think more about comforting and protecting your wife and baby than simply satisfying your sexual desires. Some men take longer than others to blend their roles as lover and father. And, some expectant dads go through a hormone change of their own. Male hormone levels, like testosterone, drop a bit, and female nurturing hormones go up, which redirect the man's thoughts more toward his mate than his penis.

Expect ups and downs. Be prepared for your wife to crave and initiate sex during the feel-better respite of the middle trimester. Some men find that during the ups and downs of pregnancy, in the first trimester she can't meet your sexual desires; in the second trimester, you maybe can't satisfy hers. For this reason, don't be alarmed if you don't always rise to the occasion.

Shift positions. Over the months, as her body changes, your positions of sexual intercourse may need to adapt. As you try new positions, it may take you a while to adjust to her changing body. The vascular engorgement and change of lubrication in her vaginal lining may make for a different fit. Be creative in changing positions during intercourse to respect your mate's changing body. See page 259 for more on this topic.

MY PREGNANCY JOURNAL: THIRD MONTH

Emotionally I feel:

_____

_____

_____

_____

_____

Physically I feel:

_____

_____

_____

_____

_____

My thoughts about you:

_____

_____

_____

_____

_____

My dreams about you:

_____

_____

_____

_____

_____

What I imagine you look like:

_____

_____

_____

_____

_____

Sharing our news. With whom? Reactions:

_____

_____

_____

_____

_____

My top concerns:

_____

_____

_____

_____

_____

My best joys:

_____

_____

_____

_____

_____

Visit to My Healthcare Provider

Questions I had; answers I got:

_____

_____

_____

Tests and results; my reaction:

_____

_____

_____

Updated due date: _____

My weight: _____

My blood pressure: _____

When I first heard your heartbeat:

_____

_____

_____

_____

My reaction:

_____

_____

_____

Ultrasound photo:

Comments:

_____

_____

_____

_____

_____

_____

_____

_____

_____

_____

_____

_____

_____

FOURTH-MONTH VISIT TO YOUR HEALTHCARE PROVIDER
(13–16 WEEKS)

During this month's visit you may have:

- An examination of the size and height of the uterus

- An examination for swelling, varicose veins, and rashes

- An opportunity to hear baby's heartbeat

- An opportunity through ultrasound to see all the organs that are now developed and possibly to watch baby move

- A test for possible prenatal genetic defects

- A weight and blood-pressure check (expect more rapid weight gain over the next three months)

- Urinalysis to test for infection, sugar, and protein

- Ultrasound screening for possible birth defects, number of babies, and placental location, and possibly to recalculate due date

- An opportunity to discuss your feelings and concerns

Fourth Month: Feeling Better

Finally! After a few months of feeling lousy, you now have a reprieve and are most likely feeling a bit more energized. This is the month when many women begin to enjoy being pregnant. While you may still have "green" days, most women can now enjoy the excited feelings of approaching motherhood. The all-day nausea is subsiding and food becomes more appealing. Since some of your energy has returned, you can now enjoy certain things, like food and sex, that you have been avoiding these past few months. During the coming weeks, both mommy and baby go through a growth spurt. Soon, that baby bump will emerge (if it hasn't already) and this pregnancy will become more obvious to those around you. The fears of miscarriage, birth defects, or genetic abnormalities (if you had genetic screening) are behind you. Your baby is now fully formed and simply growing.

HOW YOUR BABY IS GROWING, 13–16 WEEKS

By sixteen weeks, baby is about the size of a plum, weighing in at 3 or 4 ounces. Baby's arms and legs lengthen. Arms start waving and feet start kicking, yet you may not feel baby's presence until around the eighteenth week. Newly found fingers make a fist and tiny thumbs may find their way to an open mouth. Eyelids stay closed, presumably to protect the rapidly developing eyeballs. Hair and eyebrows

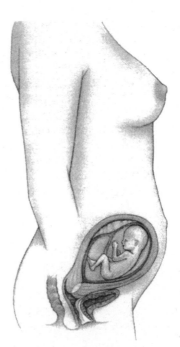

Baby at 13–16 weeks.

appear. Baby begins to "breathe" amniotic fluid in and out of tiny lung buds. Baby's beginning breathing movements may result in gentle hiccups. Hearing develops, enabling baby to react to sounds. Finally, boy babies make testosterone, and girl babies start making eggs in their tiny ovaries. More hair starts to appear on that thin-skinned scalp.

FEELING YOUR UTERUS GROW

While the height of the growing uterus varies from woman to woman, sometime between the end of the third month and midway through the fourth month you're likely to be able to begin to feel the tip of your uterus just above your pubic bone. In subsequent pregnancies you might be able to feel your uterus earlier because you know what it feels like and your abdominal muscles are looser. Try this: Empty your bladder, lie on your back, relax your abdominal muscles and gently rub your fingers across the top of your pubic bone. You might feel the tip of a little hard ball. As you can see in the illustration, by sixteen weeks that little ball feels like a baseball midway between the top of your pubic bone and your navel. By twenty weeks you will feel your softball-sized uterus around the level of your navel. The long-awaited first-felt kicks, referred to as "quickening," typically occur at around eighteen or nineteen weeks from your last period. However, they can occur a couple of weeks earlier or later, depending on the location of the placenta and your own sensitivity. Quickening often feels like a minor fluttering at first, evolving later into kicks, punches, and somersaults. Once you feel the beginning bulge inside, it's likely you'll begin to instinctively and repeatedly massage that area, as if wanting to caress your baby. Be patient; there will soon be a bigger baby bump to embrace.

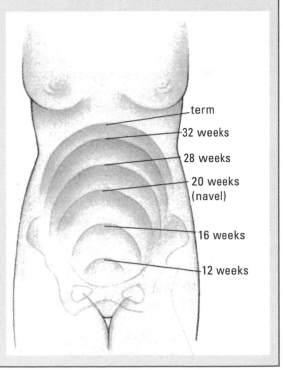

- term
- 32 weeks
- 28 weeks
- 20 weeks (navel)
- 16 weeks
- 12 weeks

HOW YOU MAY FEEL

Dr. Bill notes: *In the early years of parenting, tired moms and dads often ask me, "When will our lives get back to normal?" I smile and remind them, "This is now your normal life."*

Time to tell? While some women are still ambivalent about their changing bodies, many enjoy, and even flaunt, their fuller figures. If you have previously kept your pregnancy private, the secret may now be out—literally. Depending on your body build and the way you carry your baby, you may be showing only slightly at this stage or be more obviously in bloom. Many women find that sharing the news gives them well-deserved bragging rights and compensates for any discomforts on the inside.

Hello there! If this is your first ultrasound, the first peek may leave you speechless. Seeing your baby on ultrasound, feeling the bulge, and hearing the heartbeat all bring a heightened awareness that this tiny person has taken up residence. Your mind is likely to be more on your baby and less on yourself. These surges of love will naturally lead to a developing connection with your baby. Each day, you are deepening your relationship with your little one.

When my husband and I saw our baby on the ultrasound screen this month, we were completely blown away. It was somewhat of a visceral shock. I mean, I knew I was pregnant, but this was so real and exciting. I've been on a cloud for days.

Re-energized. You may now feel renewed energy, but remember it's all relative. You're unlikely to have your pre-pregnant level of energy. It's not that your total available energy is less, it's just that more of it is redirected to what's going on inside you.

I felt so much better that I made the mistake of plunging back into high gear, trying to do too much, too soon. Fortunately, my body wouldn't let me, as if a little voice inside prompted me to ease off the gas pedal.

No one should expect you to act like your old self and do all the things you used to do.

This is now your "new self" and your baby will periodically remind you, "Slow down, Mama!" Remember that baby is growing more during these middle three months than at any other time during your pregnancy, and there's only so much energy to go around. Biology will remind you that your baby has first dibs on mom's natural resources; you and everyone else must adjust to what is left over.

Fewer trips to the bathroom. The baby-on-bladder pressure that sent you running to the bathroom day and night last trimester will ease a bit over the next month or two as your uterus rises out of your pelvis and away from your bladder. However, in the final two months when your baby is bigger and then starts dropping, it'll be back to the bathroom again . . . so enjoy this brief respite!

Increased vaginal discharge. It's normal during pregnancy to experience a milky, uniquely odorous, egg white–like vaginal discharge. This resembles premenstrual vaginal discharge, but it is heavier and can be constant. Pregnancy hormones increase blood flow to your vaginal tissues to prepare the canal for baby's birth passage. These hormones stimulate an increase in secretions, which help nourish the stretching and changing tissues. Be prepared to change underwear several times a day or wear a panty liner to stay comfortably dry.

While most vaginal discharge is just a minor nuisance, some types may signal an infection. Notify your healthcare provider if:

- the previously egg white–like discharge becomes pus-like, yellow, green, cheesy, or foul smelling

- you experience burning or itching

- your labia (lips of the vagina) become swollen, red, or tender

- you experience burning pain while urinating

Bleeding gums. Just as the tissue around your breasts and reproductive organs needs more blood flow to nourish your baby, blood flow increases throughout your whole body. This causes exposed tissue, like gums, to bleed more easily when you brush your teeth.

The healthier your gums, the healthier your baby, plain and simple. In recent years doctors have come to appreciate the correlation between good gums and good health. When pockets of bacteria get trapped beneath the gums, they can cause infection, leading to pain, swelling, and bad breath. These bacteria can then worm their way from your gums into your bloodstream and trigger inflammation or infection elsewhere in your body.

Get a checkup from your dentist or dental hygienist. Your dentist may require a letter from your provider before doing deep cleaning, even though the research is clear that cleaning is recommended. Your provider will be happy to give your dentist the OK and alert him/her of any concerns. Here are some tips on caring for your gums and teeth:

- Be good to your gums in a gentle way. Use a soft toothbrush or, if you have a favorite toothbrush, run the bristles under hot water to soften them before brushing. In addition to brushing your teeth, focus on cleaning your gum margins, the groove (called the sulcus) between teeth and gums where there is swelling and bleeding and where bacteria tend to collect.

- Using a proxy brush (resembling a toothpick with Christmas tree–like bristles at the end), brush the gum line between and around the teeth. Pack a proxy brush in your pocket and give a few gentle jabs between teeth after each meal, especially if you eat something sticky or chewy.

- It is best to use a water flosser when pregnant. To respect your sensitive gums you may need to adjust the intensity of the jet a bit. Gentle water flossing is more likely than dental floss to clean out gum lines around the whole tooth — so it's helpful to your tender gums.

- If using dental floss, angle the floss in a "C" around one tooth and slide it away from the gum. Then angle the "C" against the next tooth and repeat. Don't force floss too deeply between tooth and gum because it may damage the sensitive tissue, causing it to bleed and forcing bacteria down into the groove.

- Use a tongue-scraper before bed each night. Scrape as far back on the tongue as you can without gagging, since that is an area where food residue tends to collect.

- Swish with warm water after each meal and before you brush. After-meal swishing is a good habit to get into and it leaves your mouth feeling fresh. You can even try swishing with soothing chamomile tea.

- Feed your gums the best foods. Avoid sticky foods, such as caramel, and eat foods with gum-nourishing nutrients, such as those containing vitamins C and D, calcium, and folic acid. Nutrients that are good for the bones are also good for the teeth. Note: Don't buy chewable vitamin C tablets. Vitamin C is ascorbic acid, which, if allowed to settle on teeth, can eat into the enamel. (Learn more about bone-building nutrients on page 48.)

SCIENCE SAYS: MAINTAIN HEALTHIER GUMS, DELIVER A HEALTHIER BABY

Researchers at the University of North Carolina enrolled a thousand women in a study and compared the birth outcome of those with and without gingivitis, or periodontal disease. Mothers with moderate to severe periodontal disease more than doubled their risk of delivering a premature baby. Obstetrical and dental researchers believe that inflammation of the gums causes a general increase in blood levels of inflammatory chemicals that may trigger preterm labor.

Nosebleeds. Hormones can also cause nosebleeds to occur, especially during forceful blowing or sneezing, or even occasionally without these triggers, because the exposed blood vessels lining your nasal passages are more fragile. When experiencing nasal congestion, it is important to respect the tiny blood vessels in the lining of your nasal passages. Try to blow gently, one nostril at a time; don't pick your nose; and keep your nasal passages well humidified. (Keep reading for information about a do-it-yourself "nose hose" and "steam clean.")

Congestion. Keep a tissue handy these days! Pregnancy hormones cause everything to swell, including the membranes lining your nasal and breathing passages. Allergy sufferers may suffer more during pregnancy, and postnasal drip may become drippier. When it comes to congestion, here's where the skills-instead-of-pills model that you learned about in chapter 9 is really helpful. Unless advised otherwise by your healthcare provider, avoid prescription and over-the-counter decongestants, antihistamines, and cortisol nasal sprays. While at modest doses most of these products are not dangerous, they are not going to help much anyway and there is no reason to expose your baby to unnecessary medications. It's better to relieve your nasal stuffiness naturally:

• Make your own saltwater nose drops (½ teaspoon of salt dissolved in 8 ounces of water) or buy a ready-made saline solution. Drop or spritz a few drops into your clogged nasal passages and *gently* blow, one nostril at a time.

• Don't blow your nose forcefully or hold both nostrils tightly while you blow, as this can cause nosebleeds and can push nasal secretions up into the sinus cavities, triggering a sinus infection.

• Try a "nose hose." A neti pot is a gentle way to unclog stuffy noses and drain congested sinuses. This Aladdin's lamp look-alike allows you to pour warm saltwater through the spout of the pot into the upper nostril while your head is tilted, allowing water to flow through one nostril and out the other, flushing out the gunk. Be sure to clean your neti pot thoroughly between uses.

• Savor a "steam clean." Use a facial steamer while reading a book or watching TV, enjoy a before-bed steam clean in a warm shower, and run a vaporizer at your bedside. In winter months, turn down the central heat in your bedroom and turn up one or two vaporizers. The warm mist from the vaporizer acts as a healthier heat source, protecting you from the dry air caused by central heating, which can further thicken the secretions in your breathing passages.

CONCERNS YOU MAY HAVE

Dizzy and Feeling Faint

Feeling lightheaded? Why? You're pregnant! Normally when you quickly change positions — for example, when you hop out of bed or jump up from out of your chair — the brain tells the heart to quickly adjust the blood pressure to maintain steady blood flow to the brain. Yet during pregnancy, this mechanism becomes quirky. The heart becomes slower to respond to the needs of the brain when you change positions because the enlarging uterus with its passenger is competing with the brain for that momentarily needed extra blood volume, and baby wins. When you rise too fast, the blood flow to your brain momentarily slows and you feel dizzy. This is called *postural hypotension,* low blood pressure due to change in position.

Orthostatic hypotension can also occur. When you're standing or even sitting for a long time, blood pools in the lower half of the body, stealing blood from the brain and leading to lightheadedness. This may get worse later in pregnancy as the lower half of your body grows larger and therefore needs more blood.

Your growing uterus can also press on the major blood vessels in the abdomen, slowing blood flow to the upper half of your body, especially when you are lying on your back or on your right side (see our suggested positions on page 84).

If feeling faint becomes more than just an annoyance, discuss the issue with your healthcare provider. There may be medical reasons that cause you to feel this way, such as low red blood cell count, called anemia, or low blood sugar. These can be diagnosed by assessing changes in your eating habits and by a quick finger stick in the doctor's office.

To help you feel less faint during your pregnancy:

- Change positions slowly, especially as you get out of bed or after lying or sitting down for a long time. Any movement that changes blood flow to your brain can cause dizziness or a headache.

- Shorten the time you stand by taking frequent sitting breaks.

- If you feel faint during a change of position, lie down immediately, preferably on your left side.

- Hydrate! Dehydration aggravates dizziness, so be sure you drink at least eight glasses of water a day. If you sweat a lot, a certain amount of salt (think: chicken soup) is helpful.

- Don't sit or stand still. If you must sit or stand in one place for a long time, flex your feet and pump your leg muscles frequently to keep the blood moving upward. While sitting, elevate your legs on a footstool to avoid blood pooling in the lower half of your body.

- Lie on your left side when resting or sleeping.

- Graze on nutritious snacks (see page 22) and eat iron-rich foods to build up your blood sugar and blood cells (see page 47).

Dr. Linda notes: I never cease to be amazed by pregnant women who come into my office, or even to the hospital, complaining of dizziness; when asked about food and fluid intake, they say they haven't had anything to eat or drink for many hours. You and your baby need lots of fluid and nutrients!

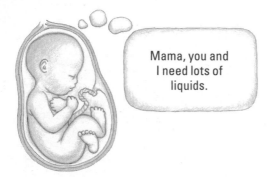

Mama, you and I need lots of liquids.

Feeling Warmer

Do you feel as though your body is heating up as it grows? Thank your baby and all the supporting tissue that she needs to grow. Similar to the feeling you get during exercise, the increased blood flow to all those tissues throughout your body bring along increased heat and sometimes extra sweating to release it. Besides feeling warmer all the time, some mothers feel periodic hot flashes and even night sweats. You might even see a temperature role reversal with your bed partner. While you may have been used to stealing the covers at night (most women are naturally cooler at night than men), now you may be the one who turns down the thermostat and shrugs off the blankets.

You are walking around with a body temperature one degree warmer than usual, courtesy of your pregnancy hormones. This is similar to the slight increase in temperature that you get when you ovulate. Keep in mind that you are a marvelous biological machine working overtime in high gear, so it's going to get hot. Try these strategies to keep cool:

- Drink extra fluids to replace those lost through perspiration.

- Wear loose-fitting cotton clothing — cotton is "breathable" and will keep you cooler.

- Layer your tops so that you can easily peel off layers as you heat up.

- Take a shower or bath. Instead of drying completely, leave a thin layer of water on your skin to evaporate.

- Go for a swim — the water naturally cools you.

- Enjoy your outdoor exercise in the cooler part of the day rather than in the heat. Fitness classes that cater to pregnant women usually have the air-conditioning turned up or heat turned down a few degrees. Of course, if you feel your body overheating to the point of discomfort, it's time to slow down and cool down.

I feel pretty warm all the time. I notice I sweat more at even the slightest exertion. I go around in short sleeves even though it's the middle of winter, and sometimes I even want to put on shorts. I also feel warmer at night, so I don't use a blanket. Sometimes I get so hot I have to put my feet out from underneath the sheet. It's as though I carry around my own personal furnace inside.

Skin Changes

The skin of a pregnant woman looks and feels different because of what's happening beneath it. The increase in blood volume, which peaks during the second trimester, brings more blood to the skin, giving the areas that are already highly vascular — mainly the face — a rosier appearance. The many glands that lie beneath the skin work overtime in a pregnant body: oil-producing glands produce more oil, pigment-producing glands produce more pigment, and sweat glands cause you to perspire more. The skin changes you see during your pregnancy depend a lot upon the kind of skin you have. The darker your skin, the more changes you can expect; the lighter your skin, the more visible all changes are. Increased hormones, especially estrogen and progesterone, stimulate pigment-producing cells so that dark areas become even darker.

Shortly after delivery you will get your former skin back, for the most part; some veins and stretch marks may linger, but even those fade eventually. Consider these skin changes the mark of motherhood.

My body got back to normal, but some stretch marks remain. I believe my stretch marks are a badge of honor for creating life, and I wear them proudly.

Be sure to treat your skin right by following the pregnancy skin-care basics on page 183. Here are some of the different kinds of skin conditions you might experience:

The pregnancy "glow." Sometime during the second trimester, you may find yourself gazing at a different face in the mirror. The glow that others notice isn't just an old wives' tale; interestingly enough, it has a biological basis. The increased volume of blood causes the cheeks to take on an attractive blush, because of the many blood vessels just below the skin's surface. On top of this redness, the increased secretions of the oil glands give the skin a waxy sheen. People experience the same flushed face when they get excited, cry, or do anything that increases their heart rate.

The pregnancy mask, or more appropriately called "the blotch," occurs because the hormones estrogen and progesterone stimulate the melanin cells in the skin to produce more pigment, but do not act on these cells uniformly. You may look like you have a blotchy tan. Brownish or yellowish patches, called *chloasma,* can appear anywhere on the face but are seen most commonly on the forehead, upper cheeks, nose, and chin. Darker-skinned women, who already have more pigment in their skin, may notice more darkening, such as circles around their eyes. You can minimize the intensity of these blotchy, darkened areas by limiting facial exposure to ultraviolet light (i.e., sunshine), which further stimulates melanin production.

The pregnancy itch. Are you beginning to itch, especially over areas of skin that stretch a lot, such as your abdomen, hips, and thighs? Besides itching, caused by all the hormonal and blood volume changes in your skin described above, some areas of the skin can be dry and flaky. Here are our remedies for soothing dry, itchy skin:

- Make an anti-itch oatmeal bath by adding ½ cup (uncooked) quick oatmeal to warm bath water.

- Enjoy a soothing soak by adding 1 cup cornstarch and ½ cup baking soda to a half-filled tub of warm water.

- Add 1 tablespoon cornstarch and 1 tablespoon baking soda to 1 quart warm water, soak a towel in it, and drape it over the itchy areas on your body.

- Try skin-soothing products (see page 183).

(For more anti-itch tips, review the pregnancy skin-care basics on page 183.)

Pregnancy acne. You may have thought your blemish-prone days were a thing of the past, but hormonal surges similar to those of adolescence may leave their mark on your skin. The good news is that acne will subside after pregnancy. Try these anti-acne remedies:

- Avoid the abrasive scrubs you may have used during adolescence when your skin was thicker and less sensitive.

- Try oatmeal-based facial scrubs, which are milder on supersensitive pregnancy skin. Gently massage the scrub in a circular motion around the areas of acne to remove the excess oil and some of the weaker whiteheads.

- Use water-based cosmetics instead of oil-based ones, which tend to aggravate acne.

- Let the sun in. Gradually increase your exposure to sunlight to fifteen minutes without sunblock to enjoy the natural healing properties of the sun on pimply skin.

- Avoid prescription acne drugs, such as Accutane and retinoid-containing creams, which have been linked to birth defects. Your dermatologist or obstetrician can give you guidance on which drugs are safe to use.

Pregnancy body breakouts. You might experience itchy, pimply, raised red patches on your thighs, buttocks, abdomen, and extremities. Called pruritic urticarial papules and plaques of pregnancy (PUPPPs), this skin nuisance comes and goes during the second half of pregnancy and disappears shortly afterward. Interestingly, it is more common in women carrying baby boys than girls. PUPPPs is harmless but can be terribly annoying. If the skin measures we have already suggested don't work, ask your caregiver for suggestions about additional over-the-counter or prescription remedies.

Pregnancy tags. In areas where skin rubs on clothing or against itself (under the arms, neck folds, or bra line), some women develop tiny polyps called skin tags. Skin tags are thought to be caused by hyperactive skin cells that grow in response to being irritated by friction rubs. Like most other skin conditions of pregnancy, they disappear after delivery, but can be painlessly excised by your dermatologist if they bother you.

Pregnancy redness. Don't be alarmed if the soles of your feet and the palms of your hands become reddened. This curious condition, due to increased blood flow, will disappear once you deliver your baby.

Pregnancy lines. Even before pregnancy, many women have a barely visible line called a *linea alba* running from the top of the pubic bone to the navel. As your belly blossoms, the stretched abdominal skin and other pregnancy skin changes may cause this line to darken. The line might migrate upward toward your breastbone. This is the *linea nigra* and may be darker in darker-skinned women. Old wives' tales say that this line helps the baby find the way to the breast after birth when placed on the mother's abdomen. Just another transient badge of pregnancy, this line naturally lightens a few months after delivery.

Pregnancy pigmentation. Pigmented areas of the body become darker, and new areas of darkening skin may appear. This is due to increased secretion of a hormone called melanin, which, interestingly, is involved in seasonal color changes in some animals. You can expect moles to become larger and darker, and to develop more freckles, since hormones cause these normal skin blemishes to get bigger and browner. Many of these changes will go away, but some will not. Be sure to have your caregiver check out any unusual skin changes. Though rare, skin cancers can occur during pregnancy.

Pregnancy spider veins. The combination of increased blood flow, enlarged blood vessels, and hypersensitive skin is a recipe for the appearance of squiggly red or purple capillaries just below the surface of the skin branching out like tiny spiderwebs. These will pop out even more on your face or in your eyeballs during the intense pushing phase of delivery. They can appear anywhere on the body, but are common on the legs and face. If they bother you, try using concealer to cover them up.

Caring for Skin during Pregnancy

Pampering your hypersensitive skin is good practice to prepare you for caring for the sensitive skin of your newborn, who, like most babies, will probably be prone to prickly-heat pimples and diaper rash. Not only are lotions and potions you put *onto* your skin important, but so, too, are the nutrients you put *into* it. Try these skin-care tips:

Feed your skin. As you learned on page 30, omega-3s are natural and safe anti-inflammatories that can slow down overreactive eruptions and calm hypersensitive skin. The 5-S diet you learned about on page 44 is chock-full of natural skin smoothers and softeners, again because of the natural anti-inflammatories in seafood, salads, smoothies, spices, and supplements. The pregnancy supersalad (see page 38) and the pregnancy supersmoothie (see page 24) are just what the dermatologist ordered.

Hydrate your skin. Hydrate your skin by drinking lots of water and humidifying the air. If you work in an office or sleep in a centrally heated bedroom, use a humidifier in the warmer months. In the winter months, turn down or off the central heating and turn on a couple of vaporizers to warm and humidify the air and your skin.

Moisturize your skin. To moisturize particularly dry, patchy, and flaky areas, we recommend what we call the "soak and seal" method. After your bath or shower, gently blot your skin with a towel, but leave a thin layer of water to soak into your skin. Apply a moisturizing cream, ointment, or oil to seal in the moisture. When using this treatment at bedtime, many moms notice fewer scaly patches and less itching when they awaken the next morning. Moisturizers are a double helper: they contain oils that seal in moisture and humectants that hydrate the skin from beneath by drawing up water to the surface of the skin. Use lip balms if you find your lips become supersensitive, irritated, or dry. (See AskDrSears.com/skincare for a list of the moisturizers we recommend during pregnancy.) We discourage powders, which tend to cake in skin folds and can actually aggravate rashes.

Care for your creases. Your skin will have more folds during pregnancy — for example, in your groin, armpits, beneath your breasts, and in any areas that are prone to friction rubs from clothing or other skin. These areas are particularly sensitive to pimply, itchy eruptions. Here's where emollients, such as Lansinoh (which you may use on sensitive nipples later on), are particularly helpful. Loosen your bra straps and apply an emollient under them, especially under the bottom band of your bra, to minimize friction irritation.

Cover your skin comfortably. Instead of synthetic fabrics, such as polyester, which tend to trap moisture, wear loose cotton clothing that allows your skin to breathe. Avoid pantyhose, which may aggravate prickly-heat types of rashes on your buttocks, thighs, and pubic area.

Select and apply skin-care products wisely. Avoid alcohol-containing cleansers that dry the skin and highly fragranced products, which can offend your heightened sense of smell. Remember, your sensitive skin may react to products that were previously skin-friendly. So, before buying anything, apply a test-dab of the product to the inside of your forearm and wait twenty minutes to see if your skin gets red or swollen. Avoid harsh abrasives, skin peelers, and oily pore-plugging facial creams. Instead, try softer emollients, such as oatmeal-based products, and apply them gently in a small, circular motion. Apply moisturizers and emollients liberally and frequently, especially in areas where your body rubs against itself or your clothes.

Don't overbathe. While water is generally kind to the skin, too much time in the tub can deplete the skin's natural oils.

Use soap sense. Since soaps generally dry the skin by removing its natural oils, use a soap that has built-in moisturizers, such as Dove. Too much soap used too often can dry out and irritate pregnant skin. Use soap sparingly on your face. Most important, avoid using soap on your sensitive nipples. Many mothers find leg-shaving especially irritating and need to shave with conditioner, a moisturizer lotion, or a gel instead of a soap-based shaving cream.

Don't get too much sun. Vitamin D–rich sunshine is generally therapeutic to skin as long as you don't overdo it and burn. Most women can get sufficient vitamin D by exposing bare arms and legs to sunshine for fifteen to twenty minutes daily. Be particularly careful if you are fair-skinned. Because of overactive pigment-producing cells, the skin of a pregnant woman is ultrasensitive to the ultraviolet rays of the sun, and this extra sensitivity may remain for about three months after delivery. Increase your vigilance to the sun:

- Use a sunscreen or sunblock of at least SPF 15 if you will be out for longer than twenty minutes, or if you tend to burn easily. Apply the sunscreen at least thirty minutes prior to sun exposure. We have used and recommended the facial sunscreen Aloe Kote for more than fifteen years. It contains the natural moisturizer aloe and SPF 25 sunscreen.

- Wear a wide-brimmed hat that shades your entire face. Even after delivery, continue to protect your face from excessive sunlight exposure for about three months.

- Avoid tanning salons, which can damage your already-sensitive skin.

Soften your makeup. Some women give up their previous makeup routine during pregnancy so as not to cover up their natural glow; others prefer to even this glow out; and still others, bothered by uneven blotches, use more makeup. Try water-based makeup while you are pregnant, which is gentler on your skin than makeup containing oils and alcohol. Don't forget to remove your makeup carefully at night to allow your skin to breathe.

Treat your skin to a soothing touch. Dubbed "vitamin T," the caress of a gentle massage is soothing not only to pregnant skin but also to the pregnant psyche, which is important since many moms find that their rashes flare up as their stress level does.

(See "Make Your Personal Care Products Safe for Baby," page 101.)

Working while Pregnant

Many women find themselves juggling the inside "job" of growing a baby and the outside job of working for pay. For some, especially those who do not suffer from morning sickness, work is a welcome way to wait out the nine months. These mothers want to work right up until the first contraction. Other women may need a month or more before the birth to prepare their nest and focus on the life inside. Some mothers, due to pregnancy complications, need to leave in the early months. Whatever your situation, here is some advice on how best to handle your news for you, your family, and your company.

Telling your employer. As soon as you learn you are pregnant, start planning when and how you will tell your boss. If you intend to stop working after your baby comes, you need to give your employer plenty of time to find a replacement, and yourself enough time to finish up important projects. Tell your boss when you plan to leave and ask how you can help make the transition a smooth one.

If you want to return to your job after the baby is born, you must be careful. You want to keep your options open for a satisfactory maternity leave and at the same time protect your position. While it is illegal to discriminate against someone who is pregnant, the corporate world is often confused when a worker becomes a mother. A promotion for which you are in line may be jeopardized by your pregnancy. You may be given less challenging assignments because of your "condition." You may be uncertain about how your coworkers will handle the news. Some may be sympathetic to your occasional memory lapses and your first-trimester miseries. Others may be worried about having to "cover" for you on days when you aren't at your best.

When should you tell? The best time to tell your employer and coworkers is just after people begin to suspect you might be pregnant and before they are sure. Although you are excited about your news, most women recommend against revealing a pregnancy in the early months.

Be careful not to wait too long to tell, either. You don't want to give your employer any reason to think you are untrustworthy; any suggestion that you concealed your pregnancy for your own gain may make you look as though you are not a team player.

Don't expect to function every day on your job at the same level as you did before you were pregnant. If you want to stay employed but find your current position too strenuous, ask for a temporary transfer to a less demanding job. Better to be honest with your supervisor than disgruntled and inefficient. If you don't want to change jobs, ask if you can work part-time, do some of your work at home, or have flexible hours so that you can work harder or longer on more comfortable days to make up for the less productive ones.

How to best negotiate your maternity leave. Do your homework before you negotiate, and you're likely to be happier with the maternity-leave package you end up with.

Know what you want. Interview yourself. If you truly know what you want, you are more likely to get it. Determine what you can afford and what's best for your pregnancy and your family. Can you grow a baby and do your job? Do you want to? Bear in mind that complications or situations during your pregnancy or after delivery may make some of these decisions for you. Explore your options. Unless your doctor determines otherwise, could you work through most of your pregnancy? Would you rather start maternity leave early? Do you want to continue your job on a part-time basis from home? After the baby is born, do you want to come back to your present job or to one that is more compatible with family life? Do you want full-time or part-time work?

Try to anticipate as best as you can your feelings toward motherhood, your financial needs, and your parenting philosophy. No career decision lasts forever. You can always change your hours, quit, or get a new job.

Know your rights. Know what your company's maternity-leave policies are and what the laws allow (see page 189). If you know and trust a coworker who previously negotiated a leave package with your company, ask what she did, what she got, and what she'd advise you to do. If you do not have a copy of the maternity-leave policy, get one from your Human Resources director. (Be aware, however, that he or she may inform your boss.) If your company does not have a maternity-leave policy and is small enough not to be legally required to have one, you may have to be a pioneer, negotiating the policy for the benefit of your future coworkers. If you can, check out the maternity-leave policies of other companies before you talk to your supervisor.

When reviewing your company's policy, be sure you understand the following:

- Is your maternity leave paid, unpaid, or partially paid?

- Pregnancy is legally considered a medical disability. Does your company have a medical disability insurance policy that pays a portion of your salary while you're on leave? Find out which forms you have to complete and where to send them, and follow up: Has the appropriate office received, processed, and finalized your application? Be sure your doctor has signed and completed the appropriate forms stating when you will be able to return to work.

- Does your company's policy guarantee that you can return to your same job or to one that is equivalent in pay and advancement possibilities?

- How much time off are you allowed?

- Can you use your present benefit days (sick leave, personal leave, vacation time) to extend your paid maternity leave?

- What is the possibility of continuing your present job part-time at home during and after your pregnancy?

- What options are available should medical complications or maternal desire necessitate a change in plans?

- Is your medical insurance plan still in effect while you are on extended leave, and does it provide partial or full coverage? How long will your company keep you on its medical insurance policy at full and partial benefits? Do you have to share the cost?

Who to tell at the office. Officially, you should tell your immediate supervisor first, before she or he hears about your pregnancy from the company grapevine. Or, you may want to talk to the Human Resources department, if it typically handles such matters or if you have real reason to fear discrimination from your boss. If you want to tell close coworkers a bit earlier, be sure they have your best interests at heart.

If you have a choice of supervisors to tell, select the one who is most likely to be sympathetic. The supervisor's own parenting experience and philosophy matter more than his or her gender. Find out ahead of time if your supervisor has previously had to juggle working and parenting. If your supervisor is female, find out if she is a parent, the ages of her children, and if anyone knows about her maternity leave history. If your supervisor is male and has children, find out what kind of package his wife had. The more you know about your supervisor's parenting situation, the better insight you have into how he or she will approach your situation.

The best way to break the news. After selecting the time and person to tell (preferably when that person is having a good day), present your case. How to break the news depends upon your pregnancy, your job, your wishes, and the reception you imagine you will get from your supervisor and coworkers. As in any negotiation, consider where the other person is coming from. Your supervisor wants to know when you are leaving, when you are coming back, and how best to fill the gap while you're gone. Be ready with those answers. Realistically, your supervisor is more concerned with the company's operations than with your personal needs. Your employer must consider the possibility that you may later decide not to return to work. (Incidentally, studies show that attractive maternity leave policies and a family-friendly workplace make it more likely that women will return.)

While listening to you, your supervisor will be trying to sense your current level of commitment to your job, though he or she is probably wise enough to know that the company can't fight the pull of motherhood. In presenting your case, first convey that you are committed to your job (if you really are) and that you are committed to working out a maternity leave package that considers both the needs of your family and the needs of the company. Opening with "The law allows me..." is likely to put your employer on the defensive and get you only what the law allows — which in some states and some companies is precious little. If a special situation later arises and you need to ask for more than the law allows, you want your boss on your side and some leftover negotiating power. It is better to open your dialogue in the spirit of cooperation. To show your commitment to your job and your respect for the needs of the company, include in your plan specific ideas on selecting and training your replacement. Depending on your familiarity with your supervisor, you may even interject comments such as, "I know you've been faced with these decisions before yourself, and I'd appreciate your help," or "Did your wife take a maternity leave? What worked for her and her company?" Remember that the company is more likely to extend your maternity leave beyond what its policy or the law allows if you show your willingness to extend yourself as well.

Get the right maternity leave package for you. Only you can figure out how much maternity leave time you will need; only your company can guess how much time it can afford to be without you. Remember, your bargaining power depends not only on how you present your case but also on your value to the company. If you have a unique skill required for the job, you'll have more clout than if there are many others within the company who can do your job just as well. Be realistic about your needs, your negotiating power, and the needs of your company; but remember, too, that companies want to be seen as family-friendly in their maternity leave policies.

Stay plugged in while on leave. If you are in the middle of a project or have specific knowledge or skills that the company relies on, show your commitment to the company and strengthen your negotiations by offering to be available by phone, fax, or email. Fax or email allows you more choice about when to respond to what's needed. Leaving your employer with the message: "Feel free to call me if you have any questions or need my help" is more likely to leave your supervisor feeling that he or she does need you.

Ease the transition. Offer to help select and train your temporary or permanent replacement, if any. Remind your supervisor of your availability by phone, fax, or email in case your replacement runs into a glitch that requires your expertise.

Leave with a clean slate. When leaving your present job, either temporarily or permanently, show your desire to tie up loose ends. Finish the jobs that need finishing or be sure you have appropriately delegated them.

Keep your doors open. Be sure to address the many what-ifs of pregnancy and parenthood. What if a medical complication during your pregnancy or after delivery requires a doctor-mandated period of bed rest or extended maternity leave? What if you have a special needs baby who, for medical reasons, requires a full-time mother? What if you get hooked on motherhood and can't bear to leave your baby after those magical six weeks are over? (Maternity leaves of six weeks reflect the needs of commerce rather than the needs of the family; there's nothing in maternal biology or infant development that marks six weeks as a good time for mothers to return to work.) Many a career train has been derailed by the lure of a precious baby.

Dr. Bill notes: Many doctors are willing to write notes for mothers to extend their maternity leave. Oftentimes, mothers come in with a six-week-old infant, pleading for just two more weeks at home…and then two more weeks…and so on. For a mother who works for a less family-friendly company, many doctors are happy to oblige by offering a variety of reasons to extend her "disability" leave.

Put it in writing. Outline your desired maternity leave package on paper and present it to your supervisor during your negotiation. Include specific dates and desired compensation. If your supervisor sees exactly what you want, you are more likely to get it. Of course, a prudent negotiator always asks for a little more than she needs as a built-in

hedge toward getting less. To be sure there are no misunderstandings, it is wise to run the written plan by a knowledgeable friend or attorney before you and your employer sign it.

Consider your personal needs, too. Besides being fair to your employer, be fair to yourself. If you do not plan to return to your present job, save as much money as you can during your pregnancy and get used to living on one income. Be sure you collect all of the benefits that you are owed, such as pay for unused vacation days. Talk to Human Resources about extending your medical insurance through the completion of your pregnancy and beyond.

No matter how carefully you map out the rest of your maternity leave plan for after the delivery, *pencil in* the date when your leave ends. Maternal instincts and baby protests can change your plans. When the reality of motherhood hits and you feel a baby at your breasts, you may push back the date you return to work for weeks, months, or years.

What the laws allow. Surprisingly, current federal laws do not guarantee the right to maternity leave for all women in all companies, and state laws vary. In 1978 Congress passed the Federal Pregnancy Discrimination Act, which applies only to federal workers and companies with fifteen or more employees. This act states that "women affected by pregnancy, childbirth, or related medical conditions shall be treated the same for all employment-related purposes, including receipt of benefits under fringe benefits programs, as other persons not so affected but similar in their ability or inability to work." This act does not entitle you to special treatment because you are pregnant, but it does entitle you to the same disability rights as any other employee in your company. Pregnancy is treated as a medical disability under the law to ensure that women are not denied medical or other workplace benefits.

A company cannot:

- Deny you a job because you are pregnant.

- Fire you because you are pregnant. Your employer may change or terminate your job only for business-related reasons (such as downsizing or failure to perform), not just because you are pregnant.

- Force you to take maternity leave if you are still able to do your job.

- Terminate your employment on the grounds that your job will harm your unborn child. You have a legal right to stay on the job even if your employer maintains (correctly or not) that it is unsafe for you or your baby.

- Deny pregnancy-related benefits that are offered to married women if you are not married.

- Treat your pregnancy disability differently from any other employee disability or medical condition. For example, if employees unable to perform a job because of disability are transferred to other jobs, you have the right to likewise be transferred. If their jobs are held for them, your job must be held for you. Depending on company policy, you may not be eligible for benefits if it is determined that you were pregnant prior to being employed by your company.

The Family and Medical Leave Act (FMLA) of 1993 permits you to take unpaid, job-secured leave to meet the health needs of your family. This law requires that:

- Companies with more than fifteen employees provide their employees with twelve weeks of unpaid leave in the case of the birth or adoption of a child or the care of a foster child; or in the case of the need to care for a child, spouse, or parent (or yourself) with a serious health condition. (The company may choose to offer some or all of the twelve weeks as paid leave, but this act does not *require* any paid leave.) Eligible employees include regular full-time employees with at least one year's service, and part-time employees with at least 1,250 hours of service during the twelve months before the beginning of the leave. The employer may require that you first use your paid vacation or personal time for any part of the twelve-week period.

- The employee must be returned to the same job or a job equivalent in pay, benefits, and other terms and conditions of employment.

- The employer must maintain your preexisting health benefits for the period of the leave.

An important exception to this act is that if you are among the highest-paid 10 percent of employees and if the employer can prove "substantial and grievous economic injury" to the company by your absence, he or she can deny you the same job when you return. (For more about what the law allows, see "Resources for Working Women's Rights," page 191.)

RESOURCES FOR WORKING WOMEN'S RIGHTS

To learn more about your rights to a safe workplace and job protection while pregnant, consult the following resources:

- The Women's Bureau, U.S. Department of Labor, dol.gov/wb. Search for information on the Family and Medical Leave Act and download the publication "A Guide to Women's Equal Pay Rights."

- Your regional office of the U.S. Department of Labor, dol.gov/dol/location.htm.

- The Federal Equal Employment Opportunity Commission (EEOC) for information about the federal Pregnancy Discrimination Act, eeoc.gov/eeoc/publications/fs-preg.cfm.

- The National Association of Working Women, 9to5.org.

- "Sex Discrimination in the Workplace: A Legal Handbook," available from online bookstores.

MY PREGNANCY JOURNAL: FOURTH MONTH

Emotionally I feel:

_____

_____

_____

_____

_____

Physically I feel:

_____

_____

_____

_____

_____

My thoughts about you:

_____

_____

_____

_____

My dreams about you:

_____

_____

_____

_____

_____

MY PREGNANCY JOURNAL: FOURTH MONTH

What I imagine you look like:

_____

_____

_____

_____

_____

My favorite exercises:

_____

_____

_____

_____

_____

My top concerns:

_____

_____

_____

_____

_____

My best joys:

_____

_____

_____

_____

_____

Visit to My Healthcare Provider

Questions I had; answers I got:

_____

_____

_____

_____

Tests and results; my reaction:

_____

_____

_____

_____

_____

Updated due date: _____

My weight: _____

My blood pressure: _____

Feeling my uterus; my reaction:

_____

_____

_____

_____

How I feel now that I am starting to show:

_____

_____

_____

_____

_____

Sonogram photo or side-view photo of my pregnant belly:

Comments:

_____

_____

_____

_____

_____

_____

_____

FIFTH-MONTH VISIT TO YOUR HEALTHCARE PROVIDER
(17–20 WEEKS)

During this month's visit you may have:

- An examination of the size and height of the uterus

- An examination of your abdomen to feel the top of the uterus

- An examination of your breasts and skin

- An examination for swelling of hands and legs and enlargement of veins

- A weight and blood pressure check

- Urinalysis to test for infection, sugar, and protein

- An opportunity to hear baby's heartbeat

- An opportunity to see baby on ultrasound, if indicated

- An assessment of fetal activity — how often your baby moves and what it feels like

- An opportunity to discuss your feelings and concerns

Fifth Month: Obviously Pregnant

Well, moms, this is the time you've been waiting for! For many mothers, this is the feel-best month of their pregnancy, physically and emotionally. Most moms are awestruck. Last month you heard the sound of your baby's heartbeat and perhaps also saw the reassuring ultrasound that confirmed his presence. This month, feeling your baby move is the amazing proof that you are indeed mothering a little person inside. Your pregnancy is certainly obvious to you, if not to all onlookers. On the roller-coaster ride of pregnancy, this month is most certainly an emotional "high."

I remember the first time I felt my baby really move — I had a visceral reaction: there's someone in there! Even though I'd known intellectually that I was pregnant, feeling such clear evidence of another person's presence was a thrilling shock.

HOW YOUR BABY IS GROWING, 17–20 WEEKS

During this month you can feel your cantaloupe-size uterus ascend to the level of your navel. Your baby weighs in at around 12 ounces and is now half as long as she will be at birth, or about the length of a banana. From head to toe a lot is going on. As baby swallows amniotic fluid, it goes through the rapidly maturing intestinal tract. Hiccups are now so pronounced you may feel them. Hair and eyebrows grow in more and baby has unique fingerprints. Bones get stronger, as do

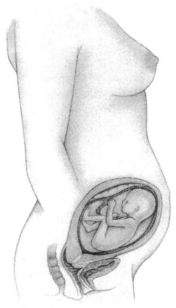

Baby at 17–20 weeks.

197

the muscles that propel those kicks. The bones of the middle ear connect better with the brain, and baby can now hear sounds. How much can baby hear from the outside world? We'll preview this on pages 206 and 254. Baby's delicate skin becomes covered with a protective coating called *vernix caseosa*, which functions as a sort of wetsuit to protect the skin from getting chapped after being in the amniotic swimming pool so long.

HOW YOU MAY FEEL

More steady emotionally. A major hormonal shift is now occurring in your body. In the first half of your pregnancy, your endocrine system had to work feverishly to make the hormones your uterus and your baby needed to grow. Since they weren't used to this new role, you may have felt that they overreacted at times. During the second half of your pregnancy, your placenta is now big enough to take over the production of most of these hormones. Your emotional roller-coaster may settle down, and most mothers describe this stage of their pregnancy as one with way fewer bad feelings and more good ones.

My baby is the best gift my body's ever given me.

Enjoying the perks of being pregnant. Now that your pregnancy is even more public, you can start enjoying the perks that come with your status. The close circle around you, even some of your previously apathetic friends, will make you feel special, because you are! Friends, even strangers, are likely to be more attentive, for example, by offering to carry things for you. Most people

are particularly polite or considerate around a pregnant woman. While you may get tired of the occasional gawker, you will generally sense others' esteem and respect for you by the tenderness they demonstrate.

I'm enjoying this stage so much, feeling so queenly and elegant with my newly emerging maternal profile. The biggest boost comes from my husband, who doesn't miss a day of coming up and putting his hands on my belly and telling me how beautiful I am to him.

Overwhelmed with advice. Be warned, though, that not all the attention and advice you will get will be welcome. At times it may seem the whole world wants to help you grow your baby! Seeing a pregnant woman can bring out the busybody in some folks, and they'll bombard you with their own personal opinions. It is important to protect yourself from those who want to share negative observations and experiences. It's OK to keep your guard up. Oftentimes your first impression will be the most accurate in guiding you through the conversation. If the person's demeanor and advice immediately make you feel good and you think, "This experienced mom could help me and my baby," then be open and attentive. On the other hand, if the word choice or body language raises your pulse and triggers your upset button, tune it out. This is practice for the constant "listen and try" versus "tune out and ignore" skills you will need after baby comes. Remember, it's normal to be hypersensitive to irritating and unwanted comments, so the quicker you can muster up your "tune out" skills, the easier it will be later on. You can always use your doctor as a scapegoat, saying "It's OK, my doctor says…"

or just "Thanks, I'll look into it." Use a positive tone and then change the subject as soon as you can.

Introspective and meditative. Now that your body has settled down a bit, your mind may naturally become preoccupied with getting to know that little person moving inside you. You may want to be alone more to meditate or just think about your baby. You will probably enjoy long periods of doing nothing more than feeling baby's kicks. You might zone out into motherly thoughts and baby imaginings at inappropriate times, such as in the middle of a conversation or during a meeting. These mental digressions are normal and necessary, as they help you prepare to prioritize for baby in the coming months.

Staying near your nest. Once you can see, hear, and feel the life inside you, your instinct might urge you to retreat into the comfort of your home and the company of a few favorite people. While many women find that keeping busy with work or social functions helps them get through their pregnancy, even the busiest pregnant woman will have times when she yearns to be among familiar things and people. Even if you are usually outgoing, you may now prefer to keep to your nest, like a sweet mama-bird.

People keep telling me, "Go out now to a movie or dinner while you can — once the baby's born, you'll be stuck at home." But I just feel like staying at home these days.

"Mommy brain" begins. Your brain is currently so focused on being pregnant that it may have a hard time switching to other decisions not related to baby. You may find yourself grasping for the right word at the right time. Feeling forgetful or "spacey" may initially scare you. While this stage may not pass as quickly as you want it to, it can improve slightly; however, it is likely to continue well into babyhood. Take heart that these momentary memory lapses rarely interfere with the ability to do your job — in and out of your home. Even the most scattered mothers-to-be are able to click into think-clearly-and-decisively mode when they need to. This mental fuzziness cannot be blamed entirely on hormones. Your brain and your body are often just plain tired. (See more about pregnancy brain on page 74.)

FEELING FIRST KICKS

Get ready to feel your little kickboxer. While first kicks are as variable in timing and action as first steps, here's what most pregnant mothers experience:

When you may feel them. The more often you've been pregnant, the earlier you can feel first kicks. Second-time moms may feel those first nudges as early as thirteen weeks, since their uterine tissues, and their memories, have been primed for what to feel; first-timers usually feel movement by twenty weeks. However, a few babies normally delay observable first kicks until

(continued)

twenty-four weeks. And thin women may experience movements earlier and stronger than well-padded moms. So, while baby has been stirring for the past couple months, it isn't until the average time of eighteen weeks that baby's arms and legs are able to really reach out and get your attention.

Dr. BJ notes: I didn't feel my baby move until almost twenty-one weeks, and I was beginning to get concerned. Of course, once his movement was clear, I realized that I had been feeling movement; it was just fainter.

During the first week of feeling kicks, you are likely to be the only one who can feel them, an intimate secret between you and baby. By twenty-four weeks anyone else permitted to touch your tummy can usually feel them, too. As the frequency and intensity of the kicks grow, so does your bonding with baby.

What you may feel. Those tiny legs don't yet have the muscle mass or bone strength to wake you up, so first kicks may feel like nothing stronger than a little nudge. If this is your first pregnancy, these movements may be mistaken for "gas." When these "gas bubbles" get stronger, you know they're the real thing. While these first movements are miniature, they are precious, unique to you, and often indescribable to anyone else. Mothers use words like "flutters," "bumps," "flicks," "twitches," "bubbles," and "little nudges." As the kicks get stronger, they graduate into thumps and punches strong enough to wake you up. In the last month

or two, you will not only feel them, you will be able to see them, as if baby is visibly trying to get your attention.

How often you may feel them. As baby grows, not only does the intensity of the kicks grow, but so does their frequency. However, there may be some weeks when the kick count is lower than others. The number of kicks is as variable as baby's personality, ranging anywhere from 50 to 1,000 kicks per day, with an average being around 200 in twenty-four hours. You are most likely to feel your baby moving when you are resting. Babies are often more active when mommy isn't, perhaps a prelude to baby's getting the days and nights mixed up. Research shows that babies in the womb move most between the hours of 8:00 p.m. and 8:00 a.m., probably because during the day they are lulled to sleep by mother's movements. In addition, when you are busy or preoccupied, you are less likely to notice them. Within a month or two, baby is likely to surprise you with stronger movement, even when your mind is engaged in something else. It's as if he is saying, "Mom, stop what you're doing and pay attention to me!"

Where you might feel them. You may feel kicks in every part of your uterus, since there is still plenty of room for baby to move around in the womb and do his gymnastics routine. Once space gets crowded, your baby will settle into the most comfortable position, with his back to your left and head down. Then, you are likely to feel the most jabs toward the center of your belly or in your lower ribs to the right.

CONCERNS YOU MAY HAVE

Vision changes. Every organ changes during pregnancy, and the eyes are no exception. The necessary increased fluid retention throughout your body actually changes the shape of your eyeballs, and with it your vision. You may find yourself squinting to focus; far or near objects may not be as distinct. Your contact lenses may feel uncomfortable or you may think you need a change of prescription glasses. Don't rush to your eye doctor yet (unless the visual changes seem extreme), as your eyeballs will return to their original shape along with the rest of most of your body after delivery. However, if you find three or four months of hazier vision unsafe or intolerable, a temporary change of eyeglass prescription, or even getting glasses temporarily, may be just what your eye doctor orders. This is probably not a good time to begin wearing contacts if you haven't done so before.

Another common, albeit temporary, visual nuisance is dry eye syndrome. The normal change in estrogen decreases the moisture in your eyes, which not only can be an uncomfortable irritation, but can increase your sensitivity to light and cause your eyes to itch, burn, and turn slightly red. You may need to use over-the-counter artificial tears to continually moisten your eyeballs. (An added benefit of the extra fish oil you are eating is that it increases the oiliness of tears.) Since your eyes may be highly sensitive to sunlight, you might find it more comfortable to wear sunglasses whenever you are outdoors. These minimal and gradual changes are normal during pregnancy, yet sudden and drastic changes, such as bleeding, severely bloodshot eyes, increasingly blurred vision, or double vision (especially if accompanied by headaches) can indicate high blood pressure. Notify your doctor if you experience any of these symptoms. Because the eyes are actually an extension of your brain, they are one of the main organs affected, for better or worse, by nutrition. (See page 30 to learn why seafood is see-food.)

Unhappy feet. If it seems as though your shoes no longer fit, you are not imagining things. Here is why your feet may change during pregnancy:

- That extra fluid you collect all over your body does settle in your ankles and feet, especially after long periods of standing.

- The pregnancy hormone relaxin that starts loosening your pelvic ligaments also loosens the ligaments that bind your foot bones together, causing them to loosen and widen. Consequently, your ankles and arches might be less supportive.

- Your extra weight, and change in the balance of the weight bearing, puts extra pressure on the already stretched structures of your ankles and feet.

Most women require shoes at least a half-size larger for the second half of their pregnancy, and some may even find that these larger shoes fit better for many months after delivery. Heed the warning, though: don't overbuy since, like your clothes, what fits now will be too loose in about six months.

Here is some advice to set you on the path to happy feet:

- Elevate them as much as possible.

- Avoid standing or sitting for long periods without a break.

- Do foot exercises: flex your toes and then pull them toward you as you point the heel away from you. Extend your leg, point your toes up, and make a circle with your toes, rotating your whole foot and ankle. This is also good for exercising the calf muscles.

- Ask for a foot massage: the masseur holds the aching foot in both hands, places her thumb just under the ball of the foot, and moves along the arch, massaging in slow circular strokes.

- Nurse swollen, painful, day's-end feet in cool water.

- Wear cotton socks to allow your feet to breathe.

- Wear proper footwear. Choose shoes with wide, low heels or wedges (no higher than 2 inches). Nonskid soles make you more sure-footed. Try soft leather or canvas shoes, preferably without laces, since sooner or later you won't be able to bend over to tie them. Shop for new shoes at the end of the day, when your feet are most swollen. Unless you are very knowledgeable about shoes, ask a salesperson's advice on proper fit. Be sure the front of your shoes is wide enough to allow your toes to fan out comfortably, and that your shoes support your feet, even if you have to sacrifice looks. If loose ligaments are causing your ankles to roll, you may have to stick to shoes that lace up since they provide more overall support. Pregnancy is not a good time to sprain an ankle.

- Insert gel heel cushions (available at most drugstores) into your shoes beginning this month.

BE SHOE SMART

Lower your heels. High heels encourage a swayback posture, which is already encouraged by your off-center baby bump. Both high heels and totally flat shoes can strain back muscles. Best are medium heels no higher than 2 inches. Put away your pumps and flip-flops temporarily, and save your knees and back, and the rest of your body, from a fall.

If your arches are painful at the end of the day, take it as a signal to stay off your feet more or try orthotic inserts — plastic arch supports that fit into your shoes. These are available at most shoe stores and pharmacies or can be custom-molded by a podiatrist. If you had flat feet prior to pregnancy, they are likely to feel even flatter in the coming months; this might be a good time to treat your feet to proper-fitting orthotic inserts.

My feet took a real beating during pregnancy. My increasing weight and the stress of chasing and carrying a toddler produced heel pain and other foot discomfort. As long as I wore my sturdy running shoes with the well-padded heel, it was bearable; but a Sunday morning in pumps guaranteed the afternoon and evening would have to be spent in very sensible shoes. And there was no going barefoot that summer. My feet needed constant protection.

Happy hair and nails. Here's one amazing side effect of your pregnancy hormones: they actually nourish your hair and nails. They lower the rate of hair loss and often leave your hair feeling thicker and looking more lustrous. You may notice less hair on your brush, and it's common to be complimented on your hair during pregnancy.

While you may have more hair, it may look and feel different. Some women report that their hair feels more dry; others report it feels more oily. Curly hair may become straighter, and straight hair may curl.

Keep in mind, though, that this lustrous season of happy hair and nails may not last long. Sometime in the early months after birth you may notice extra hair on your brush and pillow as your hair returns to its pre-pregnancy state. Interestingly enough, the hair perks of pregnancy last longer when you breastfeed.

Finally, hair growth may increase in areas you wish it didn't, namely, the face, abdomen, back, and legs. Blame this on the extra bit of male hormone you get when you're pregnant. This unwanted hair is often the first to be shed after delivery.

Here is a list of hair tips we've gathered over the years:

- Choose a style to complement your hair and face. For example, if your hair is thicker and your face has become fuller, a longer hairstyle that embraces your face may be more becoming. On the other hand, if your already long hair has become drier or more brittle, a shorter hairstyle may be more flattering and easier to take care of. A straight style can show off the luster of oilier hair; a layered look can hide flyaway dryness.

- Experiment with different shampoos. If your hair is dry, shampoo less frequently, and use a mild, low-detergent shampoo that does not wash away natural oils from the scalp. Also, use a moisturizing conditioner. If your hair is oily, shampoo more frequently.

- Towel-dry instead of using a blow-dryer.

- While standing in the shower, treat yourself to a gentle scalp massage, using your fingertips to stimulate the circulation in your scalp.

- For unwanted body and facial hair, shaving, electrolysis, and waxing are safe, but avoid bleaches and chemical hair removal, both of which can irritate your skin.

COLOR TREATMENTS WHILE PREGNANT

When your body image needs a lift, a change of hairstyle can help. But be cautious about color changes. While research has generally concluded that hair dyes are probably safe to use during pregnancy, they are not advised. Some laboratory studies show that coal-tar derivatives in dyes may cause cancer and chromosomal damage in animals. Also, the unique characteristics of "pregnant" hair can make the hair-coloring process unpredictable. It seems prudent to avoid

(continued)

exposure to hair dyes at least during the first trimester, and thereafter stick to rinses or foils that involve minimal scalp exposure and absorption.

If you can't live nine months with your present hair color, use a temporary color rather than a permanent one, and have your hair colored with applications of bleach or dye along the shaft of the hair so it's painted on rather than washed in. (The possibly dangerous dye gets into the bloodstream through the scalp, not through the hair.) It may be safest to enjoy the hair color nature gave you and to promise yourself a new look after you have given birth.

(See more green precautions on page 97.)

Since hair, skin, and nails share the same embryological source, all these seem to change together. Just like your hair, your nails are likely to grow faster. While some women find that they grow stronger, others notice they become more brittle and break more easily.

Try these nail-care tips:

- Cut your nails frequently and keep them short so they don't get a chance to break unevenly on their own.

- Take gelatin capsules to strengthen your nails — they're safe during pregnancy.

- Apply moisturizing and protective creams to your hands and nails at bedtime.

- Avoid nail polishes, which can damage your nails, and acetone-containing polish-removal products, which may not only harm your sensitive nails but give off potentially harmful fumes. If you must chemically treat and color your nails, do so outdoors, or at least in a well-ventilated room.

- Wear protective gloves when washing dishes, using household cleaners, and gardening.

(See more green precautions on page 101.)

Belly button changes. As your uterus presses outward beneath your navel, it may hurt slightly. And your belly button may pop out and become an "outie" for a while, only to become an "innie" again a few months after delivery.

Breast changes. Be aware that nipple sensitivity may increase. Your breasts may be particularly sensitive while lying on them during sleep or when they rub against your clothing. You may experience leaking colostrum, the golden yellow supermilk that your newborn will eventually enjoy. This is just one more sign of how your marvelously changing body is preparing to nourish the little life inside you.

Not feeling motherly. Here's a story from one of our parent educator/L.E.A.N. coaches:

"A mother talked to me often about how concerned she was that she did not have that 'motherly feeling.' She was afraid she wouldn't be a good mother because she did not have the same feelings that other pregnant women were talking about. She was fearing the worst and not actually allowing herself to enjoy the pregnancy. She was feeding her fear by constantly focusing on it instead of on the miracle of life she was carrying. Each time I spoke with her I would ask if she was eating right, exercising, talking to her babies (twins), and so on, and the answer was always yes. I would reassure her that she was doing everything she could to ensure the health of her babies, and that alone proved how much she loved them. I told her that not everyone has the same experience and emotions, but that did not mean she would not be a good mother. When her babies were born and she saw them for the first time, the love was overwhelming. She could not believe that she ever doubted she would love them."

Dr. Linda notes: *Mother love can come gradually. I remember being worried about my sister-in-law who had experienced several miscarriages and did not seem to be very vested in her pregnancy. She eventually became a fabulous mother to three sons. Your parental love will be there, but not every woman experiences a warm glow in pregnancy.*

Pregnant while mothering other children—help! Being pregnant while you have a toddler or preschooler in tow can be both challenging and exhausting. However, this is a "family pregnancy," so involving older children in your pregnancy can be a lot of fun for everyone. It is essential to prepare them as much as possible for life with a newborn.

Play show-and-tell. In the early months of pregnancy, even toddlers can sense that mommy is different, at least emotionally if not yet physically. As a general guide, the older the child, the sooner you can tell. Younger toddlers may not have a clue about a baby "growing in your tummy." Because they can't see it, they won't be able to understand much of the explanation. In your ninth month, when you are big as a house, your older baby will realize that it is harder for her to sit on your lap. Arrange to be around very young babies a lot so that your toddler will hear how they sound, see what they look like, observe you holding one now and then, notice that they need comforting, and learn about nursing. Once your belly is really big (around eight months), talk about the new baby, letting your child know that the baby will belong to her, too: "your new sister." Let her feel the baby's kicks, help her talk and sing to baby, and encourage her to stroke your belly. Show her simple children's books about new babies, such as *Baby on the Way* and *What Babies Need* (William Sears, Martha Sears, and Christie Watts Kelly). Show her pictures of when she was a tiny baby and tell her about all the things you did for her. Say things like "Mommies hold tiny babies a *lot* because they need that."

Once a toddler is older, closer to two years, most families elect to let him in on the big news much sooner. Depending on the age and level of understanding, tell your child why you are feeling so tired, grouchy, short-fused, impatient, or whatever else you are feeling: "Baby needs a lot of energy to grow, and that's why Mom is tired and sleeps a lot." Show your child pictures of what the baby looks like inside, especially once you're far enough along to make the baby seem real.

Martha notes: *One day four-year-old Matthew saw me lying down and asked me if I was giving the baby a rest. How neat that when he looked at me he saw baby, too.*

A time to let go. Growing a baby while raising a toddler can be exhausting. It's good for your toddler or preschooler to learn to be somewhat less dependent on you. Though he may be frustrated, not being the center of attention all the time helps him mature. This is known as "individuating," a necessary childhood developmental stage in the normal process of going from oneness to separateness. Your child learns that he can wait his turn, soothe himself sometimes when you are busy, and even assist you with your needs. As he moves into this next stage of development, you'll experience an important aspect of parenting — the gradual release of the child to whom you have been so attached. These transitions can be scary for you, so it helps to know you've given your older child what he needed when he was little. Remember, if you are anxious about letting go, your child will be anxious, too, so try to relax and embrace this transition, even if it is challenging.

You will *have enough love to go around.* Every mother expecting her second baby wonders how she'll ever be able to love another child the way she loves her first. She wonders whether there will be enough love to give to someone new. Or she wonders whether the new baby will somehow come between her and that very special toddler or preschooler. Set your mind and heart at ease about these fears. Yes, of course, you'll have enough love for your second baby, and you won't understand how it happens until it does. Love just seems to multiply — the more you give, the more you have.

Offer kids a hands-on demo. Usually by the fifth or sixth month, older children can feel their baby brother or sister move. During the times of the day or evening when your baby typically moves the most, lie down and invite your children to feel the show. Let them guess which body part they are feeling. You can show them how to be patient, and how to place their hands quietly right at the place where the kicks are coming.

Encourage baby bonding. Invite your children to talk to and about the baby. If you already know the gender and have chosen a name, encourage them to use it when referring to the baby. Or you can welcome the baby nicknames your child invents. Babies can hear at around twenty-three weeks, so this is a good time for the kids to start talking to the baby so she gets to know them. After about three months of this, their voices will be very familiar to the baby still in utero, and bonding will already be under way. Studies show that babies tend to turn toward voices they recognize right after birth.

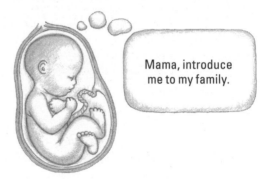

Mama, introduce me to my family.

Tyler sang three songs to the baby every night. After birth she recognized the songs. We enlisted his help with choosing names — suggestions only, leaving the final say to mom and dad. Tyler wanted to call his sister Hunca Munca.

Know your limits. Realize that while you're pregnant it's impossible to give other family members the same degree of attention they are used to. Sooner or later the children will realize that they must share Mom with another tiny taker in the family. Fortunately, pregnancy provides you with plenty of time to prepare your older children for what life will be like after the baby arrives. Getting them used to helping you while baby brother or sister is still inside is a good tool for bonding. The children will have invested their time and energy even before baby comes, and the baby will have more personal value to them.

As your pregnancy progresses, and especially in the third trimester, you will naturally become more preoccupied with your pregnancy and less willing to put up with the antics of your children. This is a good time for Dad to take over much of the childcare. Alternatively, try employing a teen helper.

The farther I got along in my pregnancy, the less tolerant I was of what I would otherwise have regarded as normal childhood behavior. I learned to address this problem on two levels: first, I made more time for myself to rest and relax, limiting my work to what had to be done; and second, I placed limits on the behavior I no longer wanted to tolerate. When my limits were defined clearly (for myself and for my children), we were all happier.

Be a positive model. While you have every reason to make excuses for how you act and feel, try not to overdo it. Be positive. You want your children to look upon your pregnancy as a joyful family enterprise, not a scary time when mom is secluded in the bedroom and bathroom. Even older children can be frightened by mom's unavailability, and seeing her sick can exacerbate their natural worries about a new baby. You especially want your daughters to understand that pregnancy and childbirth are normal parts of life and not medical conditions to be treated.

I would catch myself complaining and sometimes put on a happy face even though

I felt miserable. I didn't want my daughters to grow up in fear of having babies.

We're in this together. If your child is included in many of the practical preparations for baby, this time of waiting can be a way of deepening your bond with him even as you help him connect prenatally with the new baby. Picking out new toys together and buying clothes for baby ("these are just the ones baby will like") will get your child thinking of baby as a person who will have preferences. Getting out his old stuff can be nostalgic for you and reassuring for your child: "Oh, I remember you used to love this toy." Extra cuddle time is a great way to ease any guilt you may be feeling and any worry your child may be having. Try to nap together, since you both need the rest anyway. A retreat into your arms can go a long way toward settling insecurity.

We're in this together: involving a distant dad. Fathers-to-be recognize "their" pregnancies with varying degrees of personal involvement. Some are gung ho from the start (maybe even more so than mom) and others are likely to back away, as though they would be happy to opt out of this "woman thing" entirely and just show up for the birth. Here are some tips for both kinds of dads, but especially for dads who are unhappy with your pregnancy or are just plain distant.

Share the pregnancy. Include your parent partner when talking to family and friends about the pregnancy. "We're having a baby" is a better boast than "I'm pregnant" if you need to win over a dad-to-be who is feeling left out.

Take baby steps. Give him time to warm up to these big changes. Don't overwhelm a less-than-bubbly dad-to-be with all the decisions you have to make and the stuff you need to buy. Talk about major decisions and lifestyle changes one issue at a time, and don't do it all within the same conversation.

Don't worry, be happy to hubby. Try to find something to be cheerful about even when nausea and fatigue get your body down. What kind of pregnant person does your husband see? While some "green" days are a fact of pregnant life, weeks of complaining are bound to put off even the most sympathetic partner. Are you happy to be pregnant? If so, let your mate catch your spirit. Unfair as it seems, it might be better to unload your misery on more sympathetic female friends than on your husband. His behavior may at times feel incredibly selfish to you. Take heart! Becoming a father is one of the fastest ways for a man to stretch and grow emotionally.

Make decisions together. Involve your partner in all of the important obstetrical decisions: choosing a healthcare provider, childbirth class, and birth place, and all the decisions about routine (and not so routine) procedures. He loves you and your baby and wants the best for you; he will probably relish the chance to help you navigate the range of options in prenatal care. However, involving him in decisions about tests and technology can be a mixed blessing. On the one hand, you may find that your mate contributes valuable insight into the safety and necessity of a procedure. On the other hand, some men are enamored of the medical technology used in pregnancy and childbirth because it takes much of the mystery out of baby-growing. Thus, you may find your husband nudging you into accepting more

testing (and other interventions) than you want or feel you need. Be that as it may, the more involved your mate is in these decisions, the more likely he is to be involved throughout the pregnancy.

Go to school together. Try to attend childbirth classes together. Your partner will be amazed how much there is to learn about the miracle that is taking place! Seeing pictures and videos and getting feedback from veteran dads will open the eyes of even the most reluctant husband. With appreciation of pregnancy and birth usually comes a deep respect for the mother-to-be and involvement in her care.

An additional benefit to attending childbirth classes is that your husband will have the chance to share *his* pregnancy experience with other men. Getting together with other couples going through pregnancy can be very helpful. However, pick these couples carefully; avoid those who insist on overdosing you and your spouse with their scary birth stories.

Do your homework together. Help your husband understand why you feel and act the way you do. Read this book together, research questions together. Make learning a team endeavor! Make sure he feels needed. Your husband needs to know that his baby is likely to grow better if he nourishes you.

Enjoy a photo shoot. A series of as-you-grow portraits, artfully highlighting your blossoming belly, is a treasure well worth capturing on film. If photographing your pregnant body does not appeal to you, consider taking pictures of family, friends, your home, baby's nursery, and so on, and working with your husband to create a photo journal or other memoir of your pregnancy that you can present to baby later in life.

Invite hands-on care. Ask for a daily rubdown from your husband-turned-massage-therapist. Show how much you like and need his touch. Make these sessions special with soothing music, soft lighting, and an attractive setting, such as in a room warmed by natural sunlight. Regardless of what follows these soothing massage sessions, they are an opportunity for loving touch and expanded intimacy, two key ingredients to a healthy physical and emotional relationship.

Develop a bedtime ritual. At around twenty weeks, most dads can feel the baby move. Hearing the heartbeat and seeing baby on ultrasound are one thing, but feeling baby move is enough of a thrill to hook even the most distant father-to-be. After lights-out, as you bid each other good night, include your baby.

Martha notes: A nightly custom we enjoyed with our pregnancies is one we called the "laying on of hands." Beginning around the sixth month, before going to sleep, Bill would lay his hands on my abdomen each night to feel our baby move. He would also talk to our baby and pray a blessing. This made a double impression on me: I felt his commitment both as a mate and as a father.

Dr. Bill notes: These were precious moments for me — to feel our baby kicking inside Martha. Initially, I felt kind of foolish talking to a tiny baby whom I couldn't see and could barely feel. Then, after a while, I got to enjoy this nightly ritual, and somehow I felt baby did, too. I'll never forget those sensual bonding sessions.

Make sure he feels needed. While a few husbands instinctively know their wives' desires before they have to ask, most need to have the request made directly. Besides sending him on odd-hour treks to the supermarket to satisfy your food cravings, kindly let your partner know specifically what you need from him: help with housework, shopping, or caring for the other kids on days when you have barely enough energy for yourself and baby. Many men are more willing to help if you give them specific requests. Instead of a general "I need your help," try "I need you to do the grocery shopping today." This is good preparation for later on when he learns that "nursing" means baby comforter. While only mothers can breastfeed, father can also "nurse." Another thought: father "feeds" the mother, while mother breastfeeds baby.

Work out for three. Try exercising together. A brisk, half-hour morning or evening walk is not only a time to tone your body, it's also an opportunity for communication and connection between the two of you.

Make a date for your next prenatal visit. When you visit your practitioner, especially on visits that include exciting procedures like hearing baby's heartbeat or seeing baby on ultrasound, invite your partner along to share the experience. Ask for a souvenir ultrasound photo for him.

Share feelings. It is so important for both of you to share your feelings about the pregnancy. Knowing that you will listen to him in a nonjudgmental, accepting, and caring way can help your husband explore some of the feelings that may be putting a distance between him and the baby or between the two of you. By the same token, be careful not to let a controlling partner keep you from expressing *your* feelings. Developing a solid, trusting, comfortable pregnancy dialogue is a good warm-up for the couple talks you will later need when you become a threesome. If you find it difficult to share feelings, a professional counselor can help you learn to do so. Time and energy spent in counseling now (even just a few sessions) can make a difference in how the two of you move into parenthood together. Start working on unresolved conflicts so your couple relationship will be more ready for the stresses of life with a newborn.

When all is said and done, what your baby needs most is two happy parents who are committed to each other and to baby. It is well worth the effort it may take to draw your husband out and involve him in ways he would otherwise not manage on his own. Then prepare to watch his face light up when his newly born baby recognizes his voice and turns toward him. Once he realizes he's a *daddy,* he's likely to act like one.

GIRL OR BOY? DO YOU WANT TO KNOW?

The technology of ultrasound makes it possible for you to know your baby's gender before birth. But do you want to know? It's up to you to decide if you can't wait and must know, or if you want to be surprised at the moment of birth.

Knowing now. Knowing your baby's gender ahead of time cuts the name-choosing task down by 50 percent. Some couples feel that knowing baby's gender promotes prenatal bonding. By giving baby a specific name (rather than "the baby" or "Peanut"), they find it's easier to relate to the baby and imagine what he or she will be like. Knowing baby's gender makes your daydreams more meaningful. This knowledge also makes decorating the nursery and outfitting baby's layette easier.

My husband had his heart set on having a boy. I wanted to know our baby's gender beforehand because if our baby turned out to be a girl, I couldn't bear to see his look of disappointment at the moment of birth. Ultrasound showed we were having a girl, and this gave Daddy a few extra months to look forward to holding his daughter.

Waiting to be surprised. Other couples prefer to wait until delivery to know their baby's gender. They enjoy the mystery and the surprise and feel it gives them something to look forward to throughout labor, an added bonus at the moment of birth. If you're having an ultrasound or amniocentesis, be sure to tell your doctor or the technician ahead of time that you don't want to know whether you're having a son or a daughter.

Dr. Linda notes: Don't read too much into your caregiver's use of "he" or "she." Realize that your doctor may have trouble remembering the gender of a baby delivered two days ago, much less your ultrasound from two weeks ago.

Testing for gestational diabetes. Sometime between the fifth and sixth month your healthcare provider may test you for gestational diabetes (also called pregnancy-induced diabetes), especially if you have risk factors such as overweight, poor lifestyle and nutritional habits, or a previous history of this condition. A high blood sugar alerts you to change your diet and lifestyle habits to lower and steady your blood sugar, and it prepares your birth attendant for possible complications, such as prematurity and a more challenging delivery. Your healthcare provider may focus a lot on helping you maintain a steady blood sugar during your pregnancy. Continued exposure to high blood sugar during pregnancy may prompt baby to make too much of his or her own insulin. Baby is then born in a state of what is called hyperinsulinism, which can cause the blood sugar to drop dramatically soon after birth, a condition called neonatal hypoglycemia.

Once upon a time an oral glucose tolerance test (OGTT) was performed to detect gestational diabetes. Mother would drink 50 or 100 grams of a sweetened beverage and her blood sugar would be checked at one hour, and sometimes two or three hours, after drinking this glug of sugar. Two problems with this older test have led to its decline in use recent years. First, abnormal results can cause unnecessary worry. Second, OGTT may not be a medically wise test. As one mother said to us, "I did not want to take the OGTT. If I don't eat like that anyway (meaning she never consumes 50 to 100 grams, or 10 to 20 teaspoons, of pure sugar), what do the results mean in my case?" We believe that she has a valid point. In medicalspeak: Doing a test in an abnormal situation is likely to give you abnormal and not useful results. Many obstetricians have concluded that the routine use of OGTT causes more worry than benefits.

Should you get an oral glucose tolerance test? In our opinion, usually not. A 2006 study in the *American Journal of Obstetrics and Gynecology* tested women for gestational diabetes in various ways: fasting blood sugar level, fasting insulin level, and the three-hour 100-gram oral OGTT. The fasting blood sugar level test demonstrated the best accuracy, as did the fasting insulin level test. The conclusion of these researchers was that fasting blood sugar alone or in combination with insulin level is more sensitive than the OGTT, especially for women who would like to avoid the unnatural and upsetting biochemical imbalance of drinking 100 grams of pure sugar. Many healthcare providers rely on the fasting blood sugar and/or the insulin level tests and no longer put mother through the outdated OGTT. (See the section on gestational diabetes, page 413.)

Dr. Linda notes: A lot of women don't want to have a glucose screening test. This is fine if the woman is in her twenties, thin, and physically active. Often the women who want to avoid the test reason that they have healthy diets. When a thirty-nine-year-old woman is 40 pounds overweight, there is a lot of denial here. While testing is open to debate, it is important to recognize the toll that diabetes can take on mothers and babies, and women need to listen to their doctor's or midwife's advice.

MY PREGNANCY JOURNAL: FIFTH MONTH

Emotionally I feel:

_____

_____

_____

_____

Physically I feel:

_____

_____

_____

_____

My thoughts about you:

_____

_____

_____

_____

My dreams about you:

_____

_____

_____

_____

What I imagine you look like:

_____

_____

_____

_____

My top concerns:

_____

_____

_____

_____

_____

My best joys:

_____

_____

_____

_____

Visit to My Healthcare Provider

Questions I had; answers I got:

_____

_____

_____

_____

_____

MY PREGNANCY JOURNAL: FIFTH MONTH *(continued)*

Tests and results; my reaction:

_____

_____

_____

_____

Updated due date: _____

My weight: _____

My blood pressure: _____

Feeling my uterus; my reaction:

_____

_____

_____

How I feel now that the whole world can see I'm pregnant:

_____

_____

_____

_____

How I felt when I first felt you move:

_____

_____

_____

MY PREGNANCY JOURNAL: FIFTH MONTH

How I feel now that I am wearing maternity clothes:

_____

_____

_____

_____

What I bought when I went shopping:

_____

_____

_____

_____

Sonogram photo and/or photo of my blooming:

Comments:

_____

_____

_____

_____

_____

_____

_____

SIXTH-MONTH VISIT TO YOUR HEALTHCARE PROVIDER
(21–25 WEEKS)

During this month's visit you may have:

- An examination of the size and height of the uterus

- A weight and blood pressure check

- Urinalysis to test for infection, sugar, and protein

- Oral glucose tolerance test, screening for gestational glucose intolerance, if indicated

- Vaginal culture, screening test for beta strep infection, if indicated (learn more about Group B Streptococcus on page 412)

- An opportunity to hear your baby's heartbeat

- An opportunity to see your baby on ultrasound, if indicated

- An opportunity to discuss your feelings and concerns

15

Sixth Month: Feeling Baby Move

This month your baby will go through a huge growth spurt, gaining about one pound! Naturally, as your baby grows, so will you, probably putting on 4 or 5 pounds yourself. As baby's little muscles get stronger, you will feel more and more of those magnificent movements. Not only can you feel your baby move more, so can everyone who has the privilege of laying their hands on this active little bundle. Your uterus expands above your navel and the baby bump shows in all its glory. Enjoy gazing at your new profile in the mirror!

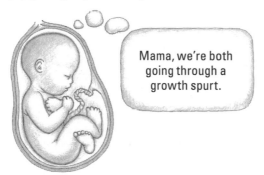

Mama, we're both going through a growth spurt.

HOW YOUR BABY IS GROWING, 21–25 WEEKS

Baby is now around a foot long and weighs about a pound and a half. By the twenty-fourth week, baby's nostrils open and her face is more baby-like. In fact, this month baby truly looks like a tiny baby. Baby's sense of taste is more developed and here is when researchers believe, with a bit of scientific support, that mother's diet influences the flavor of the amniotic fluid, which begins shaping baby's tastes for food later on. (Breast milk has this taste-shaping feature, too.) Toward the end of this month, actual breathing movements begin. Even though baby's lungs still lag behind the other organs in development, tiny air sacs, called alveoli, start blossoming out like flowers and now stay open a bit, though not enough to sustain breathing on their own outside the womb. In fact, many babies born at six months survive and do quite well, obviously within the modern neonatal intensive care unit and on assisted breathing until the lungs mature. Baby's skin is now completely covered with a thin layer of whitish paste, called vernix. The skin is still loose and wrinkly because the subcutaneous fattening up hasn't yet begun. Baby's bone marrow also starts making more blood cells. If you could sneak a peak, you might see baby experimenting with more hand and face play: thumb-sucking or face-rubbing. How darling!

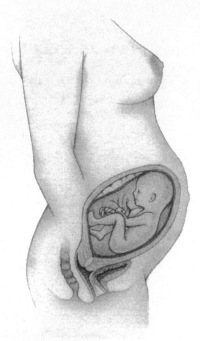

Baby at 21-25 weeks.

How baby is growing emotionally.

Around five or six months, prenatal researchers believe that babies are more connected to what's going on outside. For example, baby may startle in response to a bright light blinking at mother's abdomen. At this time, baby and mother begin to share emotions. What mother feels, baby may in some way "feel" (happy, calm, angry, frightened). Baby may also now start reacting to the tone of mother's voice. Soothing tones calm baby; angry or anxious tones can upset him.

HOW YOU MAY FEEL

Most women continue to enjoy the middle trimester. They delight in feeling pretty darn good most of the time and although they are big enough to look pregnant, they aren't so large that their bodies become unwieldy.

Enjoying more kicks. The gentle twitches and soft kicks of the last month give way to little jabs now — all over the bump. In fact, you'll have fun chasing baby around to feel those little thumps.

One night as I lay on my left side and snuggled close to my husband, our son kicked and kicked for thirty-five minutes. Finally, my husband looked at me and said, "Just roll over, please." I remember thinking, "Is this an insight into my son's personality?" My son is four years old and he is very strong willed, and I would not have him any other way.

Feeling these little kicks can be fun for the whole family. Once your other kids get a feel for baby's movements, get ready for those curious little hands to constantly be on your abdomen. Enjoy a before-bed or morning ritual of feeling and talking to baby. Your kids will get a "kick" out of this and may eagerly anticipate baby's active times. To help your child feel baby move, place her hand where you last felt a lot of movement and hold it there with some gentle pressure for a while. If your child does not show particular interest in the kicking yet, don't worry. It may be too abstract to her; it doesn't mean she won't be interested in the baby. Record in your pregnancy journal the "kick quotes" of your children's reactions to feeling baby move.

You may also begin seeing baby's movement from the outside. While sitting at your desk you may look down and see something jump beneath your clothing. As you lie down you can watch areas of the bulge "bubble up" from beneath. Anticipate that next month this amazing sight will be even more noticeable.

When my husband first felt our baby kick (the twenty-third week), he finally made the connection with our baby that I had waited for so longingly. To be able to feel movements highlights the reality of baby's presence in such a beautiful way. When baby starts to move, I suddenly realize that he is awake and conscious on some level that we are only starting to understand. If he is awake, is he aware of us, too — our voices, our movements, our hands pressing over the place where he kicks? Is he getting a message back from us?

Feeling your uterus "move." Around the end of the sixth month you may start feeling "minicontractions." These are called Braxton Hicks contractions (also dubbed "false labor" or "practice contractions") and indicate that your uterus has started flexing its muscles as a warm-up for the big event. In reality, your uterus seldom rests, as these muscles actually contract and relax a lot, even though you may not always feel them. Some women even feel these little squeezes as early as the fourth or fifth month. Unlike the real thing, Braxton Hicks are short, relatively painless, irregular, and may feel like mild-to-moderate menstrual cramps. Many women describe them as a "tightening sensation" in their uterus. Unlike these practice squeezes, true labor contractions are longer, stronger, more frequent, and definitely more uncomfortable, and they follow a consistent pattern.

These practice contractions are thought to tone up your uterus for the strenuous work it will soon have to do. Think of it as prenatal exercise for the uterus. Expect them to become more frequent and uncomfortable in the eighth or ninth month, as baby enters, shall we say, the homestretch.

When you feel the squeeze coming on, rehearse the relaxation skills you are learning in childbirth classes. This warm-up helps you prepare for the real thing, when you will need a lot more mind-over-contraction focus.

Need to slow down. On the days you overdo it, you will know it. After a busy day, you will need some catch-up rest that evening or the next day. Exhaustion is your body's reminder that there is just not enough energy, emotional or physical, to continue a busy lifestyle *and* grow a baby. If you feel that you need to keep busy to get through your pregnancy, try to balance physical exertion with rest, mental stimulation with mindless relaxation, work that makes the time fly with leisure that allows your mind and body to catch up.

Sleepier. Getting bigger is likely to make you feel sleepier. One reason for this is that it's becoming more challenging to take a deep breath, and so the biochemical sleep-inducer, carbon dioxide, builds up. If you find you're dozing off at inconvenient times, such as during work, take several deep breaths to perk yourself back up. (See the deep breathing tips on page 255.)

New Aches and Pains

Even though the middle trimester is a relatively peaceful and comfortable season of your pregnancy, as your uterus grows, you'll probably experience new discomforts.

Leg cramps. Just as you're likely to feel little bumps in the night, be prepared to feel little cramps. Toward the end of the middle trimester and throughout the last one, many women are awakened by knot-like cramps in their calf muscles or feet. These cramps are sometimes blamed on an electrolyte imbalance of calcium, phosphorus, magnesium, or potassium. An additional explanation is that circulation decreases to the most active muscles in your legs. Pressure of the uterus on major blood vessels, as well as standing, sitting, or lying for a long time, can slow blood supply to these muscles, causing them to cramp up.

Preventing leg cramps. You can help prevent leg cramps by both improving the circulation and decreasing the swelling in your leg muscles:

- Wear support stockings during the day. Avoid standing or sitting for long periods.

- Exercise your calf muscles before going to bed: try the foot exercises described on page 202. The cramp-relief exercises described below are also good preventive measures. Do them about ten times on each side.

- Have your mate massage your calf muscles before you go to bed.

- Elevate your legs on a pillow at night.

- Lie on your left side in the sleeping position shown on page 85.

Relieving cramps. Besides the standard cramp cures of massage, rubbing, and getting up and moving around, try these:

- Standing calf stretches. Place the leg with the cramped muscles one foot or so behind your other leg. While keeping your back straight, gently bend the knee of the noncramped leg so that you are leaning forward while keeping the cramped leg straight and its heel on the floor. (The forward leg also keeps its heel on the floor.) Without bouncing, stretch gently. You may find it easier to balance if you press your hands or forearms against the wall while doing this stretching exercise.

- Wall push-ups. Place your hands flat against the wall and step back until your arms are fully extended. Keeping your feet flat on the floor and your back straight, lean in toward the wall while bending your elbows. You should feel your calf muscles stretch comfortably. If it's too much of a stretch, stand closer to the wall.

- Sitting leg stretches. Sitting on the floor, stretch the cramped leg out to the side, foot flexed. Fold your other leg in, foot toward your crotch. While keeping your outstretched leg straight, bend forward and reach toward your toe. Hold this stretched position for a few seconds. Don't point your toes straight out and pull your heel toward you since that contracts the muscles that are already cramped.

- Bed stretches. Sit up in bed, grab the toes of your cramping leg, and pull back on them while keeping your leg straight. If your tummy bulge prevents you from bending forward enough to grab your toes, straighten your leg, pressing the back of your knee into the mattress and flexing your foot, toes pointing toward you.

Remember to stretch *gradually.* Avoid lunging or bouncing movements, which only aggravate the cramp and may even injure the muscles. While an electrolyte imbalance is likely to be the cause of your leg cramps, if they continue despite all these measures, consult your healthcare provider for a nutritional makeover. Reread page 48 to be sure you're getting enough calcium, potassium, and magnesium. While these stretches are targeted to relieve leg cramps, you can also do them daily as part of your general exercise routine to help prevent cramps.

Numbness and tingling in your hands.
The carpal tunnel is a narrow space between your wrist and the base of your palm where the nerves and tendons cross over the wrist bones and tunnel into the carpal bones of the hand. Any swelling in this area can pinch the nerves that supply sensations to the thumb, the first two fingers, and half the ring finger, causing them to feel numb or tingly. The extra fluid that seems to accumulate during pregnancy can settle in the sheath beneath the ligament running across your wrist. And when you overuse swollen tissue, you're likely to feel it.

A full 25 percent of pregnant women experience tingling in their hands toward the last half of their pregnancy. This pins-and-needles or burning sensation may be accompanied by pain in the wrist that can shoot all the way up to the shoulder. Sometimes you may feel soreness when you press the inner surface of your wrist. This condition is known as "carpal tunnel syndrome."

Carpal tunnel syndrome is a common repetitive strain injury among those who work with their hands a lot (such as checking groceries at the supermarket, playing the piano, or working on computer keyboards). Symptoms are most likely to occur during the night, after a daylong accumulation of fluid in the wrists, or when you wake up in the

morning, especially if you sleep with your arm under your head.

To ease carpal tunnel syndrome discomfort, try these strategies:

- Rest your hands more during the day.

- Soak your hands in cool water to reduce swelling.

- If you work on a computer, type with your wrists in the neutral position or flexed slightly down rather than with your wrists curved up. Use a wrist rest to help you maintain this position. There are ergonomic keyboards designed for this condition.

- Elevate the affected hand(s) on a pillow at night.

- Wear a plastic splint (available in drugstores, or your doctor can prescribe a custom-fitted one) at night to immobilize your wrist in a neutral position.

- If repeated phone use triggers these discomforts, use a headset or speakerphone so you don't have to use your wrists as much.

- As often as you can, elevate your hands.

- If the pain is getting more frequent and severe, your doctor may refer you to a specialist for cortisone injections, which will immediately relieve the swelling. This is safe during pregnancy.

As with nearly all the muscle aches and pains during pregnancy, carpal tunnel syndrome goes away after delivery. Some breastfeeding mothers need to continue to use their splints until the body's fluid balance adjusts to lactation, in about four to six weeks. The use of the wrists is important for positioning the baby properly at the breast, and long periods of time spent holding the baby in one position for nursing can aggravate carpal tunnel syndrome. A lactation consultant can help you with special positioning tips, for example, by using pillows to help you hold baby correctly without stressing your wrist.

Shooting pains in your lower back and legs. You may feel pains in your back and legs due to swelling tissue. As your baby and your uterus grow, the center of gravity from your whole midsection shifts, straining your back, hips, and legs. You may occasionally feel shooting pains, tingling, or numbness in your lower back, buttocks, outer thighs, or legs. These occur when your loosened pelvic joints, the baby's head, or your enlarging uterus press on the major nerves that run from your spine through the pelvis and toward each leg. Sudden, sharp pain that begins deep in the buttock on one side and travels down the back of that leg is due to pressure on the sciatic nerve in your lower back; hence the name "sciatica." Sciatica is aggravated by lifting, bending, or even walking. Tingling numbness and pain along the outer thigh is caused by stretching of the femoral nerve. Here are some strategies to help you with aches and pains:

- Change positions often. Shifting your center of gravity shifts all those organs that are "getting on your nerves." Try the knee-chest position (see page 72), which shifts the pelvic organs away from these nerves. Keep experimenting to find a position that alleviates the pain.

- Enjoy a warm bath.

- Place ice packs at the site of the pain.

- Try alternating ice packs and a heating pad at the site of the pain.

- Enjoy a back massage.

- Work it off: doing pelvic tilt exercises (see page 71) several times a day tends to stretch and relax the aching tendons and joints.

- Swim it off. As you swim, you rhythmically and naturally change the center of gravity, and therefore all those pelvic pressure points, so swimming may be just what the back doctor ordered.

- Move more slowly. Sudden twisting or reaching movements are likely to fuel the fire of these pains.

- Sleep in the "position of comfort" as shown on page 85.

- If back pain and/or sciatica pain become severe enough, ask your doctor or midwife for a referral to a physical therapist, preferably one trained in maternity care.

In the later months your backaches may become more than just an occasional annoyance and you will need additional measures to be kind to your back (see page 222).

Soothing a backache. To soothe your aching back:

- Stand in a shower with a jet of warm water focused on the painful area, or enjoy the warm-water jet from a Jacuzzi, being careful not to overheat your body (see page 68).

- Place alternating hot and cold packs on the painful area.

- Assume the knee-chest position to bring your uterus forward a bit, easing the pressure against your spine (see illustration, page 72).

- Ask hubby for a back massage in the side-lying position. It's good practice for the new masseur to help ease the pain of back labor. Have him try this technique:

    1. Massage down each side of your spine, using his thumbs to apply pressure along the way.

    2. Extend the massage along both sides of your lower back.

    3. Have him knead your neck and shoulder muscles, then massage down your backbone and across your lower back.

Ten ways to prevent backache. During the second half of pregnancy, as baby grows more and more, many mothers have that daily, even hourly, feeling of "Oh, my aching back!" What's good for your back also helps alleviate pains in all the joints below the back, especially your hips and knees:

1. *Practice the best posture for pregnancy.* Your overstretched abdominal muscles, pulling you forward, force you to rely on your back muscles to pull you backward to maintain your balance. Eventually, the overworked muscles and back ligaments protest in pain.

2. *Head up.* You probably spend much of your day looking down, either using a computer, reading a book, or watching where you walk so you don't stumble. This bent-over position causes extra strain on the neck and back muscles, causing some pregnant women to have the stooped-over appearance of old age. To give your neck and back muscles a lift, look up to the sky as often as possible. Even while walking, look down with your eyes, not your head.

3. *Stand smart.* Try these exercises to help strengthen the structures of your back:

- Bend your knees slightly instead of locking them. Feel how your thigh muscles flex as they absorb some of the weight from your knee and back joints.

- Tilt your hips and pelvis slightly forward, tucking in your buttocks. To do this you may need to tighten your buttock and abdominal muscles. Feel how this straightens your back, which is overarched by your protruding abdomen.

- Place one foot on a stool or step while standing to lessen strain on your back.

- Take standing breaks at work if your job requires sitting most of the day. Periodically stand up and, while inhaling deeply, slowly stretch your hands to the ceiling. This exercise extends the bones of the lumbar spine that have been compressed by prolonged sitting.

4. *Sit smart.* If your lumbar spine bones could talk they would say: preserve your curve. The curve of your back decreases by as much as 30 percent when you sit down. Many mothers find that a lumbar cushion is their back's best friend.

- No matter where you are sitting, preserve your curve with a rolled-up towel or even your mate's folded jacket.

- Use an adjustable chair, especially at work. Sitting in a chair that is too high increases swayback, but one too low flattens the lumbar spine. It is best to keep your feet flat on the floor or on a footstool and your knees level with, or slightly higher than, your hips.

- Avoid the common habit of crossing your legs while sitting, as this contributes to poor circulation and promotes varicose veins.

- Avoid sitting for long periods of time and then suddenly springing up, which stretches and strains your ligaments. While sitting, do foot-flexing exercises to increase circulation.

- Descending bottom first onto a hard chair jars the sensitive lumbar bones. Ease slowly onto a cushioned seat. Do not sit on a hard seat while driving on a bumpy road.

- Adjust your car's seat position relative to the steering wheel so that your knees are raised. Support your lower back with a lumbar cushion.

5. *Lift smart.* To avoid lower back strain — and pain — use your legs, not your back, as a lever. Squat instead of stooping over. Never bend your back without first bending your knees. Instead of bending at the waist to pick up heavy objects (you shouldn't be picking up heavy objects while you're pregnant anyway), bend your knees and keep your back straight. Pull the object close to your thighs; then gradually stand up, allowing the legs to bear most of your

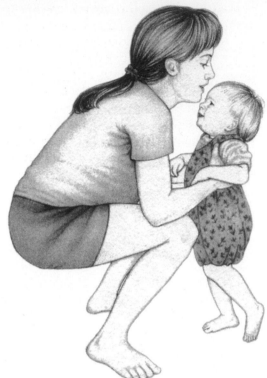

Lift smart.

weight. When moving heavy objects off a table, don't bend at the waist; instead keep your upper body perpendicular to the floor and the heavy object as close to your body as possible. Avoid lifting heavy objects above the level of your elbows. As a general guide, anything over 35 pounds is too heavy for your sensitive back muscles.

6. *Carry smart.* Have someone else carry heavy bags for you. If you have to carry heavy grocery bags yourself, try to distribute the weight evenly on both sides, in the same way you would hold barbells of equal weight in each hand.

7. *Don't twist or you'll shout.* Avoid sudden twisting, especially when getting out

of bed in the morning. During prolonged sleep, lumbar disks swell, making them prone to injury from sudden torques. Instead, roll over onto your side, use your hands to push your upper body into a sitting position, place your feet on the floor, and then stand. When getting into a car, ease yourself into the seat backside first. When exiting the car, open the door, turn your whole body to plant your feet on the ground, then hold onto the door for support as you slowly stand up.

8. *Be deliberate with your moves.* When shifting from standing to sitting, lower yourself gently. Extend your arms behind you, bend your knees, and let your thighs do most of the work. Resist the temptation to simply fall into a chair. While it certainly won't hurt the baby, it could, in later months, cause you to strain some already loose ligaments. To stand from sitting, once again make the most of your leg muscles. With your feet well under you, push up from your calves. Take care not to jerk yourself forward; it may be faster, but it can wreak havoc on your lower back. In fact, any kind of movement while pregnant is best done a bit more deliberately than you're used to. Be particularly vigilant when lifting a young toddler out of a car seat. After unbuckling the car seat, turn the seat toward you before you lift your child out. An older toddler can help himself down after you unbuckle his harness.

9. *Enjoy back-building muscle exercises.* Traditional back-builders require lying on your abdomen, which, of course, you can't do. Try this favorite yoga back exercise instead: Get on all fours. Raise your right arm and left leg, pointing them straight out. Tighten your abdominal muscles while keeping your head down in line with your back. Hold for ten seconds, then use the opposite arm and leg. Repeat this cycle three times. Feel your back muscles tighten and strengthen as you raise each leg. Do the pelvic tilt exercises shown on page 71.

10. *Tread lightly.* Fortunately, most women don't walk like men, who are heavy-heeled pounders walking in a clump-clump-clump way. As much as possible, don't jog or even walk on hard surfaces, such as concrete or asphalt, which can jar the sensitive joints, especially the spine. Walk on natural surfaces like grass, earth, or sand. Finally, wear pregnancy-appropriate shoes. High heels accentuate the forward curvature of the spine and aggravate the back. Pain will be minimized by wearing flat or relatively low-heeled shoes with arch support. (See also our recommendations for wearing heel cushions while pregnant, page 202, and selecting shoes, page 202.)

I've now developed the "pregnancy sway." When I walk I swing my arms and my belly gets its own momentum going, separate from my body. If I don't catch myself and correct my posture, my back goes into an extreme sway and my shoulders slump forward. This posture causes my back and hips to ache, so I try to keep my pelvis tilted and my shoulders square.

CONCERNS YOU MAY HAVE

As you've read, swelling tissue causes many changes. Here are some conditions you might experience this month:

Enlarging veins. Pregnancy hormones relax and widen your veins, contribute to swelling of tissue around them, and increase blood volume. While you may notice veins all over your body getting larger, such as little knots in the veins along the sides of your neck, the tissue around your vagina, and elsewhere, your legs are the most visible host to varicose veins. Your expanding uterus puts pressure on the pelvic blood vessels, and this in turn puts pressure on the veins of the legs and often causes blood to pool in them. Large veins, especially those of the neck and legs, have one-way valves to keep the blood flowing toward your heart. This flow of blood is impeded by all the pressure, causing these valves to weaken, and leading to the bulging, knotty, bluish-purple areas you see and even feel under the skin. The good news is that in a few months, delivering your baby will deliver you from this problem. To reduce the unwanted appearance and annoyance of varicose veins:

- Avoid standing or sitting for long periods of time. Gravity is a particular foe for varicose veins.

- When sitting, elevate your feet and avoid crossing your legs.

- Lie and sleep on your left side, as shown on page 85.

- To keep the blood moving and not pooling, keep your legs and feet moving by doing the leg pumping exercises described on page 179.

- If you need to stand in line for a long time, pace a few feet in each direction and do leg-pumping exercises. If pumping your legs throws you off balance while standing, lean on your mate or a willing bystander. A nearby mom will understand and will often lend a shoulder to lean on.

- Wear loose-fitting clothing. Avoid tight pants, tight waistbands, and tight socks, which can restrict circulation in your legs.

- Wear support hose. Put them on before you get out of bed in the morning, before gravity gives your veins a chance to pop out. Avoid knee-high support stockings, since the band at the top can constrict blood return.

From Martha's journal: I marvel at the incredible changes my body has gone through to accommodate this pregnancy. It's as though my whole abdominal structure is being remodeled, brought on by relentless inner changes. My body is really not my own anymore — it has been taken over by a process and a presence that draws everything it needs without regard to how I might be affected. I can only stand by and watch it happen and realize the consequence of sharing my body with someone else. The takeover is not pleasant at times, yet these discomforts are a small price to pay to welcome our baby.

Hemorrhoids. Varicose veins appear not only in the legs, but also around the inside of your rectum, causing rectal pain and streaking of bright red blood that you may notice on toilet paper. Yes, you can blame those little pains-in-the-butt on the same pressures that cause varicose veins in your legs. Additionally, the constipation that often accompanies pregnancy can further aggravate these nuisances. Hemorrhoids occur around the anal opening and look like pea-sized clusters that bulge out, bleed, itch, and sting, especially during the passage of a hard bowel movement. (During the downward pressure of delivery, these little "peas" swell up like grapes.) Hemorrhoids are usually at their largest — and most uncomfortable — in the eighth and ninth months. However, some women find them at their worst after the downward pressure of pushing while giving birth. Like all those other big vessels around your body, they too will shrink after delivery.

Preventing hemorrhoids. While it's difficult to completely prevent these little pains-in-the-behind, here are things you can do to reduce their occurrence:

- Prevent constipation (see pages 22 and 150).

- Graze according to the rule of twos (see page 21).

- Exercise a lot.

- Avoid sitting or standing for long periods of time to keep blood from pooling.

- Practice your Kegel exercises (see page 68).

Treating hemorrhoids. If these swollen blood vessels occur, here's how to manage them:

- Wipe gently after a bowel movement, using more of a patting motion than a rubbing one. Consider using moistened wipes instead of regular toilet paper.

- Apply cool or cold compresses: crushed ice in a clean sock will shrink the vessels and alleviate the pain. Lie on a thick towel to keep water from soaking your sheet.

- To relieve itching, take a short soak in a warm bath to which a half cup of baking soda has been added. (While warm water can soothe an itchy bottom, it can also dilate blood vessels and further aggravate bleeding, so don't stay in for more than a few minutes.)

- Place a cotton ball or gauze pad soaked in cool witch hazel (or a medicated pad recommended by your healthcare provider) against the hemorrhoids to help shrink them and ease the discomfort.

- If you find the hemorrhoids extremely irritating or painful, assume the knee-chest position (see the illustration on page 72), which takes pressure off the swollen blood vessels momentarily while you await relief from the witch hazel or other remedy.

- If you must sit on a very sore bottom, buy a rubber doughnut to place on your sitting surface. Some women, though, find the pressure the doughnut puts on the buttocks aggravating. Alternatively, sit on a pillow, or lean to one side while sitting.

- Check with your doctor before using an over-the-counter hemorrhoid medication. Though there is little evidence that these ointments are dangerous to baby, some of them are absorbed through the rectal tissue and into the bloodstream.

Leaking urine. Yes, it's that pelvic pressure again! You may notice that every time you sneeze, you have to cross your legs or else you wet your pants a bit. Don't worry — this problem should go away after the baby is born. When you sneeze, cough, or belly-laugh, your diaphragm contracts and pushes your abdominal organs and uterus down onto your bladder, causing you to dribble urine if your bladder is full or your pelvic-floor muscles are weak. To avoid this nuisance:

- Keep your bladder as empty as possible by urinating frequently and practicing the triple-voiding technique: grunt and bear down three times to completely empty your bladder.

- Open your mouth when you cough to avoid building up pressure in your chest and abdomen.

- Strengthen the muscles that control urination by practicing Kegel exercises (page 68). Contract and release these muscles between bathroom visits, as if you were trying to stop urination. But don't stop urinating once you start, as this could cause urine to reflux back up into the kidneys, leading to a urinary tract infection.

- Wear a panty liner or maxipad to absorb leaks.

Later on, you may worry that leaked urine is really amniotic fluid leaking, but you will be able to tell the difference by the telltale odor of urine — and by the fact that amniotic fluid doesn't stop once it starts leaking.

My mother advised me to bend my knees and lean forward slightly if I have to sneeze or cough while standing — a big help.

Abdominal muscles separating. This is a unique pregnancy occurrence. While you may think that you have a hernia in the middle of your pregnant belly, you don't. Normally, the two bands of muscle that run down the middle of your abdomen from your ribs to pubic bone separate as your uterus grows, leaving your belly button pooching out. If you run your fingers across your belly button, you may feel a gap where the muscles have separated, and the gap will get bigger in the next two months. The muscles will come back together and fill in the gap a few months after delivery. Be prepared for your lower abdominal muscles to be a little looser and droopier with each pregnancy.

MEN: FEELING PREGNANT

Yes, guys, your hormones do change as part of the "we're pregnant" duet. You may feel morning sickness. It may be the first time in your life when you lose some libido. Dubbed "couvade syndrome" after the French word *couver* ("to hatch"), as many as 50 percent of dads share some of the quirks of their pregnant wife. While there are many theories, this is probably a side effect of the physiological bonding many couples experience during "their" pregnancy.

As mom's sexual hormones take a downturn as delivery day approaches, so may dad's. Her body's priority is to prepare for the birth of your child, not to procreate more just yet. Your hormones may also make a switch: your sex-wanting hormones dial down while your fathering hormones dial up. How perfect for mother, father, and baby. You can see that the advice "go with the flow" is biologically correct.

Traveling while Pregnant

Air travel. You both may want to treat yourself to a getaway before baby arrives. This may be the last time for a couple of years that you can travel without luggage full of diapers and toys. The ideal time to travel is in the middle trimester when you're likely to feel less tired, less nauseated, and more romantic — and thus have more fun. If possible, try to get all travel (business or pleasure) in by the end of your seventh month. After that, you're likely to be too tired and too off-balance to be traipsing around the world, and besides, the airlines won't let you on the plane. Be sure your healthcare provider clears you for takeoff. Follow these safe and comfortable travel guidelines:

When to fly. Foreign airlines prohibit air travel after thirty-five weeks, domestic airlines after thirty-six weeks. Don't count on flight attendants being trained midwives. If you look more pregnant than the guidelines allow, airlines will require an estimated due date note from your healthcare provider.

Where to fly. The shorter the trip, the less risky and the more comfortable. On the one hand, a nonstop coast-to-coast flight cuts down on takeoff and landing queasiness and the hassle of airport transfers. On the other hand, these long trips don't give you as much chance to stretch out and walk around. If you're planning a vacation, especially if you have any risk factors for premature labor, avoid travel to any place that is not equipped with newborn intensive care facilities. If possible, avoid hot, humid climates that simply aggravate what's going on in your pregnant body. If the place you're going to is not air-conditioned, you should probably scratch that off your list. Also, those blood-sucking mosquitoes love the luscious pregnant body, so it may be best to avoid mosquito-prone areas, since these pesky insects carry disease.

Where to sit. Different fliers have different needs. Pregnant women have various seat preferences. Here are some considerations:

- Choose a seat as far forward on the plane as possible, where the air circulation tends to be better and it's easier to get on and off the aircraft.

- Or choose a seat as close as possible to the bathroom, which is often at the rear of the plane.

- Opt for a window seat to minimize queasiness.

- Or opt for an aisle seat, which makes it easier to stretch your legs occasionally, and to get up and go.

- A bulkhead seat has the most leg room, yet the armrests cannot be moved up and so can restrict your sideways mobility and prevent you from stretching out, should the adjacent seat be vacant.

- Obviously, you will not be allowed to sit in the exit rows because in the event of an emergency people would be helping you rather than vice versa.

- If traveling with a companion, request an aisle and window seat. The kind and observant booking agent may leave the middle seat vacant to give you extra space for maneuvering.

- If you have extra credit card mileage to upgrade to first class, now is the time to pamper yourself, especially on long flights. Seats are wider, air circulation is better, the bathroom is closer, and getting on and off the plane is easier. Plus it's just plain nice to get the VIP treatment.

- If there are last-minute no-shows, parade your pregnant self up to the agent's desk and ask for the most favorable seating. You may be lucky enough to find a sympathetic ticket agent who has been pregnant herself to seat you more comfortably.

How to sit. Ask for a pillow so you can cushion your lower back. If you are in one of the bulkhead seats, you can elevate your feet. On long flights, expect your feet to expand a size no matter what you do. Once you remove your shoes, you may not be able to get them back on, so be sure to take along a roomier pair, or even a pair of safe slippers. To enhance circulation in your legs, do leg-pumping and feet-flexing exercises several times an hour. Fasten your seatbelt comfortably below your belly.

KEEP YOUR CIRCULATION CIRCULATING

Pregnancy puts you at increased risk of blood clots, which can result in thrombophlebitis in the legs. Immobilization of the legs during air travel increases these risks. Ask your doctor or midwife about specific precautions. For most pregnant women, simple precautions include the leg exercises we mentioned above, frequent walks around the cabin during air travel, and support hose. See page 37 for a natural remedy for decreasing the risk of blood clots.

How to go — to the bathroom. Empty your bladder by triple voiding (see page 228) just before boarding. Take as many "walks to the bathroom" as you can. The best time to get up and go is just before starting descent, since after landing there may be traffic congestion that requires the plane to sit on the runway, and you in your seat.

How to deal with dry air while you're up in the air. Be sure to drink to your thirst's content, and more! The humidity of cabin air is only around 7 percent, which dries the mucus membranes of the mouth and nose. Drink a lot of caffeine-free, nonalcoholic fluids before, during, and after the flight. Enjoy a "nose hose" — bring along a tiny bottle of saline nasal spray and spritz some into your nose every hour or so. If you're very careful you can try this vaporizing trick: carefully hold a hot cup of water while inhaling the steam.

How to eat. Review the rules of grazing (page 21), which are even more important when traveling by air when pregnant. The combination of airsickness and morning sickness is a double whammy that you want to avoid if at all possible. Pack your own tummy-tested munchies, especially if you're in the first trimester. Because the low cabin pressure can cause intestinal gas to expand and contribute to uncomfortable bloating, keep your tummy settled with these munchies.

What planes to avoid. While nearly all airplanes are now pressurized to compensate for the lower levels of oxygen at high altitudes, some smaller, older commuter crafts are not pressurized, since they usually fly below seven thousand feet. While a short time spent in an unpressurized cabin above seven thousand feet is unlikely to lower baby's oxygen level in the womb (it's already slightly lower than mother's), it can reduce the oxygen level in your blood, causing you to feel lightheaded or faint. If you feel lightheaded or disoriented, ask the flight attendant for some oxygen.

HELP! I'M PREGNANT

Be kind, yet assertive, when asking for help while you're pregnant. Let someone else lug your luggage. Above all, never try to lift even a slightly heavy piece of luggage into the overhead compartment. That's a setup for a severe back injury. Take advantage of your pregnancy and avail yourself of the kindness of others around you. You deserve a helping hand! You are a VIPP — a very important pregnant person!

What to avoid at the airport. Many pregnant mothers worry, and rightly so, about the possible hazards of the total body scanners to themselves and especially to their more radiation-sensitive baby inside. While the slight bit of radiation used in the total body scanners is probably safe, in our opinion, these scanners, especially those scary cages that completely encircle you, fall in the "when in doubt, leave them out" category. You can ask for a personal pat-down by a female TSA agent instead.

When to vaccinate. The good news is that while some vaccines may be recommended, most are no longer required for the countries that are safe to visit while pregnant. If you must go to a high-risk area, see the Centers for Disease Control and Protection International Travelers' website (wwwnc.cdc.gov/travel/page/vaccinations.htm) or consult your healthcare provider. If absolutely necessary, pregnant women can safely get the following vaccines: tetanus, pertussis, rabies, hepatitis B, and gammaglobulin. (To learn more about getting vaccines while pregnant, see AskDrSears.com/topics/vaccines.)

PREGNANCY TRAVEL RECORDS

Put together your personal travel kit, especially for international travel:

- List of medical issues, including medication allergies

- Medical insurance card

- Email addresses and phone numbers of home contacts and your healthcare provider

- Any notes or prescriptions your healthcare provider gave you to take along

- List of vaccines you have recently had

- Address for the CDC's Travelers' Health website: cdc.gov/travel

- Address for the International Association for Medical Assistance to Travellers' website: iamat.org

---

Martha advises: When you travel to an unfamiliar land, avoid taking any unwise risks. Accidents are more common on strange turf. Now you have another life to consider, so travel wisely — you're traveling for two.

Cruising while pregnant. A cruise can be one of the most relaxing and romantic vacations for a pregnant couple. Your dining and entertainment pleasures are always just a short walk away. Remember, though, ships move and hotels don't, so try these cruise-comforting tips:

Which ship to choose. If possible, choose a larger and newer ship, which will have more state-of-the-art stabilizers that lessen side-to-side rolling. And, the larger the ship, the less likely you are to sense the craft's up-and-down motion and side-to-side roll. In calm seas, if you don't look out the window you may even forget you're at sea. Choose a nonsmoking ship if possible; if not, dine outdoors. (Be sure to check to see whether the cruise line has a policy regarding how late in your pregnancy you will be allowed to cruise.)

Where to sail. Upset seas usually mean upset queasy tummies. Choose a shorter voyage in calmer waters, especially if you are not a seasoned sailor.

Where to sleep. Choose a midship cabin on a lower deck where there is the least ship motion. If possible, choose a balcony cabin with sliding glass doors, giving you access to fresh air.

TAMING TRAVELER'S DIARRHEA

Besides being unsettling to mother, traveler's diarrhea is potentially harmful to baby. Diarrhea depletes your body of necessary nutrients, salts, and fluids, all of which you need more of during pregnancy. Severe and prolonged diarrhea can dehydrate mother and reduce blood flow to baby. To avoid the foods and germs that cause diarrhea while traveling, take the following precautions:

- Drink only boiled or bottled water. Use ice cubes made only from bottled water.

- Consume only pasteurized dairy products.

- In countries with a reputation for traveler's diarrhea, avoid uncooked fruits and vegetables. Eat fresh fruit and vegetables only if you wash them in clean water yourself and then peel them.

- Avoid undercooked meat and fish. Don't eat fish from waters known to be mercury-contaminated.

- Dine only at restaurants that appear to have high standards of sanitation.

If, despite these ounces of prevention, you still get traveler's diarrhea, your main goal is to keep yourself from getting dehydrated. Here are ways to treat your diarrhea:

- If the diarrhea is severe (more than six watery stools per day), take small, frequent sips, adding up to a quart or two a day, of an oral electrolyte solution. (This solution replenishes the salts and minerals you are likely to lose during diarrhea. It is available at pharmacies without a prescription.) Call your doctor or midwife.

- Some over-the-counter antidiarrheal medicines are safe during pregnancy, while others are not. Antidiarrheal agents that contain salicylates and bismuth (e.g., Pepto-Bismol) are not safe to take while pregnant: some animal studies have shown them to be harmful to babies in the womb. Prescription antidiarrheal medications containing atropine and narcotics are certainly not safe. Consult your doctor about which antidiarrheal medicines are safe to take while pregnant.

- Be prepared. Before your trip, ask your physician or midwife what medications to take along and what you should do to prevent dehydration.

Car travel. Now that there are two people in the driver's seat, even though your baby is well protected, here are some precautions to take while driving:

Listen to your body. Since you are driving under the influence of pregnancy hormones, you may be more prone to lack of concentration, falling asleep, or even dizzy or fainting spells. Listen to your body and let it advise you when it's safe to drive and when it isn't. If you need to drive during a time of the day when you're the most queasy or sleepy, you may want to change your appointment time or leave the driving to someone else.

Take safer roads. When possible, drive during off-peak hours on the least crowded and polluted roads, and try to take the shortest distance between two points.

Adjust the seat for two. To leave more room behind the wheel as your little passenger grows, gradually move the seat back to maintain a distance of 10 or 12 inches between your chest and the steering wheel. As your pregnancy progresses and you need to move the seat back farther, your feet may have trouble reaching the pedals, so you can install a pedal extender.

Buckle up for baby. Without the protection of the seatbelt, in the event of a sudden stop or crash, your baby would come between you and the wheel. Be sure to wear your seatbelt correctly. Place the lap belt as low as possible underneath your uterus and snug across your upper thighs and hip bones just under the bulge. If the belt presses uncomfortably on the bulge, insert a pad between the belt and your lap. Place the shoulder belt above the bulge and between your breasts, over your shoulder, but not against your neck. Be sure neither the lap nor the shoulder belt is across your uterus, but rather beneath and alongside it. Don't worry that the seatbelt will squeeze your uterus or harm your baby in the unlikely event of a crash. Baby is in a natural fluid bag, like an airbag, for protection. Studies have shown that mother and baby are more likely to be unharmed in a crash when secured and properly positioned in a seatbelt.

Don't turn off the airbag. It's more likely to protect than hurt you and your baby during an accident.

When to seek medical attention. If you're involved in an accident, even though your baby is well protected by the muscle of the uterus and the amniotic fluid, there could be injury to the placenta. Signs that warrant immediate medical attention are leaking of amniotic fluid; vaginal bleeding; severe pain or tenderness in your abdomen, uterus, or pelvis; onset of contractions; and/or a change in the amount and intensity of fetal movements.

Dr. Linda notes: Your doctor or midwife will most likely want to monitor you in the hospital for several hours if you are involved in a motor vehicle accident, and may do blood work and possibly an ultrasound to check for any signs of internal bleeding. For women with Rh-negative blood type (see page 424), it may be especially important to check for an exchange of maternal and fetal blood, which could require administration of Rh immune globulin to prevent Rh sensitization.

Be comfortable. Use a pillow in the curve of your back. Take along easily reachable snacks and a water bottle, and try to make short, frequent stops during long trips to use the bathroom and stretch your legs.

Martha notes: Our family hobby is sailing, but the last place I wanted to be while pregnant was on the sea. Bill suggested that

if I took the helm I was less likely to get seasick. It really worked. I also noticed that I felt less nauseated when I was the driver instead of a rider in a car. Keeping my eyes engaged while driving also kept my mind off my tummy.

Choosing a Childbirth Class That's Right for You

You will want to take a childbirth class for the same reason you are reading this book: the more informed you are, the more safe and satisfying your pregnancy and birth are likely to be. Furthermore, a satisfying birth will get your parenting career off to a confident and joyful beginning. Childbirth classes can also provide a support group to help you through your individual questions and introduce you to friends you can call on after your birth. You may also learn from experienced parents in the class who share their previous birth and parenting experiences and express what they want to do differently this time around.

One of our childbirth educator friends says that some of her clients also go to meetings to find breastfeeding information and encouragement. La Leche League International, International Cesarean Awareness Network (ICAN), and Attachment Parenting International, for example, organize such meetings. You could also arrange lunch with your new pregnant friends, or have a prenatal potluck.

The relationships you begin in your childbirth class network can lead to years of friendship and family activities together. A fun part of the childbirth class Martha taught was what we called the "show-and-tell" night. A month or so after the last couple gave birth, everyone gathered for a reunion to show off their babies. Or new parents can come to your childbirth class to present their babies, tell their birth stories, answer questions about breastfeeding, and offer parenting tips.

In addition to the social benefits of a great childbirth class, you will learn about birth mechanics, being a wise consumer of medical care, and pain avoidance/management techniques. Perhaps the most valuable lesson you will learn in childbirth classes is how to break the fear-tension-pain cycle.

Dr. Grantly Dick-Read, a British pioneer in the field of unmedicated birth, identified this cycle as a key reason many women needed drugs during childbirth. Dr. Dick-Read demonstrated that most women do not have to choose between suffering or being heavily drugged to give birth. He found that he could help educate parents and thus eliminate the fear of childbirth (especially the fear of the unknown). His wife, Jessica, taught the classes, and she told women how their bodies worked in labor and why they felt the way they did. The Dick-Reads taught relaxation techniques to counteract the tension in mind and muscle produced by fear. They showed women how to work with rather than against their bodies in labor. Dr. Dick-Read's book, *Childbirth without Fear* (Pinter and Martin, 2013), is a classic that has continued to be revised and updated.

When choosing a childbirth class, you should consider more than its proximity to your home or its schedule. Take a class that supports your birth philosophy. Do some reading and talk to veteran parents.

When to sign up. If you can find an "introduction to pregnancy" class, consider taking it sometime in the first few months of pregnancy. A class like this helps you learn about the birth philosophy of the instructor or method, helps you form your own birth philosophy, and makes your later choice of a class easier. You may see a film and receive information on basics of relaxation, exercise, nutrition, and questions you can ask when visiting doctors or midwives. You may be able to start checking out books from the class library and see the childbirth workbooks and materials you will be using.

Most childbirth educators design their regular classes for couples nearing the end of their second trimester. These classes generally run from six to twelve weeks in length and ideally end a week or two before your due date, or include free weekly reviews until birth so the knowledge you gain will be fresh in your mind when you go into labor.

Independent teachers may start a new class series only every few months, so it is better to contact the teacher you want early rather than just at the time you'd like to start taking the class. Big institutions, such as hospitals and community colleges, tend to have more teachers and to start classes more frequently, but their groups may be large and they may not afford opportunities for close relationships with teachers and classmates. Hospital-based childbirth classes may include a tour of the maternity area. Doing your homework before you choose a class will help you to select a class that fits your needs.

What the class will teach you. Besides helping you to explore the various birth options available to expectant couples and to work out your particular birth needs, a complete childbirth class should cover the following:

Eating right for two (or more): For many couples, this is the first time that they have ever had a "course" on nutrition, and it may also be the first time they have been motivated to eat healthy.

Exercise: You'll learn when, what, and how much to do to prepare your birth-giving muscles and to increase your overall stamina.

Stages of labor: You will learn how to recognize your body's signals at each stage of labor.

Relaxation and pain-management techniques: Birth brings some of the most intense sensations you will ever experience. You will learn that pain has a purpose in labor, and unbearable pain is a signal to do something differently. A good childbirth class will not only explore relaxation skills and self-help methods such as verbal encouragement, massage, counterpressure, movement, and use of showers or tubs for labor; it will also explain the effects of different medical methods of pain relief. That way you go into labor equipped with a whole toolbox of pain-prevention or management skills and the knowledge of which ones are best in your situation.

How your partner can help: Once dads appreciate what's going on inside the bodies of their pregnant wives, they become more sympathetic and helpful. They also learn a lot from other pregnant couples in the class. Remember this: "We're pregnant" so "we" take the class together!

Breastfeeding tips: Successful breastfeeding depends on a good start; the more you know

ahead of time, especially about positioning and latch-on, the easier the transition will be. There are great classes led by certified breastfeeding educators and board-certified lactation consultants, and education/support groups like La Leche League, as well as audio-visual aids and books, handouts, and other teaching materials to help you. (See our resource list on page 429.)

Postpartum concerns: A great childbirth class not only helps you have a safer and more rewarding birth; it helps prepare you to adjust to the many changes a baby brings to your family. You'll learn about various parenting styles that help you better bond with your baby. You'll cover whether to leave your baby boy "intact" or have him circumcised, and ideas on introducing the new baby to the whole family. You can work out an approach on how to get the basic duties of family meals, laundry, shopping, and housework managed. You will have an understanding of what to expect from your postpartum body and emotions. The class may even touch on the basics of newborn care, such as bathing and diapering. Different couples will choose different approaches to childbirth education. Following is information on the three best-known organizations: ICEA, Lamaze, and Bradley.

The International Childbirth Education Association (ICEA). This organization trains and certifies teachers who incorporate the best of several methods into their instruction in keeping with the organization's motto: "Freedom of choice through knowledge of alternatives." The ICEA is a credible source of information for expectant couples and childbirth educators. They hold national conventions, operate an online bookstore for parenting, pregnancy, and childbirth education resources, and put out some of the best-researched childcare pamphlets in the business. For more information on resources from the ICEA or on how to find your nearest ICEA instructor, visit ICEA.org.

Lamaze International. Though its original focus included techniques to divert a woman's attention from her contractions, in the past decade or so Lamaze has been teaching a wider variety of techniques for pain control, and emphasizing relaxation skills and parental choices. One useful resource is *Healthy Birth Practice 4: Avoid Interventions That Are Not Medically Necessary* by Judith A. Lothian, RN, PhD, LCCE, FACCE, available online at lamaze.org/HBP4.

Lamaze students are also taught the advantages and disadvantages of all medical options of pain relief. The Lamaze graduate is then equipped to choose either no medication, an injection of pain reliever, or epidural anesthesia without feeling that any judgment is being placed on her choice.

The other distinctive trait of Lamaze, and one of the secrets of its success, is that its teachers and its teachings tend to be less "radical" than teachings of other groups. Obstetricians generally back Lamaze programs, since most classes are hospital-based and focus more on preparing their clients to deliver within the medical system. Not all Lamaze International instructors are hospital employees and some do teach independently.

The Bradley Method. Also called "husband-coached childbirth," this method was developed in Los Angeles in the 1970s by Marjie and Jay Hathaway, founders of AAHCC (American Academy of Husband-Coached Childbirth), in association with Denver obstetrician Dr. Robert A. Bradley. Dr. Bradley practiced from the 1940s to the 1980s and wrote *Husband-Coached Childbirth* in 1965. He believed that it is healthier for a woman to be involved in the sensations of her labor than for her to try to escape from them, and that pain, rather than being a problem to get rid of, is a signal to be listened to. He believed that almost all mammals can give birth spontaneously in the absence of physical complications; animals have inborn instincts, and humans need to learn how to overcome the fear of the unknown, to prepare their bodies through good nutrition and exercise, and to practice what to do in labor and birth. They also need a doctor or midwife who is familiar with normal drug-free birth and a place to give birth where that is common. They need to know when technology is appropriate or when it is overused and can lead to other interventions.

The Bradley philosophy and the people who teach it are passionate about instructing women to trust their bodies. They believe that nearly all women, given proper education and support, can have a safe and satisfying birth without medication — and over 90 percent of Bradley grads having vaginal births do. Their cesarean rate is much lower than the national average.

Rather than using diversionary tactics to try to cover up their birth sensations, Bradley laborers are encouraged to relax, listen to their basic instincts, and work with their bodies to find their own way to labor more comfortably and efficiently. Bradley recommends more natural breathing techniques such as diaphragmatic/abdominal breathing for the first stage or opening of the cervix; and breathing techniques to aid your uterus in birthing the baby. Bradley courses tend to be more detailed and longer than most other methods and usually include a Healthy Pregnancy Class followed by twelve weeks of classes and free weeks of review if desired. The classes not only help women to be informed participants in their birthing decisions, they also equip them to be wise consumers. For more information about the Bradley Method, visit bradleybirth .com.

Dr. Linda notes: *A certain amount of flexibility can be helpful. Keep your mind open as you explore options.*

In teaching childbirth classes, Martha integrated the best of all of the above options and offered a balanced curriculum.

To increase your chances of having a great birth experience, do a lot of research to find the childbirth course that is best for you. Ask the prospective childbirth educator for names of her previous clients and check her references. Ask yourself if you feel comfortable with both her style and her course content. Talk to friends, not only about their childbirth educators, but about what they wish they had known or done differently at the time of their babies' births.

Realize there will be a huge range in the cost of a series of classes. Some hospital classes may be included in the cost of your birth package or be quite inexpensive, because the number of couples in the class will fill up a whole lecture room. In other cases, where class length and content may be many times that of the others, expect the price to be proportionally higher, especially if the number of students is low. A good class is worth every penny. (For information on hypnotherapy, see page 306.)

A note from a childbirth educator: *We birth professionals can plant seeds to help women feel good about their choices on how to birth. We believe that pregnant women have a deep wisdom about what is right for each of them and for their babies. In our classes we try to avoid the "right versus wrong way to birth" tug-of-war that causes a lot of unnecessary stress for new mothers. We also reject the myth that if you birth your baby naturally you are a true mother-woman. We're obviously all for natural childbirth, but we have seen how important medical interventions can be for some women. A lot of women put pressure on themselves if the births do not go the way they have envisioned them and feel as if they have failed as women. We are proud of these moms because they probably worked even harder than those who had uncomplicated births.*

Dr. Linda notes: *You and your caregiver (which is the term I use for birth attendant, doctor, or midwife) need to be a team. I have never understood why a woman would adopt an antagonistic attitude toward her caregiver. If you want a noninterventionist birth experience, then seek out a birthing center or home birth experience. Obstetricians and midwives delivering in hospital settings are constrained by the policies of the hospital. It is important to have an honest discussion with your doctor or midwife about what expectations are realistic.*

"NATURAL" CHILDBIRTH

"Natural birthing" means different things to different mothers. To childbirth educators, however, it means delivering a baby without drugs. Birth reformers have recently started to use a new term, "pure birth," which means no drugs or technological interventions. What you call your birth means little; it's what the birth experience means to you that matters the most. A medically assisted birth may be perfectly natural for you; and if medical assistance helps you avoid a surgical birth, you have achieved the natural phenomenon of vaginal birth.

A term we like is "physiological birth," which, in contrast to "pharmacological birth," focuses on a mother who is informed and empowered to work with her instinctive hormonal signals to birth in the healthiest way for herself and her baby. (To deeply appreciate the physiological marvels that are going on in your body during birthing, read ahead: "The Hormonal Symphony of Birth," page 324.)

We also like the term "responsible childbirth." Responsible childbirth means that you have done your homework — studied the options, worked out a birthing philosophy that suits you, assembled the right team, chosen the appropriate birth place, and educated your mind and trained your body to have a safe and satisfying birth. Regardless of whether your birth goes according to your plans, go into your labor informed and empowered and you can call your baby's birth anything you wish — and feel good about it.

For me, "natural childbirth" means going to the hospital without any makeup on.

Choosing a Hospital

As you assemble the right team to help you birth your baby, you also need to choose the right place for this special event. Oftentimes, the birth attendant and the birth place go together as a package. The doctor you choose may deliver at only one hospital. However, you might have a choice of hospitals, so it's back to doing your homework or, in this case, legwork.

Commonly the choice of a hospital is dictated either by geography, practicality (where your doctor or midwife delivers), or economics (where your insurance company covers your care). These are significant concerns, but presuming you have some choice in hospitals, focus on whether the hospital offers features you want, such as:

- A family-centered maternity unit with rooms for labor and birth. A pleasant place to labor, deliver, and enjoy the first day of your life with your baby.

- Oversized labor tubs, the newest innovation among the many natural methods to ease labor pains (see page 303).

- A birthing bed that is comfortable to labor and sleep in, yet adjusts to many positions to accommodate different stages and styles of labor.

- The latest noninvasive technology, especially the new electronic fetal monitoring by telemetry, in which baby's heart-rate changes can be monitored without mother having to stay in bed or be tethered by wires to a bedside machine.

- A "level 3" special-care or newborn intensive-care unit that has all the equipment and personnel essential to care for a sick newborn, including an on-premises neonatologist, should the baby need specialized care at the moment of delivery. This saves transferring a sick newborn to another facility and separating mother and baby.

- An anesthesiologist or nurse-anesthetist residing in the hospital twenty-four hours a day in case an emergency cesarean section or other obstetrical emergency occurs.

- Nurse-midwives or midwives who are intricately involved in the obstetrical facility, either as head nurses, labor support persons, or as the primary attendants at low-risk, uncomplicated births.

- A certified lactation consultant (or obstetrical nurses with such certification) on staff to help breastfeeding mothers get the right start.

- A flexible birthing philosophy. Wearing both a "natural" and "medical" hat is difficult, if not impossible, for most obstetrical units. Attendants assist mothers with walking during labor,

encourage delivering in whatever position is most comfortable for mother and most healthy for baby, and are open to following a mother's birth wishes and birth plan as long as these are in the best medical interest of mother and baby. On the other hand, the staff is able to click into the medical mindset should an unanticipated complication arise.

- A hospital certified as "baby-friendly," meaning that it practices a philosophy that helps the breastfeeding mother-infant pair. (See babyfriendlyUSA.org.)

Choosing a Birth Center

The main difference between a birth center and a hospital is not so much the birthing environment, but the birthing philosophy. Birth centers are generally run by midwives, and they usually attend all normal deliveries, with obstetricians available as consultants (and backup in case transfer to a hospital becomes necessary). Birth-center midwives focus on supporting the mother and the birth she wants.

Dr. Linda notes: *Many alternative options are available at a birth center, such as freedom of movement, upright laboring, warm water immersion for labor and water birth, and constant surveillance of mother and baby with limited intervention.*

Birth centers trust nature, are cautious about technology, and assume that most of the time everything will go right. Opponents of birth centers fear that the pregnant woman places herself and her baby at unnecessary risk, since emergency care that can be given only in a hospital is not immediately available. Proponents of birth centers counter that because a mother is allowed to labor and deliver in a more natural way, she is less likely to need emergency care. Most birth centers are now located near maternity hospitals. Birth centers focus on physiological birth rather than pharmacological birth.

A professionally staffed, properly accredited birth center is a safe alternative to a hospital birth for women with uncomplicated pregnancies. In 1989 one of the most reputable medical journals, the *New England Journal of Medicine,* published a study of twelve thousand women admitted for labor and delivery to eighty-four birth centers in the United States. The cesarean rate for women in this study was 4.4 percent, far below the national average. There were no maternal deaths, and the neonatal death rate was well below average. Twenty-five percent of first-time mothers had to be transferred to a hospital, and only 7 percent of women who had a previous birth needed to be transferred. The study concluded that a birth center offers a safe and acceptable alternative to hospital birth for low-risk expectant mothers. So if you are low-risk and have a "proven pelvis" (i.e., you have previously delivered a baby vaginally), delivering in a birth center is an alternative to consider. If you are a low-risk, first-time mother, you might consider a birth center, but do your homework about hospitals and get to know your backup obstetrician in case a transfer is necessary. This way, you can combine the environment and birthing philosophy of a birth center with the option of having a satisfying birth in the hospital, should it become necessary.

Dr. BJ notes: While many hospitals call their labor and delivery units a "birth center," some of these hospital units have staff and procedures much like traditional labor and delivery units. Real birth centers are organized as a center specializing in the care of women that have a low-risk pregnancy and follow a philosophy that enhances natural birth. They provide a personalized and intimate setting for women who have an uncomplicated pregnancy and no anticipated risk to vaginal birth. They usually provide a more labor-friendly atmosphere, such as the ability to walk during labor without continuous monitoring, eat and drink as tolerated, water immersion for labor, and often water birth. They are furnished with birth balls, squat stools, rocking chairs, large water immersion tubs, and large beds. Midwives are specialists at providing care for women without the cumbersome technologies of traditional settings.

Birth centers are accredited by the Commission for the Accreditation of Birth Centers (CABC), and some states require them to be licensed as well. Accreditation ensures that the birth center provides care that is consistent with the standards for low-risk pregnancy, labor, and birth. The CABC standards do not allow the use of Pitocin in labor or epidural anesthesia, as these procedures may put mother and baby at risk.

Many insurance plans now provide birth centers as a benefit of maternity coverage. The midwifery model of care recognizes the normalcy of pregnancy, labor, and birth and provides continuity of care to carefully monitor labor and birth. One of the hallmarks of the midwifery model of care is "labor sitting," which means that the midwife (or physician) must be present with the woman during labor as well as at birth. Midwives at birth centers provide a "high-touch" approach with some "high-tech" procedures available should they be required. The providers and staff are certified in procedures such as neonatal resuscitation and have all the equipment for emergencies should they occur. Birth centers provide a safe and satisfying location where your birth plan will be respected.

Here are some points to consider when choosing a birth center:

- Is the birth center nationally accredited and/or state licensed?

- What is the philosophy of the birth center?

- Can you tour the birth center and learn about the care provided there?

- Who attends the birth at the birth center?

- Does your insurance cover the cost of the birth center? If so, find out how to get authorization for this facility fee to be covered.

- Does your midwife have a backup physician at a nearby hospital?

- How far from the birth center is the referral hospital?

- Does the birth center have transfer agreements with the physician and hospital to ensure easy transfer, should it be necessary?

WHAT IS YOUR "RISK"?

We downplay the medical term "high-risk pregnancy". While this classification is often needed in medical charts to alert the staff to possible complications, a mother should never fearfully wonder "High risk of what?" Remember, one of the central messages of our book is to take the fear out of childbirth. Better terms of endearment are "challenging," "special circumstances," and any laboring language that conveys to the mother that because of special obstetrical circumstances she needs to be "highly informed" and "empowered," and take extra care of herself to birth a healthy baby. Even terms like "uncomplicated" and "complicated" can be less scary.

Choosing a Home Birth

Home sweet home! In recent years the home birth movement has been gaining momentum. According to a 2011 study that analyzed birth records between 2004 and 2008, home births increased by 20 percent. In 2008, some twenty-eight thousand home births occurred in the United States.

Home birth can be a safe alternative for a woman with an uncomplicated pregnancy who has an educated birthcare provider. While the American Congress of Obstetricians and Gynecologists (ACOG) continues to advise against home birth, there is good evidence that planned home birth is a safe option. The American College of Nurse-Midwives believes that home birth is safe when a pregnancy is low-risk and the home is a safe environment. Women who are considering a home birth should interview their birth team to ensure that the midwife or doctor is experienced in birthing at home, has the appropriate equipment to bring to the home, and is connected with other medical support, such as a local hospital, so that there is no delay in providing care for the mother or baby should it be needed. Home birth can be as safe as hospital birth when there is a plan in place for every eventuality.

If the birthing model in North America were similar to the model in European countries, where home births are the rule rather than the exception, home birthing would be considered safe by organizations such as ACOG. In European countries obstetricians and midwives work together, there is an efficient transport system in case of emergencies, and obstetricians and hospitals provide backup for midwives attending home births. A 2009 study published in the *Canadian Medical Association Journal* compared the safety and complication rate of planned home births attended by a certified midwife and planned hospital births attended by a midwife or physician between the years of 2000 and 2004 in British Columbia, Canada. The conclusion was that the outcomes were essentially the same in home births and hospital births. However, we can't translate studies from other countries into a judgment on whether home birth is safe in the United States because there is such a wide degree of competence among home birth attendants. It's not that home birth itself is unsafe, it's that the current maternity-care system in the United States is not set up for home births.

Noting that home births unattended by a certified birth attendant are associated with a higher rate of complications for mother and baby, ACOG advises these safety precautions when considering a home birth:

- Prior cesarean is an absolute contraindication to planned home birth.

- The midwife or home birth attendant should be appropriately trained and certified under local and state laws. All midwifes should be certified by the American Midwifery Certification Board.

- The home should be within easy access to a hospital that has a maternity unit, and the home birth attendant should have preexisting ties and transport protocols set up to ensure safe and timely transport to the hospital.

Suggested checklist for choosing a home birth:

❑ First, interview yourself to be sure you really are a candidate for home birth. Do you really want to deliver at home, or are you just afraid of hospitals?

❑ Do you trust your body to work for you better at home? While it's normal for all women to carry some fear into birth, regardless of the birth attendant or birth place, you need an especially positive attitude for a safe home birth. If you're at all afraid to have a home birth, you shouldn't have one.

❑ · Do you have a proven pelvis? Have you previously delivered safely at home or had an uncomplicated birth in a hospital or birth center?

Knowing that in the past your body worked well for you helps you feel it's more likely to come through for you again. That feeling takes much of the fear and riskiness out of home birth. (Consider, however, that no two deliveries are the same, and unforeseen complications can occur with any pregnancy and delivery, even if there was no previous history or warning.)

❑ What is your history of handling stress and pain? Remember that epidural anesthesia that your friend raved about so much in her near-painless birth? Epidurals are not an option for midwife-attended home births, though midwives do know a great deal about nonmedical pain relief, such as positioning and relaxation, and one advantage of home births is that the bathtub can be used for pain relief.

❑ Do you have a licensed and certified midwife in whom you have unquestionable confidence? Does she have obstetrical backup?

WHY SOME EXPECTANT MOTHERS CHOOSE A HOME BIRTH

• It's a family affair. Appropriately aged children (usually three years and up) can experience the excitement of birth. Family bonding naturally takes place without having to wait for routine hospital procedures.

• Labor is often faster, less painful, and more efficient.

• The drive to a hospital in labor can be painful and anxiety producing.

• Some mothers feel that hospitals and all the routine technological tests and monitoring can disturb the normal birth process.

• They are more comfortable at home. No birth center can compare with the comfort of your own home.

• They can labor at their own pace, without being hurried by the system.

• They want to enjoy a midwife-attended birth, especially if midwives cannot deliver babies in their local hospitals.

• They simply feel that a home birth is less complicated and more user friendly than a hospital birth.

• They believe in the benefits of the "friendly germ environment" and no separation from baby.

• They can enjoy water labor in their own bathtub or a rented birthing tub, which may not be allowed in some hospitals.

• They are more relaxed, and a more relaxed mother enjoys an easier birth.

The disadvantage of a home birth is that if unanticipated problems arise, the delay in expert medical interventions could compromise the health of mother and baby.

Note from Dr. Bill and Martha: *In our own family, at this writing, we have been blessed with seventeen births, eight of Bill and Martha's (one by adoption, at whose birth Martha was the labor coach), and nine grandchildren. Of these seventeen, four were born at home, three in a birthing center, and the rest in a hospital. Most of the births were attended by both obstetricians and midwives. We are blessed with the outcome: no surgical births, one obstetrical challenge, and seventeen healthy babies. The information and empowerment package we provide in this book works. Be sure to go through the safety checklist above to help guide you to the best and safest decision for you and baby.*

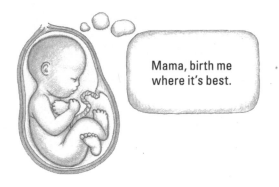

Mama, birth me where it's best.

MY PREGNANCY JOURNAL: SIXTH MONTH

Emotionally I feel:

_____

_____

_____

_____

_____

Physically I feel:

_____

_____

_____

_____

_____

My thoughts about you:

_____

_____

_____

_____

_____

My dreams about you:

_____

_____

_____

_____

_____

What I imagine you look like:

_____

_____

_____

_____

My top concerns:

_____

_____

_____

_____

My best joys:

_____

_____

_____

_____

Visit to My Healthcare Provider

Questions I had; answers I got:

_____

_____

_____

_____

Tests and results; my reaction:

_____

_____

_____

Updated due date: _____

My weight: _____

My blood pressure: _____

Feeling my uterus; my reaction:

_____

_____

_____

_____

How I feel when I feel you kick:

_____

_____

_____

_____

How Dad feels when he feels you kick:

_____

_____

_____

MY PREGNANCY JOURNAL: SIXTH MONTH

What I bought when I went shopping:

_____

_____

_____

We started taking childbirth classes at:

_____

_____

_____

Our teacher is:

_____

_____

_____

_____

The method we chose is:

_____

_____

_____

_____

Because:

_____

_____

_____

_____

We decided to give birth to you at:

_____

_____

_____

_____

Because:

_____

_____

_____

_____

_____

The main person who will help me deliver you is:

_____

_____

_____

_____

Other helpers I would like in the birthing room are:

_____

_____

_____

_____

Sonogram photo:

Comments:

_____

_____

_____

_____

_____

_____

_____

_____

_____

_____

_____

_____

_____

_____

SEVENTH-MONTH VISIT TO YOUR HEALTHCARE PROVIDER
(26–29 WEEKS)

During this month's visit you may have:

- An examination of the size and height of your uterus

- An examination of your skin for rashes, enlarging veins, and swelling

- A weight and blood pressure check

- Blood test for diabetes; Rho-GAM if you are Rh-negative.

- A test for hemoglobin and hematocrit, if indicated

- A review of your diet and an opportunity to discuss your weight, if necessary

- An opportunity to hear your baby's heartbeat

- An opportunity to see your baby on ultrasound, if indicated

- An opportunity to discuss your feelings and concerns

If your healthcare provider has additional concerns, she may want to check you twice a month during the seventh and eighth months.

16

Seventh Month: Bigger and Loving It

As your baby gets bigger, she makes herself known in many ways. You may be awakened by punches to your ribs and poked all day long in different places, with a knee here and an elbow there. Baby will continually remind you that she's going through a growth spurt; as she doubles her weight and lengthens her limbs, she needs more room to stretch, and your body shows it as well. You may find yourself staring in awe at where your waist used to be, and your hands seem to be drawn like magnets to this sphere filled with life. Because baby now occupies more of you, you will notice even more changes. You walk differently, eat differently, sleep differently, and sometimes wonder whether your baby could eventually take over your body.

HOW YOUR BABY IS GROWING, 26–29 WEEKS

Baby is now a complete little person, with mature enough organs to survive life outside the womb. All the organs are working, though not at their full capacity; they need two more months to reach complete maturity. Because the lungs continue to lag behind other organs, babies born at this stage would probably need assisted mechanical ventilation for a few weeks.

During this month, baby enjoys a big growth spurt. Baby doubles her weight to 2 or 2½ pounds and lengthens to around 14 inches. From head to toe baby starts fattening up. During this month, baby not

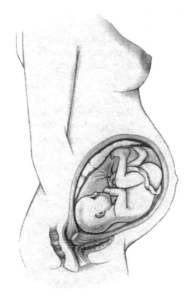

Baby at 26-29 weeks.

only gets bigger, she gets smarter. Trillions of brain cells start building myelin, a fatty layer that looks and acts like insulation on electrical wires, allowing nerve impulses to travel faster.

Baby's eyelids open and senses are now developed so highly that baby can see, hear, smell, and taste. How much baby hears is a matter of imagination. Parents and prenatal researchers claim that babies can recognize familiar voices and move to melodious tunes. Just keep talking and singing to baby, knowing that some sounds do get through. Fingers and fingerprints are fully formed and baby can now make a tiny fist. Air sacs in the lungs, called alveoli, mushroom in size and number, and the cells lining these rapidly budding alveoli begin to secrete a soapy substance called surfactant, which will keep these air sacs from collapsing — similar to the substance that keeps a soap bubble expanded. Baby fat accumulates to smooth out the wrinkly appearance of the previous stage of development. Baby's arms and feet are longer and stronger, a fact you will feel as baby makes bigger impressions on your abdomen. Naturally, as baby is going through a growth spurt so will you, gaining from 3 to 5 pounds as your uterus expands above the level of your navel.

HOW YOU MAY FEEL

Most women find the seventh month an emotionally easier time. You are now used to being pregnant and have learned to celebrate and tolerate the perks and pains that go along with the experience. You may feel that many of the emotional and physical "growing pains" of pregnancy are now behind you as you take on a new set of changes that focus on giving birth to your baby. While every woman's emotional and physical journey through pregnancy is as unique as her personality, here are the feelings many women experience:

More curvy. This is the month many women begin to really value their amazing, changing shape. They realize this is a special look they only experience when expecting.

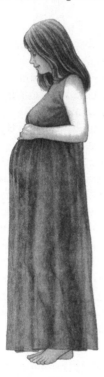

The pregnancy high. Many women describe their feelings at this stage as "ecstatic" or "euphoric." The specialness you felt in the previous month can blossom into the euphoria of looking and feeling truly pregnant. Many women revel in the pregnancy high of realizing that they're doing something extraordinary.

Resourceful. You may feel, "In a couple of months baby is going to take up all my free time. I had better tie up loose ends at work and get things done around the house that I won't have time to do later."

Forgetful. Your preoccupation with pregnancy may seem to fill all the available space in your mind, leaving little mental energy left over for daily tasks. Important events, such as birthdays and anniversaries that you have always remembered, may go forgotten. You may find yourself stuck in the middle of a sentence, forgetting the topic you had begun or how to finish it.

However, although you now have nature's best excuse for your forgetfulness, family and professional life must go on. There may be children to pick up at preschool, employer deadlines to satisfy, and many other facts of real life that you still have to attend to. If this is your first baby, see this as preparation for the multitasking of motherhood.

When you can no longer rely on your memory for your daily agenda, you'll learn to carry around a notepad, a smart phone, or something else that helps you remember healthcare appointments, birthdays, childbirth classes, and who's coming for dinner. Your calendar may have to be in a more visible place, such as pasted on your refrigerator or even on your bathroom wall. And you may as well post little sticky notes everywhere, reminding you of what you're likely to forget.

My husband calls me Spacey Gracie. Although I remembered my doctor's appointment, I forgot to pay the electric bill, left a quart of milk on the counter to spoil, left a friend dangling on the phone while I ran to the bathroom and forgot the call,

and found the checkbook even more out of balance than I was. All this seemed funny until the other day when I ran a stop sign and, in shock, realized that there are times when I really need to keep my head together.

Heart working harder. Because your growing baby and growing body need more blood for oxygen and nourishment, by the third trimester your cardiovascular system has 45 percent more blood than it did before you were pregnant. To pump this extra blood to needy tissues, your heart has to work harder and faster, and you may feel it. Because your heart rate increases by about ten beats per minute and your heart pumps about 30 percent more with each beat, you may feel "heart-pounding sensations," especially when you change positions suddenly or during exercise. These heart-pounding sensations are most prevalent between twenty-eight and thirty-two weeks and are just another reminder of all the extra work your body is doing. You will need to remember to change positions slowly.

Breathing for two. Your lungs, like your heart, are also working overtime to take in extra oxygen, so there may be moments when you feel short of breath. To accommodate this increased oxygen need, your lung capacity increases, and you will probably add a few inches to the circumference of your rib cage. Because your expanding uterus may cramp your expanding lungs by pressing upward on the diaphragm, you might experience the occasional feeling of not getting enough air. To compensate for this, you will breathe a bit faster and more efficiently. You may unconsciously sigh more often, another way of taking deeper breaths.

Here are some ways to be sure you and your baby are getting enough air when you feel short of breath:

- Slowly stand up to relieve some of the pressure of your uterus on your diaphragm.

- Slowly raise your arms outward to the side and upward while inhaling slowly and deeply.

- Lower your arms back down to your sides while exhaling slowly. Occasionally place your hands on the sides of your rib cage to make sure you are expanding your lower chest as you inhale.

- Sit smart, as you learned on page 223. Instead of slumping over, which further compresses your lungs, sit upright with shoulders back and chest lifted.

- Try sleeping semi-reclined, with your back and head propped up with pillows, or use an extra pillow under your head while side-sleeping.

Take a deep breath. During the ninth month as baby drops deeper into your pelvis and takes pressure off your diaphragm, you will be able to breathe more easily.

Thirstier. Thirst is your body's signal that you and baby need more fluid. Because thirst is not a totally reliable indicator of fluid needs, drink to your thirst's content — plus a couple more glasses of water, usually eight to ten glasses of fluids daily. If you don't, the demand for fluid is so great that your body will take it as needed from your intestines, contributing to constipation.

More swelling. The total-body puffiness of pregnancy peaks in the third trimester. You are naturally carrying around ten quarts (20 pounds) of extra fluid. Your body needs to make extra blood, increase kidney flow to wash away extra waste, and refill baby's amniotic swimming pool.

You're likely to see and feel swelling of all the tissues where gravity causes the build-up of fluid; this is called gravity edema. You might wake up in the morning with facial puffiness from fluid accumulating beneath the thinner tissues of the eyelids and around your whole face. As you stand up throughout the day, gravity causes all that extra fluid, like rainfall, to move downward, making you feel as though you're lugging around heavier hands, legs, and feet, where gravity causes fluid to settle by the end of the day.

When swelling is normal. While some pregnant mothers experience more swelling than others, here are signs that swelling is normal for you:

- The swelling shifts with gravity, with different areas of your body being swollen at different times of the day.

- Your diet is healthy and balanced and you're gaining weight normally.

- Your blood pressure and urine checks at your healthcare provider's office are normal.

When swelling is not normal. Building up excessive fluid can be a sign of a problem, such as high blood pressure or preeclampsia (see page 423). Call your healthcare provider if you notice any of the following:

- The swelling of your legs is steadily increasing, becoming excessive, and when you press on your swollen ankles it leaves a noticeable dent, called pitting edema.

- The swelling is not relieved when you elevate your legs.

- You experience a new onset of significant headaches, blurry vision, or sharp or constant pain in your upper abdomen.

To reduce the discomforts of swelling:

- Avoid standing or sitting for long periods of time and change positions frequently. Don't cross your legs when you sit as this can restrict circulation in your legs and aggravate swelling.

- While sitting or standing, flex your feet to increase circulation in your legs.

- Walk or swim to increase circulation and decrease swelling.

- While sitting, elevate your feet on a stool and elevate your hands.

- Elevate your legs at the end of the day, especially if your feet are swollen.

- Sleep on your side instead of your back to take the pressure of your weighty uterus off the major blood vessels and promote better blood return from your legs (see the best sleeping position on page 84).

Dr. BJ notes: *If you have access to a pool, sit in the pool with the water to shoulder level and soak for thirty minutes. The hydrostatic pressure of the deep water will help to push the fluid out of the tissue in your feet and ankles and back into the bloodstream so that your kidneys can clear it.*

Clumsy. Your new body is naturally off-center. Add to this a forgetful mind and you have a recipe for frequent falls. Even more so over the next two months, your less-than-graceful gait and waddle walk cause you to be naturally klutzy. The 20-plus pounds you are lugging around, as well as the loose and waterlogged ligaments in your hands, pelvis, and leg joints, can cause you to stumble on curb corners, trip over toys, or drop your fork in the middle of a meal. It is important to accept that while pregnant, you're not going to be as nimble as you used to be, and that all of your movements require a bit more caution and foresight. Be more careful when lifting hot items, carrying a toddler, and even walking on unfamiliar or bumpy terrain.

Dr. Linda notes: *This is not a trivial concern. When I am on duty in our busy tertiary care delivery unit, barely a day goes by that we are not dealing with a pregnant woman or two who have fallen, commonly twisting or breaking ankles or falling on their abdomen. I understand how it happens, but pregnant women need to use common sense, wear sensible shoes, and* pay attention. *One woman, for example, broke her leg while walking down her basement stairs with a load of laundry in one arm, a squirming toddler in the other, and wearing flip-flops. She needed surgery, a cast, and anticoagulant injections twice a day for the rest of her pregnancy.*

More baby movements. Now that baby's limbs are longer and stronger, the punches are more powerful. Studies show that babies kick the most frequently during the seventh month, and more often at night and in the early morning hours. Enjoy, or tolerate, these kicks while you can, since increasingly crowded living conditions in the womb will soon take some of the leverage out of baby's punches.

Tom and I enjoyed falling asleep with me curled around him. He'd feel the baby gently thumping him on the back. It was a nice experience for the three of us to be all cuddled up together.
    Dr. BJ notes: *In the third trimester, baby's movements change from "aerobics" to "yoga" with more stretching than kicking and punching.*

Baby hiccups. Besides the kicks and shifts you love to feel (though not necessarily at 3:00 a.m.), you may notice more fetal hiccups — short, spasmodic blips in your lower abdomen. Hiccups are usually short-lived, but they can last as long as twenty minutes. By the time you've hollered "Come feel this!" they will probably have stopped. Hiccups often occur around the same time each day, so family members may be able to catch another performance soon.
    Some mothers of babies who turned out to be sensitive to certain foods have noticed that their babies hiccupped a lot in utero. One mom actually figured this out because her baby got hiccups within an hour of mom drinking milk. This helped her focus on milk as the offending food in her own diet when her breastfed baby developed colic at two weeks of age.

CONCERNS YOU MAY HAVE

Many of the sensations you experienced in the second trimester continue or increase in intensity this month. There will probably be a few new ones, too, to keep you on your swollen toes:

Aching hips and back. The ligaments in your hips and pelvis stretch and the cartilage softens, preparing these bones to accommodate the passage of baby. These joint and ligament changes can be uncomfortable while walking and give you a looser gait, the common "waddle walk" of pregnancy.

Groin and pelvic pains. You may notice a sudden sharp pain when you cough, sneeze, laugh, change positions, or reach for something. These pains are caused by stretching of those now looser ligaments that attach your uterus to your pelvis. While putting on your underwear or getting out of bed, you might feel a sharp pain or pressure in your pelvis or groin. You might even experience the occasional sharp pain in your vaginal area, due to pressure on your cervix.

More vaginal discharge. Whitish vaginal discharge often increases, requiring many women to now use a panty liner, or even a maxipad, daily.

More practice contractions. The normal Braxton Hicks contractions you learned about on page 219 now become stronger and more frequent. They can be uncomfortable and cause you to wonder if you are going into premature labor. But true labor contractions show a definite pattern. To tell if you are really experiencing preterm labor, employ the 4-1-1 formula: if your contractions are 4 minutes (or less) apart, last at least 1 minute, and continue for at least 1 hour, you are most likely in labor. Alert your healthcare provider immediately. We tell mothers that if they are having more than six contractions per hour, they need to call.

Enjoying late-pregnancy sex. Sex in the seventh month may be slightly less passionate, less frequent, and less athletic, but also inevitably more inventive. You may be preoccupied with the prospect of giving birth and your husband may find that his own feelings are undergoing a metamorphosis — his wife's body is not just exciting and different, it is a constant reminder that life is about to change. As the abdomen reaches its full shape, couples come to the realization that they are no longer a twosome, and they begin to look ahead. Women tend to focus on birthing and nurturing the baby; men focus on their new role as father and the impact that will have in all domains of life. Your partner may worry that he's losing you to motherhood and both of you may experience ambivalence about the changes ahead. All of these anxieties can impact your sex life.

Nevertheless, many couples still do have sex late in pregnancy. As you grow, you will have to experiment with workable and comfortable positions for intercourse. The man-on-top position is usually the most awkward — it is difficult, literally, to get over the hump — and least comfortable; penetration is deepest in this position, and the man's weight on the woman's abdomen and breasts, while not harmful for baby, is uncomfortable for the woman. Besides, in the final few months, women are often uncomfortable lying on their backs. Experiment with these alternatives, which allow the woman to control the depth of penetration and the amount of weight she bears:

- Woman on top
- Man on top, but with his weight supported on his arms
- Couple side-lying front-to-front or woman's back to man's front (her upper leg supported with pillows)
- Rear entry (woman on hands and knees with partner behind her)

Use whatever position gives you the most pleasure. If the desire for sex overrides your physical discomforts and your mental distractions, you will discover new ways of coming together. The most challenging time is yet to come: enjoying sex after birth while your new baby is close by.

Dad's note: *One night in the heat of passion, when we thought we finally had a little time to ourselves, baby started crying, my wife started leaking, and milk squirted right into my face. This shock was followed by a mutual laugh.*

Worried about the what-ifs. Other mothers might want to share their personal birth stories, whether positive or negative. As much as possible, try to turn a deaf ear to people who want to tell you all the things that could go wrong, because for most parents births go right. And what about all those things that could go wrong with baby? Again, chances are greatly in your favor that your baby will be born perfectly healthy. Try not to worry about the what-ifs.

Dr. Bill notes: Don't be put off if your healthcare provider unintentionally magnifies your health worries by listing what could go wrong. Part of the job of a doctor or midwife is to inform you of all the possibilities, yet they should also be quick to inform you that birth usually goes well.

If negative conversation like this disturbs you during your prenatal visits, tell your practitioner. Don't allow health worries to rob you of the joys of pregnancy and motherhood. While it's normal to be concerned, chances are great that the two of you will celebrate Birth-Day as a healthy mother and healthy baby.

Will I be a good enough mother? Worry about the health of your baby and the quality of your mothering often go together at this stage. Ambivalent feelings are part of the package of parenthood. During your pregnancy there will be days you are excited about the big event; other days you may be nervous about all the changes baby will bring to the family. You may question whether you will be a good enough mother. These feelings are rehearsal for parenthood. There will be days when you love being a parent, and there will be days when you wonder why you got yourself into this. You have probably heard of "mother's intuition," like a sixth sense that develops as soon as baby arrives. Rest assured that whatever the magical biochemicals are that will make you the best mother you can be, they will be there for you. Some mothers are more intuitive, while others seem less adept at reading baby's cues. This is why we devote a whole chapter of this book, "The Week After," to giving you time-tested tools

to bring out the best in you and your baby. Remember that your own internal wisdom is your greatest mothering tool!

MORE CHOICES TO MAKE

Choosing a Professional Labor Coach

Soon after fathers were finally admitted into the delivery room and given the title "labor coach" (a term coined by Dr. Bradley), women began whispering a little secret to each other, one they'd never tell their husbands or their doctors (who might throw the men back into the waiting room): many dads aren't cut out to be labor coaches. Few men are completely comfortable with the role, and few women find their mate's play-by-play strategizing helpful. Childbirth methods, while still emphasizing the important function of the father at birth, have redefined the father's role as one of psychological support and reassigned the coaching task to a professional labor assistant.

Who's the coach? The labor support person, a woman and probably a mother herself, brings a relaxed, natural approach to a traditional hospital birth. Her presence means that a mother does not have to rely solely on her husband for help in dealing with pain. She can instead enjoy his emotional support and love at a time that is special, but stressful, for them both.

Dr. Bill notes: I am a very good Little League baseball coach, but I don't feel comfortable as a coach for laboring women. My first experience as birth coach was when, even after rehearsing all those breathing and stopwatch exercises, I worried at Martha's first difficult contraction. Once I dropped the role of coach and took on the role of husband, the whole process became more natural for me and better for Martha.

Though a friend can certainly be a labor support person, mothers typically have the best results when they hire a professional labor assistant, also known as a birth doula or a labor coach. In addition to providing comfort and companionship to the laboring mother, this coach has special obstetrical training as a midwife, obstetrical nurse, or educated layperson — and she has typically chosen this role because she has a passion for helping women through the birthing process. Her knowledge of and experience with birthing, and her sole focus on your needs, make her a unique and indispensable part of a hospital birth. She coaches, counsels, supports, and anchors a laboring woman, helping the process move more quickly and comfortably. She also helps facilitate communication between the parents and the hospital staff, conveying their wishes and freeing mom and dad up to focus on labor and birth.

What's in it for you? Studies show that woman-supported labors result in:

- Shorter labors (by as much as 50 percent)
- Fewer medical interventions
- Reduced need for surgical births
- Fewer epidurals, episiotomies, and perineal tears

Labor coaches are especially valuable in high-risk pregnancies where the necessary use of technology makes natural methods of pain control much harder to employ. Most important, they aid immeasurably in getting a mother to relax and work with her birthing body.

Who pays? Even though labor coaches save medical costs, insurance companies don't typically cover them. You'll likely have to pay for a labor coach yourself. Fees range from $400 to $1200. Negotiate with your insurance carrier.

I had a previous cesarean section, and with this pregnancy I wanted to do everything possible to have a VBAC. I read that having a professional labor support person would increase my chance of having the birth I wanted. So I negotiated with my insurance company. I told them about the studies showing a lower rate of repeat cesarean deliveries in births that are attended by professional labor assistants. I asked them to pay for the labor assistant if I didn't end up with a cesarean birth, and they agreed. This not only eased my mind during my pregnancy, but it was also good business for the insurance company: paying my labor support person $500 was better than paying $5,000 for a C-section. I used a wonderful labor support person, got my vaginal birth, and my insurance company willingly reimbursed me her fee.

If you're lucky enough to live in a part of the country where the use of a labor coach is standard practice, your hospital or obstetrician may have a list of them for you to call. Midwives are generally connected with the doula community and would be an excellent resource for finding an experienced labor coach. In addition, you may find a labor support person through your childbirth educator or friends.

Once you've chosen your labor coach, she will schedule a meeting or two midway through your third trimester to help you work out a realistic birth plan. Some coaches meet you at the hospital once you are in labor, but many will come to your home and help you labor there until it is time to leave for the hospital.

Dr. BJ notes: Both a midwife and labor doula can provide support for labor and birth. If a midwife is providing your care she will provide support for you in labor as well. However, the midwife will not be with you during the early phases of your labor. If you want to stay at home until you are in active labor, a doula who provides early labor support would be an option to consider. The early part of labor is unpredictable, and having a doula may reduce the number of "false runs" and frustrations that you have during this time.

Questions You May Have about Labor Coaches

Would a labor coach cause my husband to feel displaced in the birthing room?

Not likely. In our experience, fathers welcome this experienced woman with open arms. The coach does not displace the father at birth; instead she takes the pressure off him to perform as coach and frees him up to do what he does best — love his mate. In the same way, she fills in the gaps in the healthcare team and frees the obstetrician or obstetrical nurses to do what they do best. She also empowers dad, such as showing him ways to help keep mom comfortable.

I chose to employ a labor coach because, after doing my homework, I realized there was a missing person in the current maternity system. Due to economic pressures, obstetrical nurses are often overworked, and obstetricians are overloaded. I wanted more than just my next-door-neighbor friend holding my hand during delivery, and I feared my husband would panic at my first pain. After talking to other mothers about their deliveries, I realized that many first-time mothers are left alone a lot during delivery and don't really know how to interpret what's going on in their bodies. My coach was the missing link I needed, and I think she saved me a lot of pain — literally.

I'm categorized as high-risk because of high blood pressure, and my doctor is worried about toxemia. Could a labor coach help in my situation?

Absolutely! As we mentioned previously, studies and common sense show that the probability of having a satisfying birth and a healthy baby is increased by the presence of someone who provides accurate information and support, empowers a woman to work with her body, and helps her make wise birthing choices. Labor coaches really shine in crisis moments when, due to an unanticipated complication, there is a sudden change in plans, requiring decisions to be made about technology or surgery. During these situations, you often do not have a clear enough mind to understand your options completely. The coach acts as an advocate or a go-between, often interpreting the medical information for you so that you can more easily understand and be part of the decision.

Dr. Linda notes: As an obstetrician, I love labor coaches. They help relax both the woman and her spouse. If things don't go according to plan, labor coaches can really help with interventions and with understanding the physician's recommendations.

Choosing a Pediatrician for Your Baby

Forty years ago when I (Dr. Bill) was finishing my pediatric training and was about to hang out my shingle and open a practice, my professor advised me that there are three qualities parents look for in a pediatrician — the three A's: able, affable, and available. Picking the right pediatrician for you and your child is one of your most important long-term investments. Medical care is a partnership between parents and pediatrician. The first step is choosing the right physician for your family.

Depending on the healthcare needs of your child, expect to be in your pediatrician's office at least fifteen times during the first five years of your child's life. You might as well get the most out of it. Here is a step-by-step plan, as well as some insider tips, on how to choose and use your child's pediatrician.

1. Interview yourself. Before you interview prospective healthcare providers, do some soul searching. What qualities do you need in

your child's doctor? If this is your first baby, you probably do not have a lot of experience in normal childhood development and the common childhood illnesses. Do you lack confidence (as nearly all first-time parents do) and believe you will need an involved pediatrician who will help you understand normal growth and development as well as manage your child competently when sick? Are you a worrier (which many parents are) and need an empathetic listener who will take your worries seriously? Are you evaluating various options in parenting styles and need a doctor who will help you formulate a parenting philosophy? Or are you veteran parents already firmly rooted in your parenting philosophy and styles and simply want a like-minded pediatrician?

Does distance matter? Are you willing to drive farther for higher quality, or do you rely on public transportation and therefore need a doctor's office that is close to your home or workplace and easily accessible by bus or subway?

If you are a first-time mother and are adamant about breastfeeding your baby, obviously you want to choose a breastfeeding-friendly pediatric practice. Or you might have special communication needs. One of my favorite patients, Nancy, is blind, and I have learned so much from her about the power of mother's intuition. Nancy and I learned to communicate by voice and touch. During an exam I would guide her hands over her baby's body to help her develop the feel for normal skin, normal muscle tone, and help her get an appreciation for the marvels of her baby's developing body. One time she brought in her infant for consultation about a rash, yet I couldn't see it. The next day she returned to the office with her obviously spotted child.

Nancy could feel the rash the day before I could see it.

2. Get references. Talk with friends who share your parenting philosophy. Pick out the most experienced and like-minded mothers in your circle and get references about the doctors they use. Ask them specific questions: "What do you like most about Dr. Susan?" "Is Dr. Tom available when you need him?" "Does Dr. Laura give you the time you need?" "Are Dr. Alan's partners just as good?" Pick out at least three names before continuing your search. If you are choosing a pediatrician toward the end of your pregnancy, consult your obstetrician or midwife, who by now has a feel for your specific needs. It's not only important for the pediatrician to be right for your child; he or she needs to be right for the parents as well.

Insider's tip. Suppose the doctor you have chosen to be your child's pediatrician is not taking new patients. Write a brief letter personally asking the doctor to accept your child as a new patient and follow up the letter with a phone call. This nicety informs a doctor that you sincerely care that much about your child's healthcare provider, and it motivates the doctor to want to open the practice to you. As I tell my receptionist, "There's always room in our practice for nice patients."

3. Do your insurance homework. It's disappointing to have chosen Dr. Right only to later find out that your insurance isn't accepted there. Once you have a list of prospective doctors, check your insurance plan booklet to see which ones are participating members. After you have narrowed down the list, check with these doctors' offices to be sure they are still members of the plan and are still accepting new patients. If you absolutely want to go to a certain doctor who is not a member of your current insurance plan, check your options with your insurance carrier. The best insurance carriers are now respecting the valuable freedom of choice in choosing doctors and offer a "point of service" (POS) option, which allows you to see healthcare providers outside the plan, usually for an additional charge.

CHOOSING THE RIGHT MEDICAL INSURANCE FOR YOUR BABY

At no time in history has the conflict between practical economics and quality medical care been so confusing to parents. In preparing yourself and your baby for the current healthcare reform, today's savvy moms will have more questions, yet doctors will have less time to answer them. A very important medical decision — if you have an option — is what type of medical insurance is best for your family. While there are many options, here's the most important decision you will make: PPO or HMO?

Here's an insider's tip. If possible, go PPO. A PPO payment means that your doctor is able to charge according to the time your baby needs. If your baby has a challenging medical problem requiring extra time and expertise — say, a chronic condition such as diabetes or a behavioral issue such as autism — your doctor is able to upgrade the fee for this higher level of service and give you and your child the level of care you both need.

With an HMO, on the other hand, the doctor is paid a set monthly fee, regardless of the time or level of medical care you and your child need. For this reason, many HMO practices allow only five minutes per visit. And, to make the HMO practice more "cost effective," your child may be seen nearly all the time by a nurse practitioner or medical assistant (many are quite well trained and conscientious) instead of a pediatrician. Some HMO plans even "reward" the doctor with a year-end bonus for costing the HMO less in medical expenses. An exception to this "do less, get paid more" medical model is Kaiser Permanente. The original HMO, this organization has maintained a high level of medical care and is a wise choice for parents who must choose an HMO. (See how grandparents can make a wise long-term investment, on AskDrSears.com/grandparenting.)

4. Check out the office. Once you've made your appointment, arrive early for your interview appointment and browse around the office a bit. Chat with other parents in the waiting room and ask what they like, or dislike, about the office and the doctor's practice. Notice and ask the staff about how children with potentially contagious illnesses are handled. A question many first-time interviewers ask is, "Do you have separate waiting rooms for well and sick children?" This is a question they obviously got from their childbirth class or a book written by someone who has never run a pediatric office. Most doctors who have tried separate sick and well waiting rooms have found that this system does not work, because nobody wants to use the "sick" waiting room! The more practical solution to minimize the spread of illnesses is to reserve the waiting room for well children only and to usher potentially contagious children immediately into examining rooms, maybe even through a separate entrance.

5. Interview the office staff. Introduce yourself to the office staff. Are they friendly and accommodating? You're likely to have as much contact with the office staff as you will the doctor. During doctor-shopping interviews, I love to hear new parents say, "Your staff is so helpful." To maximize the time you have with your doctor, you can get many questions answered by the office staff before meeting the doctor: hospital affiliations, after-hours coverage, appointment scheduling, and anything else that is important to you.

Insider's tip: Try to schedule newborn and well-baby checkups as the first appointment in the morning or right after lunch, times when the office tends to be the least crowded and the doctor is on time.

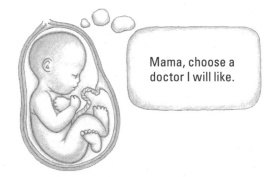

Mama, choose a doctor I will like.

6. Interview the doctor. Remember, the goal of your interview is to decide whether this pediatrician is the right match for your family. Try these interviewing tips:

• *Be brief.* Since most doctors do not charge for these interviews, five minutes is considered enough to make a "meet the doctor" assessment. If you feel you need more time due to special needs, schedule a regular doctor's appointment for a "checkup" and not an "interview," and expect to pay.

• *Be concise.* Bring a written list of your most pressing parenting concerns. This is not the time to ramble on about future behavior worries, such as bed-wetting or learning disabilities.

• *Be positive.* Avoid opening the interview with an "I don't want" list. I remember parents who opened their interview with, "We don't want to give our baby eye drops, vitamin K, newborn shots, newborn blood tests, immunizations. . . ." The negative opener put me on the defensive as I realized the mismatch between their desires and my professional beliefs. While it's good to do your homework and formulate opinions about certain routine medical practices, it's better to phrase your question positively, such as: "Doctor, what is your custom about routine immunizations?" This allows you to learn the doctor's side of an issue and opens the door to factors you may not have previously considered. Also, realize that a full discussion on this specific topic is beyond the scope of the interview visit.

• *Be impressive.* One set of first-time expectant parents who were checking me out as a potential doctor for their baby opened their interview with a line that impressed me: "This is a well-researched baby." I immediately warmed to these parents, since this statement let me know that they had thoroughly done their homework. They had carefully chosen their obstetrician and explored their birthing options, and now I was on their list of pediatric finalists. They conveyed that selecting who would be caring for their child was a high priority.

• *Avoid doctor turnoffs.* Remember, doctors take a lot of pride in being chosen by selective parents. Don't reveal that you would choose this practice "because I found you in the yellow pages" or "because you're on my insurance plan." These openers do not make for the best first impressions.

• *Ask leading questions.* To decide whether you and the doctor are of similar mindset, ask leading questions. Pick out topics that are most important to you, such as: "Doctor, I really want to continue breastfeeding my baby, but I'm going back to work in a couple of months. How will you help us continue breastfeeding?" (You want to find out if the doctor has experience helping breastfeeding and working mothers.) "If my baby wakes up in the middle of the night, what would you advise?" (You want sensitive and specific recommendations rather than the quick and easy "let him cry it out.") If you are a high-touch parent who wants to hold your baby a lot and respond sensitively to your baby's cries, watch for telltale comments such as "Now, you don't want to spoil that baby," which reveals that this doctor has not researched the science of the Attachment Parenting style. If you are planning to have a dual career and need some practical advice about juggling working and parenting, getting a lecture on the hazards of daycare is an unhelpful turnoff.

Dr. Bill advises: *Choose a pediatrician primarily on medical competence, secondarily on parenting-style compatibility.*

CORD BLOOD BANKING

Should you bank your baby's blood? Normally, cord blood is simply thrown away with the placenta, so it is often a wasted resource that could be used for your own baby or even for other family members. As you get closer to baby's Birth-Day, the subject of whether and where to bank your baby's cord blood is just another family choice to be made. Cord blood contains stem cells, which have ability to grow into different types of tissue when transplanted. These cells are being used successfully in treatment of leukemia and other blood disorders. There is lots of encouraging research going on in the use of cord-blood stem cells for the treatment of diabetes, brain damage, and many other illnesses that need tissue healing. There are other potential uses for cord-blood stem cells that continue to evolve, including treating and repairing heart tissue after heart attacks and other forms of cardiovascular disease; nerve and brain injury after strokes, trauma, or various neurodegenerative diseases; as well as rare metabolic and genetic disorders that children may be born with.

Shortly after birth the vials of cord blood are taken from the umbilical cord and stored for future use. There are two ways to store this precious resource: donate it to a public blood bank or pay for private cord-blood banking in order to save this superhealing tissue for possible use by your baby or family. If you have a family member with a disease such as leukemia who might benefit from cord blood, ask this person to ask their doctor about the ability of donating your baby's cord blood for stem cell therapy.

What about storing umbilical cord tissue? Some cord-blood banks now also offer to store a small portion of the umbilical cord to take advantage of the specific type of stem cells present in the cord. While this technology is too new to know all the possible advantages, it may be a good idea for families who are already choosing to store the cord blood. For more information, visit the Cord Blood Registry at CordBlood.com.

COMPOSING YOUR BIRTH WISH

While birth, like life, is full of surprises, the more convincingly you state your birth wishes, the more likely they are to come true. The purpose of a birth plan is not only to increase your chances of getting the birth you want but also to alert your birth attendants to your personal needs. Obstetricians, midwives, and obstetrical nurses attend mothers with a variety of birth wishes. Some mothers prefer a high-touch, low-tech, more "natural" style of birth. Others want or need more high-tech management and intervention during their labors. Your labor attendants will not know the style of birth you want unless you tell them.

(continued)

Obstetrical nurse to mother:

I've read your birth plan and know you don't want to have drugs. It would be easy for me to ask the doctor to prescribe some pain relievers, but you won't like me later. Before getting a shot of a pain reliever, let's try changing your positions.

Obstetrician to mother:

In your birth plan you stated that you wanted the epidural turned off after

transition so you could participate in and experience pushing, so I decided to use a lower dose that wears off more quickly when you seemed not to need them anymore.

Personalize your plan. Don't copy it from a book or class. This is your birth, so it must be your plan. You will learn how to compose a birth plan during your childbirth classes. *The Birth Book* (William Sears and Martha Sears) is another useful resource.

Why Are So Many Women Having Cesarean Births?

We prefer to call it a cesarean birth, not a cesarean section, because it is first a birth and second an operation. Once upon a time 95 percent of women delivered vaginally, and in many countries it's still that way. So why does the United States have one of the highest percentage of surgical births? Presently, nearly one in three American mothers have surgical births. Do American women have smaller pelvises or grow bigger babies than European mothers? Not likely. So, what is the real reason and why do nearly all other pregnancy books avoid this question? Pregnant mothers deserve an answer.

Modern technology and safer surgical deliveries have saved the lives of many mothers and babies and enabled babies to be born healthier than they would have during prolonged vaginal deliveries. I, Dr. Bill, have attended over a thousand surgical births in my forty years as a pediatrician and can attest to the fact that many babies are expertly

delivered by emergency C-section and possibly spared lifelong disabilities caused by lack of oxygen during complicated vaginal births. The good news is that there are a few basic healthcare tools that informed women can use to lower their chances of needing a surgical birth.

Surgical births have been on the rise over the past two decades, from 5 percent in 1970 to 23 percent in 2000 to 33 percent in 2009. Here are the most prevalent reasons for the increase in surgical births:

More multiples. Surgical birth for multiples is obviously safer. Modern fertility drugs have led to an increase in the number of multiple births, and therefore an increase in the number of surgical births. But this accounts for just a small portion of the increase.

More epidurals. While modern childbirth is now more scientific and in some ways safer, and "pain-free" is the goal, tampering with nature is not without its risks. For example, pain-relieving drugs that help women have more comfortable deliveries can slow down their labor, eventually making surgical birth necessary. This is true of the epidural — a pain-relieving method that many women view as the obstetrical advancement of the century.

There is legitimate debate about whether epidurals increase the cesarean rate. There are good studies suggesting that epidural anesthesia is indeed associated with rising cesarean rates, and also good studies showing that well-timed epidurals and well-managed labors do not increase the cesarean rate.

Epidurals relax the muscles in the lower pelvis and vagina. The relaxation of these muscles can allow the baby to settle into a posterior position (face up), which can delay or prevent the baby from descending into the birth canal, which is the physiological trigger that gives the mother the urge to push. Without the intense but natural sensation of the urge to push, mothers have difficulty understanding how to push in coordination with the work of the uterus; this can lead to "failure to progress" and a surgical birth.

More technology. The major technological advance that most contributes to the rising cesarean rate is electronic fetal monitoring (EFM), which can lead to false-alarm C-sections. On the one hand, this valuable tool can detect problems such as low heart rate or low oxygen in an unborn baby, and can alert doctors to intervene surgically before baby suffers the effects of these problems. On the other hand, despite its more than forty-year history, it's still not an exact science. Some of these wiggly tracings are hard to interpret: Are they simply meaningless patterns or do they mean baby's oxygen supply is being compromised? False

alarms are one reason many mothers are rushed to the operating room unnecessarily, often rightly so, since obstetrical wisdom is "when in doubt, get baby out." If there's any chance that the EFM tracing might signify insufficient oxygen to baby, the obstetrical team cannot take a chance.

The overuse of EFM is a setup for both mothers and obstetricians to be *wired to worry*. Naturally, mother may wonder, "Why am I being wired up? Is something going wrong?" Fear sets in, and the more she worries that something might go wrong, the more likely it will. The obstetrician, meanwhile, worries what those squiggly lines mean and what to do about them.

Dr. BJ notes: Research has shown that with low-risk pregnancies and labor, EFM is not often necessary and leads to unnecessary intervention — an increase in the use of medications and cesarean birth. What has been shown to reduce unnecessary interventions in uncomplicated pregnancies and labor is monitoring the baby intermittently with a Doppler device, such as the one used during prenatal visits, and the continuous presence of a professional support person. Midwives are comfortable with this type of labor sitting.

Greater fear of liability. While you'll seldom see this cesarean cause revealed in pregnancy books, it is one of the top causes for the skyrocketing surgical birth rate. I (Dr. Bill) have personally been involved as an expert witness in many cases where the obstetrician made a judgment call about the results of EFM tracings and elected not to do a surgical birth (which is a much more difficult decision, but one in which the obstetrician has the best interest of the mother and baby). Through no fault of anyone involved, baby's health was compromised and the doctor was sued. "Doctor, did you do all you could have to spare this baby damage from low oxygen?" is a common question in court. Obviously, that leading phrase "all you could do" includes surgical birth. One of our birth wishes is medical-legal reform.

Seven Reasons for Needing a Cesarean

In many ways birthing a baby has never been safer for women with challenging pregnancies. Surgical advances have made a cesarean a much safer operation, but the fact is it is still major surgery. Complications, though uncommon, do occur, and recovering from major surgery is a difficult way to spend the first few weeks of motherhood. Let's look at the seven most common reasons for a surgical birth and what you can do to influence them in your own birth experience.

Repeat cesarean. While this is a common reason for surgical birth, it is also the one you can most influence. As you will learn on page 276, the belief that "once a cesarean, always a cesarean" is no longer true, as VBAC (vaginal birth after cesarean) is becoming more sought after.

Dr. BJ notes: While VBAC is a safe option, there are obstetricians and hospitals that will not support it. The current standard requires the obstetrician to be physically present in labor and delivery when a woman who has had a prior cesarean birth is in labor. This is not the practice of many obstetricians and they will not agree to "labor sit" or to plan around the unpredictability of when a woman will be in labor. If the obstetrician is supportive, be sure to check with the hospital where you plan to give birth to make sure there are no policies that prevent you from VBAC. In other words, do your homework early rather than just assume that the hospital will accommodate your request.

Failure to progress. Most of the time when I (Dr. Bill) have been called to attend a surgical birth, I would see the diagnosis of "FTP" in mother's chart. Translation: "failure to progress" — a labor that doesn't progress according to the usual timetable. FTP accounts for around 30 percent of surgical births. Usually for unknown reasons the baby does not descend far enough or the cervix doesn't dilate enough. After years of attending FTP births, I wondered about the math. Around 10 percent of laboring mothers go on to need a surgical birth because of "failure to progress." Think about it. No other healthy system in your body "fails" 10 percent of the time. Why should your "delivery" system?

The answer to this question is that many women, through lack of information, preparation, and good labor support, do not use their body's own birth-giving system the way it was designed to be used. You will learn some strategies to help your labor progress on page 346.

Dr. Linda notes: Over the last thirty years, there is no doubt there have been a lot of unnecessary cesareans performed when "failure to progress" means "failure to get a woman in labor," which can happen when a woman comes to the hospital too soon, when elective labor inductions are overdone, or when doctors and mothers get tired of prolonged early labor and move too quickly to cesarean. On the other hand, American childbearing women have largely become older, more obese, and more likely to be diabetic. All these conditions make for bigger babies relative to the mother's pelvic structure. You can minimize your risk of "failing to progress" by being sure you are physically fit and of normal weight, and maintain excellent communication with your caregiver.

Dr. BJ notes: All women and babies have their own timetable, and "failure to progress" often means "failure to wait." When women follow the standard labor curve, it is not labeled a problem. But if they go beyond the standard labor curve, it is often labeled a problem. It is only those labors that are way beyond the average where FTP is a correct label.

Dr. Bill notes: "Failure to progress," the label given to laboring women, is more appropriately given to healthcare policymakers who fail to push for women's rights to have not only a safer but a more satisfying birth. "Failure to progress" also points to the fact that despite all the advances in obstetrical care, the surgical birth rate is increasing instead of decreasing, and the United States ranks toward the top of the list in percent of surgical births and near the bottom of the list in birthing healthy babies.

Fetal distress. The third most common situation leading to a cesarean delivery is fetal distress, a widely used term in the 1980s and 1990s that obstetricians and midwives are discarding in the twenty-first century due to its vagueness. Fetal heart patterns on the electronic fetal monitor can suggest that baby's well-being is in jeopardy unless he is delivered quickly. A fetal heart rate that is higher or lower than average can be a sign that baby is not getting enough oxygen, or not recovering well from the decreased heart rate that is normal during contractions. While some of the reasons babies receive insufficient oxygen are beyond your control, the positions you assume in labor greatly influence your baby's well-being. For example, if a mother stays in bed in the back-lying position during most of her labor, the chance that she will need a surgical birth is increased. (We will discuss this more on page 351.)

Cephalopelvic disproportion (CPD). Another reason for surgical births is CPD, when baby's head seems too large to pass through the pelvic outlet. Even though X-ray and ultrasound measurements, called a fetal-pelvic index, can indicate a smaller than usual pelvic outlet, there are specific laboring positions that you can use to widen the passage. Laboring and birthing in a more upright position, and even squatting, will enlarge your pelvic outlet as much as 20 percent, enough to allow the baby's head and shoulders to rotate normally through the dimensions of the birth canal to find the easiest way out. Enlarging your pelvic outlet by changing positions, along with baby's natural maneuvering, often allows even a small mommy to deliver a big baby. The bones in the baby's skull are all separate and are designed to "mold" to the mother's pelvis in order to pass through.

Most of the women in my family "had to" have cesareans because, they were told, their pelvises were too small. With our first child I lived up to the family history and had a cesarean. With our second baby I did my homework. I chose the right birth attendant and the right birth place, and I was not a patient but a participant in my delivery. I pushed out a healthy nine-pound baby. I let my body birth the way it was intended.

Active genital herpes. A newborn baby can contract herpes during passage through an infected birth canal, so it is necessary to deliver any baby whose mother has active herpes at the time of birth via cesarean section. Herpes infections are life threatening in newborns. If you have herpes, your doctor or midwife may recommend you take antiviral medication at around thirty-five or thirty-six weeks to minimize the risk of an outbreak occurring when you go into labor. He may want to culture suspicious lesions and will do a very careful inspection of your vaginal and vulvar tissues in late pregnancy and early in labor. Women with prior herpes outbreaks actually pass some immunity to their newborns. Women who acquire herpes for the first time during their pregnancy and have active sores at the time of delivery pose the greatest risk of infecting their babies. If you have herpes sores when you begin labor, you will need a surgical delivery.

Breech position. While around half of all babies start out bottom-down in early pregnancy, most turn head-down by thirty-four weeks; 3 to 4 percent of babies don't flip and stay in the breech position. This may be due to the uterus having an unusual shape; some women have heart-shaped or V-shaped uterine cavities, which lend themselves to keeping babies in breech position. If there is not very much fluid the baby may get caught in a bottom-first position, and ironically if there is too much fluid the baby may somersault into a breech position. Often breech positions simply happen.

The American Congress of Obstetricians and Gynecologists currently recommends surgical birth for breech babies because of the higher risk of harm to the baby during delivery. Baby might get stuck in the birth canal, or prolapse of the umbilical cord may occur as the cord slips through the cervix before baby's body and gets pinched (both situations require emergency cesarean). There may also be damage to the major nerves of the arms because of the compression put on the arms stretched above baby's head. These complications are much more concerning when baby presents feet first ("footling breech") rather than buttocks first ("frank breech"). Breech babies can sometimes be turned prior to labor in a procedure called a cephalic version, so if your caregiver thinks the baby is breech ask if this would be an option for you.

Multiple babies. Many, but certainly not all, mothers of twins are advised to have a cesarean delivery because of the chance of insufficient oxygen to two babies delivered vaginally. Triplets (and more!) nearly always need surgical births. This is a case-by-case decision based on the size of the babies, how many you are carrying, your previous obstetrical history, and other factors. By all means if you are carrying twins talk to your physician, and if a safe vaginal trial of labor is important to you, find a physician who will at least consider a vaginal delivery.

Dr. Linda notes: *There are many reasons for the rising rate in the United States of cesarean birth — some of them good, some not so good:*

- *Higher-risk women are having babies*

- *There are more multiple births due to fertility treatments*

- *More older women are having first-time babies*

- *We as a country are fatter, and overweight women have a higher cesarean rate*

- *Some women request cesareans so that they can avoid the "inconvenience" of unscheduled labor*

- *First-time cesareans are often quicker and easier for doctors to perform than sitting out long labors*

- *Breech babies are almost all delivered by cesarean*

- *Fewer women are having vaginal birth after cesarean (see page 276)*

- *Fear of lawsuits over infants with any type of difficult birth has prompted physicians to recommend cesarean births*

- *Physicians in training are not learning techniques for forceps and vacuum deliveries. Such "operative vaginal deliveries" were previously used to avoid cesarean deliveries*

The good news is most women will have uncomplicated vaginal and/or cesarean births. There are ways to empower yourself, however, to help avoid an unnecessary cesarean.

OUR BIRTH WISHES

We have a dream that birthcare reform will give high priority to the belief that the future of any culture depends upon how mothers birth their babies. Here are our wishes:

- More economic value and compensation will be given to the whole business of birth, adequately reimbursing obstetricians and midwives and other birthcare professionals for the world-enriching work they do.

- Every obstetrical practice will assign a midwife to a mother so she has the best of both birthing worlds: an obstetrician and a midwife.

- Modern birth centers will be adjacent to maternity hospitals, providing mothers a safe choice.

- Every laboring mother, upon entering the hospital, will have the privilege of having a familiar midwife attend her birth. The mother then feels safe that she has the best of both worlds: the midwife to empower her to use her best efforts to birth her baby in the way her body intends, yet just in case (which she should not dwell upon) an unexpected complication occurs, the doctor is in.

We believe that babies will be born healthier, smarter, and emotionally more stable, and that our society will benefit from better birth starts.

How to Increase Your Chances of a Vaginal Birth

Here are some strategies to increase your chances of giving birth vaginally:

Pick your caregivers with care. Before and during pregnancy, you want to be sure your caregivers have a philosophy that ensures an appropriate cesarean rate. Be sure to schedule a time with your provider early in the pregnancy to discuss this — you do not want to wait until the third trimester when your options for changing providers may not be possible. Here are some good questions to ask:

- How likely is it that you will be the one to attend the birth of my baby? If not you, how many providers cover for you?

- What is your or your group's primary (first-time) cesarean rate?

- What is your or your group's repeat cesarean rate?

- Do you have any recommendation for childbirth preparation classes? How do you manage patients who have Bradley or hypnobirthing preparation? (This will give you an insight into the caregiver's philosophy of natural birth.)

- What hospital or birth center are you affiliated with?

- Do you have the ability to perform forceps or vacuum delivery? If you yourself do not, do you have immediate access to individuals possessing these skills? How about others who might be covering for you when I go into labor?

- What is your philosophy on elective induction of labor? (See the section on inductions, page 346.)

- What is your philosophy on breech infants? Do you offer version procedures to turn breech babies?

If you have had a previous cesarean, there are additional questions to ask:

- Do you offer trials of labor for women with previous cesareans?

- What is your success rate for vaginal birth after cesarean (VBAC), also known as trial of labor after cesarean (TOLAC)?

- How many VBACs do you do a year?

There are no right or wrong answers to any of these questions, but in discussing them you will get a real sense of your caregiver's philosophy and how she responds to your concerns.

Follow the Healthy Pregnancy Plan (page 10). The better you prepare your body for the passage of your little passenger, the healthier your birth is likely to be — for both of you. Well-nourished, toned tissue stretches and changes to accommodate the forces of a vaginal birth.

Maintain an optimal weight. Just as you would have a harder time finishing a marathon lugging around 10 pounds or more of extra weight, ditto that for birth. Lots of excess body fat not only throws hormonal harmony out of balance and increases your chances of needing a surgical birth, but it also delays tissue healing, should a surgical birth be needed.

Stable blood sugar, optimal weight, stable blood pressure — plus all those hormonal influences that are mostly under your control — increase the likelihood of having a vaginal birth. When your other hormones are stable, your birthing hormones are likely to work more efficiently. Review all the tips in Part I.

Strengthen your birthing muscles. There is no exercise ever invented that even comes close to giving birth to a baby. Imagine the muscle energy needed, the focus demanded, and the endurance required to push out a baby. The more you stretch, strengthen, and rehearse the star muscles most involved in labor and birth, the more likely it is to go smoothly.

Position yourself upright for birth. The more time you spend laboring on your back, the more likely you are to need a surgical birth. During our many years of experience attending births, Martha as a labor coach and Dr. Bill as a pediatrician, here's a common scenario we saw: We stand in the doorway and watch a laboring mother lying on her back, all wired up and medicated, and unable to move much. We both think, "This is a surgical birth waiting to happen." Simply put, gravity is one of your best birthing friends. When you lie on your back, gravity pulls your baby down toward your back. When you stand, walk, squat, or assume any vertical position, gravity pulls the baby down toward your cervix. One of the most important sections in this book is "Working Out Your Best Birthing Positions," page 353).

Move more. One of the most common causes of "failure to progress" is "failure to move." The more you get up and move around, the less likely you are to need a surgical birth.

A COMMON CESAREAN CYCLE

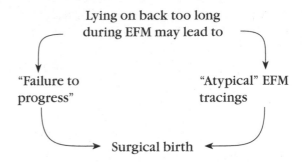

Lying on back too long during EFM may lead to "Failure to progress" "Atypical" EFM tracings Surgical birth

Use technology wisely. Discuss with your healthcare provider if and when electronic fetal monitoring (EFM) may be necessary. As you learned on page 269, EFM, while lifesaving in some circumstances, does lead to an increased chance of a surgical birth. For example, laboring on your back increases your chances of getting atypical EFM recordings, as does "continuous" versus "intermittent" EFM, and in order to apply EFM, the laboring woman is often required to stay in bed. A growing trend among obstetricians is to discourage routine EFM for low-risk mothers, because it has not been shown to improve the outcome of birth in this group of moms.

Get a coach. Want to cut your chances of having a surgical birth by 50 percent? Hire a specially trained doula, professional labor assistant, or labor coach. As we discussed on page 260, hiring labor support can not only increase your chances of having a more satisfying labor, but also greatly increase your chances of having a vaginal birth. Unfortunately, despite statistics and studies showing that this is one of the best ways to prevent surgical births, many insurance companies still do not cover this service. (See page 261 for tips on negotiating with your insurance company.) Regardless, having a labor support person attend your birth is certainly an investment in your health and your baby's.

Trust your body to work for you. Trust that your body's delivery system will work. Know that your pelvic passages are designed to birth your baby. The fear that you won't be able to go through with giving birth can be a self-fulfilling prophecy, since fear tenses the uterus into not working efficiently. Surround yourself with positive supporters. Even if many of your family members or friends have had cesarean births, know that this does not have to be your experience.

Remember, what's good for mother is good for baby. The more you follow these surgery-prevention tips, the more likely you are to be able to give your baby the needed and undivided attention after birth, and the less likely you are to have to divert your energy from mothering into healing. (For more tips on lowering your chances of needing a surgical birth, see the related section, "Thirteen Ways to Help Your Labor Progress," on page 346.)

Wanting a VBAC

If you previously had a cesarean, chances are good you'll be able to deliver your next baby vaginally. Years ago, cesarean incisions were made vertically, in the upper part of the uterus — the area most prone to rupture. Now cesarean incisions are made horizontally, in the lower part of the uterus (even in emergencies). This cut, a low-transverse incision, or "bikini cut," is

extremely unlikely to rupture. With a low-transverse incision, authorities now estimate the risk of uterine rupture in subsequent labors to be around 0.2 percent, which means that there is a 99.8 percent chance of mother going through labor without rupturing her uterus. In a survey of 36,000 women attempting VBAC, no mother died of uterine rupture, regardless of the type of prior uterine incision. In a study of 17,000 women attempting VBAC, no infants died as a result of uterine rupture. (Don't let the term "rupture" scare you — it does not mean that your uterus will suddenly explode. Instead, it means that the previous cesarean scar could gradually pull apart.) There are warning signs of this separation that can be picked up by using EFM, which will be recommended if you are having a VBAC. So the numbers are greatly in your favor — having a VBAC poses only a very small risk for nearly all women. You may not be a candidate for a VBAC if you have any of the seven reasons for needing a surgical birth listed on page 270.

Whether you are a candidate for a VBAC may depend upon the reason for your previous cesarean. If you needed a surgical birth because your baby was in a breech position, you had an active herpes infection, you had preeclampsia, or the electronic fetal monitoring suggested that baby was experiencing serious fetal distress, there is no reason to expect that you will need a cesarean again. These factors were unique to the earlier pregnancy and may not recur. If the diagnosis leading to your previous cesarean was cephalopelvic disproportion (CPD) — your baby's head was thought to be too big to pass through your pelvis — there's still no reason to worry. New studies show that this diagnosis does not lower your chances of having a VBAC. True CPD is uncommon, and in most instances the births could just as easily have been diagnosed as "failure to progress." Often one baby won't come out because he is malpositioned, and another, even bigger, baby of the same mother in a better position might just glide right out the next time! (OK, not really glide.) Studies report a 65 to 70 percent chance of successful VBAC despite a previous diagnosis of CPD. A woman's pelvic outlet usually becomes more flexible with each delivery, and various changes of position during labor can make it easier for baby to find the way out. However, don't count on the positive statistics alone to carry you through a VBAC. Get empowered:

Join a support group. ICAN (International Cesarean Awareness Network, ican-online .org) has chapters nationwide. This support group will help you deal with feelings of guilt or regret from your previous cesarean while arming you with information on how to avoid another one. You will hear helpful suggestions from mothers who have gone the surgical route once and were highly motivated to have a VBAC the next time.

Don't replay. Keep your mind on your present labor and don't allow yourself to be discouraged by flashbacks from the labor that led to the previous cesarean. Otherwise, you may panic at the first monitor alarm and forget everything you've been doing to progress through this labor.

This time around you can benefit from what you learned and be more informed and better prepared. You can follow the suggestions we have given throughout this book on having a healthy pregnancy and well-supported labor. In our experience,

many women who begin studying up for a VBAC realize, looking back, that there were things they could have done to avoid the cesarean. Mothers who can satisfy themselves that they did all they could do to give birth vaginally typically do not experience feelings of guilt and failure, because they realize they had a truly necessary cesarean. Either way, you can rejoice in your motherhood and revel in the joy of finally holding your baby.

Select a VBAC-friendly birth attendant and birth place. You will need to find a supportive birth attendant and an obstetrical system with a high VBAC success rate. A successful VBAC rate of 70 to 85 percent is acceptable. The most important issue is not the actual percentage you are quoted, but the philosophy of the doctor and a supportive infrastructure. If a physician or midwife allows only a few "ideal" women to have labor trials, their success rate may be high because they are recommending repeat cesarean sections to most of their patients. While there are some extra precautions that must be taken for a woman pursuing a VBAC (blood available, IV access established, anesthesia and immediate operating room access), you want the birth place and doctor to have a mindset that this process is normal and not terribly high risk.

Studies show that even mothers with two or three previous cesarean births have a 70 percent success rate with VBAC if they deliver in a birth place supportive of VBACs. Obstetrical centers that specialize in VBACs do not consider most VBAC candidates high-risk and treat them like normal laboring patients. In fact, they consider it counterproductive to attach the "high-risk" label to VBAC mothers because they require no additional technology, intervention, or monitoring. Beware especially of birth attendants who have a "pelvic prejudice" against small-hipped mothers wanting VBACs. Many petite women successfully push out big babies.

Don't let measurements scare you. VBAC studies fail to show any correlation between the size of the baby and the chances of uterine rupture. Moreover, estimates of fetal size and weight by ultrasound are not always accurate, especially in the final month.

Employ a labor coach. Mothers using an experienced labor coach are much more likely to have the birth they want (see page 260).

Dr. Linda notes: Many women, sadly, refuse to even consider a VBAC, even though there is roughly only a 0.2 percent risk of problems with the prior scar. Many doctors and hospitals do not offer VBACs because they do not meet the criteria ACOG has set forth for facilities offering this option. If you are interested in a VBAC, it is essential that you find a like-minded caregiver who uses a facility adequately staffed and equipped to handle possible VBAC complications.

SCIENCE SAYS: VBACS ARE SAFE, BUT THERE IS A SLIGHT RISK

A study published in the *New England Journal of Medicine* in 2004 revealed that VBACs are generally safe, but not 100 percent. Obstetrical researchers from nineteen medical centers enrolled 45,000 women who had previously had cesareans. Eighteen thousand of these women attempted VBACs. After analyzing the results, researchers concluded that the risk to a baby of getting low blood supply and oxygen to the brain during VBAC is 1 in 2,000 VBAC attempts. The authors of this study also concluded, but not everyone agrees, that while this risk is small, it is a bit greater than that associated with elective repeat cesarean birth.

Even though the risk to the baby was extremely low, these findings, coupled with legal pressures, were enough to dampen obstetricians' enthusiasm for VBACs. This study also revealed that there was a greater risk of uterine rupture when VBAC-attempting mothers were given oxytocin to induce labor, compared with those who gave birth without the use of oxytocin.

Scheduled C-Section

Scheduling surgical births, while most convenient for the doctor and the parents, and theoretically safer, is not necessarily in the best interest of mother and baby. On the positive side, it's nice to know exactly what day and around what time of day you're going to have a baby. But I (Dr. Bill) have attended many "elective cesareans," in which the baby came out unexpectedly premature because of misdating. Another option to consider and discuss with your healthcare provider is having the cesarean after several hours of active labor. The advantage: your due date is determined by you and your baby, not by the estimates of ultrasound or measurements. If your newborn could talk, she would thank you for your labor of love. The natural hormones released during labor prepare baby to adapt more easily to life outside the womb. Studies show that babies surgically delivered after mother labors a while have fewer breathing problems in the first few days after birth than babies whose mothers were not in labor.

Dr. Linda notes: *There is now enormous pressure on doctors and patients to have VBACs. This is overall a good thing, and I think it improves women's well-being. But be sure you are having a VBAC because you and your caregiver think it is appropriate. While our practice has a 90 percent VBAC trial rate and an 80 percent success rate, the other 20 percent is important to consider. It includes the 10 percent of women who, after careful consideration, decide along with their caregivers that* *this particular pregnancy may best be served by a repeat cesarean. The other 10 percent are women who end up with a cesarean despite doing all the right things.*

While the complication rate of cesarean section in laboring patients may be slightly more than that of a cesarean scheduled electively, the due date determined by Dr. Mother Nature is more precise than that calculated by technology, thus avoiding unnecessary premature births. According to the guidelines from the American Congress of Obstetricians and Gynecologists, elective surgical births are best performed after thirty-nine weeks. Therefore, important questions to ask your caregiver include: How many of your prior C-section patients attempted a VBAC? What is your success rate? If either the trial rate is under 80 percent or the success rate is under 50 percent without a good explanation, then you may want to find a group with more experience and expertise in this area.

IS LABOR GOOD FOR BABY?

If you plan to have a surgical birth anyway, you may wonder why you should put you and baby through all that work of labor. Research shows that labor is good for mother and baby. While the process of labor and birth is stressful for baby and mother, the stress has positive effects. In mothers, labor brings on the release of healthy stress and bonding hormones that help a mother cope with pain and adapt to caring for a newborn. Mother's hard work also stimulates her baby's adrenal glands to secrete high levels of the same "fight or flight" hormones that are released into an adult's system in response to a stressful or life-threatening situation to help the adult quickly adapt. Known as the "fetal stress response," this helps baby "fight" to adapt to life outside the womb. Studies have shown that newborns whose mothers went through labor had higher levels of these "helper hormones" than newborns delivered by scheduled cesarean without the benefit of labor. The fetal stress response helps baby

(continued)

make a healthy transition to life outside the womb in these ways:

- *Facilitates breathing.* These hormones increase secretion of surfactant, a chemical that helps keep the lungs expanded. Also, some birthcare providers believe that the hormones of labor help stimulate breathing.

- *Increases blood flow to vital organs.* Stress hormones direct the blood flow to baby's heart, brain, and kidneys.

- *Increases the newborn's immunity.* Adrenal hormones increase the number of infection-fighting white blood cells in baby's bloodstream.

- *Increases energy supply to baby* by providing nutrients for baby to use

during the transition from placental feeding to breastfeeding — tiding baby over until mother's milk comes in. Labor also stimulates the milk-making hormone prolactin.

- *Makes bonding easier.* A high level of labor hormones helps newborns be more alert and responsive to interaction with caregivers.

The fetal stress response is further testimony to how mothers' and babies' bodies are beautifully designed to cope with birth and begin a new life together.

(To learn more about how labor hormones help mother and baby, see "The Hormonal Symphony of Birth," chapter 18.)

Healing after Cesarean Birth

Because of modern obstetrics, surgical births, though unfortunately more common, are also safer. Cesarean delivery is still major surgery, though, so there are things you can start doing now to help your body heal faster and ease your transition into motherhood.

For tissues to heal better and hurt less they need:

- Nutrients to repair and grow

- Adequate blood flow to deliver these nutrients

- A strong immune system to prevent and fight infection

- Clean food and a clean environment, free from "anti-medicines" — chemicals that hinder healing

While you learned much of the information on helping your body heal earlier, here's our Healthy Healing Plan in a nutshell:

- Remember the five S's of healing foods: seafood, salads, smoothies, spices, and supplements (see page 44).

- Proteins and healthy fats provide the basic structure of your healing tissue.

- Healthy carbs provide energy to help your tissues heal.

- Vital vitamins and mighty minerals nourish healing tissues.

- Antioxidants act like anti-wear-and-tear nutrients to help these tissues stay healed.

- Review the top twelve pregnancy superfoods you learned about in chapter 3; these can appropriately be called "healing superfoods."

- Reread the following sections: how hormonal harmony promotes healing (page 324); how exercise helps your body heal (page 59); how managing stress helps your body heal (page 73); and the healing properties of healthy sleep (page 79).

The earlier in pregnancy you start practicing our Healthy Healing Plan, the faster you're likely to heal from childbirth.

(See the related section on "How to Help Your Body Heal from Childbirth," page 393.)

Making the Best out of a Cesarean

"I've been scheduled to have a cesarean section. I know that in my situation it's best for my baby, but I'm disappointed. I wanted so much to have a natural birth. Besides, I'm scared of surgery." These feelings are why we call it surgical *birth* or cesarean *birth,* not just a surgical "section." It is first a birth, second an operation. It's good that you know about the surgery ahead of time, rather than having to fight disappointment at the time of birth. You can also plan ahead — there are things you can do to create a positive experience for yourself and your baby.

Having your baby born surgically will be no less of a joyful celebration than having a vaginal birth.

Because cesarean births are so common, one of your childbirth classes may be entirely devoted to it. Here are some ways you can make your baby's birth personal and meaningful:

- Have a regional anesthetic. A spinal or epidural anesthetic is safer for both mother and baby; only rarely is a general anesthetic necessary. Your anesthesiologist or nurse-anesthetist will discuss the pros and cons of the anesthetic choices in your particular situation.

- Have Dad or a supportive and calm friend or family member sit next to you at the head of the operating table. If Dad is hesitant, remind him that the actual procedure takes place behind a sterile curtain. Neither of you will see anything unsettling.

- Ask your obstetrician to lift baby high enough so you can see her right after delivery. It is a beautiful sight to see your newborn lifted "up and out" during a cesarean birth.

- Immediately after your baby is out and quickly checked over (for temperature, breathing and pulse, and heart rate), ask that baby be brought to you to be held and hugged. You will need some help since you could be a bit groggy and one arm will be immobilized by an intravenous. This mother-father-baby bonding is an ideal time for pictures, and in many cases, someone will act as a photographer for you.

- While your uterus and abdomen are being sutured closed (this takes about thirty minutes) and the operation is finished up, your husband can accompany baby to the nursery so she will not be alone with strangers. This extra father-baby bonding time will have a deep impact on both of them.

• To decrease postoperative pain, ask your anesthesiologist about using a long-acting pain medication given via the tubing used for the spinal/epidural. This medication will provide continuous relief for about twenty hours so that you do not need additional pain medications. Another option is to have medication through an IV that you can control, called patient-controlled analgesia. Just turn the pump on and off as you need relief. This medication is completely safe for your breastfeeding baby.

• In most cases your baby will stay with you in the recovery room and go to your room with you when you are both stable. If your husband or a nurse can be with you in your room, and baby is healthy, it's even possible for a cesarean-birthed baby to room-in with you. The best postoperative pain reliever is an injection of baby in your arms.

• Plan ahead for some long-term help at home; remember, you'll be recovering from major abdominal surgery.

MY PREGNANCY JOURNAL: SEVENTH MONTH

Emotionally I feel:

_____

_____

_____

_____

_____

Physically I feel:

_____

_____

_____

_____

_____

My thoughts about you:

_____

_____

_____

_____

_____

My dreams about you:

_____

_____

_____

_____

_____

What I imagine you look like:

_____

_____

_____

_____

My top concerns:

_____

_____

_____

_____

My best joys:

_____

_____

_____

_____

Visit to My Healthcare Provider

Questions I had; answers I got:

_____

_____

_____

_____

MY PREGNANCY JOURNAL: SEVENTH MONTH

Tests and results; my reaction:

_____

_____

_____

_____

Updated due date: _____

My weight: _____

My blood pressure: _____

Feeling my uterus; my reaction:

_____

_____

_____

How I feel when I feel you kick:

_____

_____

_____

_____

How Dad feels when he feels you kick:

_____

_____

_____

Reactions of your brothers or sisters when they feel you move:

_____

_____

_____

_____

What I bought when I went shopping:

_____

_____

_____

_____

Photos (sonogram of baby and/or me in bloom):

Comments:

_____

_____

_____

_____

_____

_____

_____

EIGHTH-MONTH VISIT TO YOUR HEALTHCARE PROVIDER
(30–33 WEEKS)

During this month's visit you may have:

- An examination of the size and height of your uterus

- An examination of your skin for rashes, enlarging veins, and swelling

- A weight and blood pressure check

- Urinalysis to test for infection, sugar, and protein

- A test for hemoglobin and hematocrit, if indicated

- A review of your diet and an opportunity to discuss your weight, if necessary

- An opportunity to hear your baby's heartbeat

- An opportunity to see your baby on ultrasound, if indicated

- An opportunity to discuss your feelings and concerns

If your healthcare provider has additional concerns, she may want to check you twice a month during months seven and eight.

17

Eighth Month: Almost There

Now that the end is in sight, many mothers get more introspective. You will probably begin to slow down your busy lifestyle and focus your thoughts more on life with your baby. As your maternal instincts intensify, you may wonder what your baby will feel like when you finally have her in your arms and can gaze into her eyes. You may create mental pictures of your baby, imagining what she will look like and act like; what her hair and eye color will be; and what her cries will sound like. You may even fast-forward past this vision, imagining her kicking a soccer ball or dancing in a recital in the years to come. It is natural to begin focusing almost entirely on the life within you.

Of course, you may still want to play supermom and multitask right up until you go into labor. But since there is no "job" as important as this one you are doing, every so often try to sit down, put your feet up, close your eyes, and pat yourself on the bump for accomplishing one of humanity's greatest undertakings and most profound privileges: growing a human being.

HOW YOUR BABY IS GROWING, 30–33 WEEKS

When you look down, it might be difficult to imagine getting bigger, but you and baby still have some growing to do. Over the next eight weeks, baby is likely to double in weight, but don't worry, you won't grow that much; baby's living space just gets more crowded. By the end of this month baby will likely weigh close to 4 pounds and measure 16 to 18 inches long. Most babies gain around a half pound and a half inch each week between now and Birth-Day. During this month, baby fat deposits double, especially under the skin, giving baby a more filled-out appearance. Hair grows longer, and the silky, fur-like hair all over his body begins to shed. Baby can now blink his eyes in reaction to outside light. Since this is the stage of most rapid brain growth, be sure to feed yourself, and therefore your baby, more "brain foods" (as listed on pages 22 and 24).

Baby flips. For the first six or seven months baby tends to be in the breech position (butt down) because it's roomier for his head,

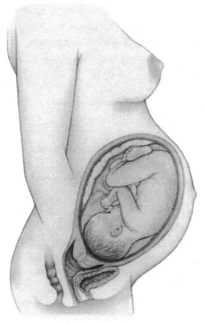

Baby at 30–33 weeks.

limbs, and torso at the top of the pear-shaped uterus. Babies can change position fairly easily during early pregnancy because they are relatively small and there is enough amniotic fluid to allow somersaults. By thirty-four weeks most babies will flip to a head-down position, contributing to the difference in location and intensity of kicks. Obstetricians and midwives don't worry too much about the position of the baby until the last few weeks of pregnancy, unless you go into preterm labor.

Feel baby dropping. Toward the end of the eighth month, or early in the ninth month (especially for a first-time pregnancy), baby settles downward into your pelvis, as though maneuvering into a position to "get out," changing what you look like on the outside — the bump looks lower — and how

you feel on the inside. Many second-time mothers find that their babies don't drop until a week or less before labor begins, because the pelvic muscles have already accommodated a baby passing through and so no warm-up is needed. While baby dropping relieves pressure on your stomach (less heartburn) and diaphragm (easier breathing), baby now puts more pressure on your bladder and pelvic tissues, causing you to leak urine and triggering the urge to urinate more frequently. (See page 227 for tips to minimize leaking.)

HOW YOU MAY BE FEELING

While your body is obviously growing outward, your mind is turning inward toward baby. Here are some typical eighth-month emotions:

Impatient. You might think, "Why does it take so long just to have a baby?" or "I've been gradually bulging out for seven months — and I still have two more long months to go? Let's get this thing over with!" The remaining two months can seem like an eternity. It's natural to grow tired of being pregnant and eager to hold your baby.

When you consider how your body has to adapt to grow, carry, and birth a baby, you can appreciate why nature takes its own sweet, though sometimes uncomfortable, time. If your bones, muscles, ligaments, and all those baby-bearing tissues grew and stretched quickly, it would really hurt! This nine-month "slow stretch" allows tissue to gradually accommodate the baby with relatively minor aches and pains along the way. The tissues of the vagina, for example, need to gradually soften and stretch to accommodate the birth of a baby. Try to savor these last two months and remind yourself that this is the last chance you'll have for a while to sleep in, go to a movie without paying a sitter, and make love without the interruption of baby's cries. Enjoy the next two months "off duty."

Needing to rest and nest. For many mothers during the eighth month, the brain tells the body to slow down, put your feet up, close your eyes, rest, and nest.

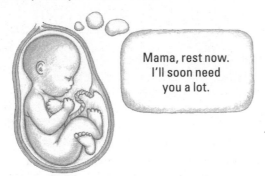

Mama, rest now. I'll soon need you a lot.

Replaying a previous birth. Each birth is as individual as your baby's personality. If you've given birth before, you may begin to think a lot about your previous birth(s), recalling the sequence of events and emotions. How will this labor and birth be different? Will it hurt more or less? Will it be shorter or longer? This is also a good time to process the lessons you learned from your previous labor and delivery. What aspects do you want to re-create this time around? What do you want to do differently? Will you use the same pain-relieving techniques? The same labor and birthing positions? You are much wiser this time around; put your experience and your wisdom to work for you.

Feeling bigger. Obviously you're feeling bigger because you *are* bigger. The good news is that this is about as high up as your baby is going to get. Next month baby will begin to drop lower into your pelvis. Being bigger might also bring more to complain about. It's harder to move around. Your joints ache and your feet swell. It may even be more of a chore to bend over to tend to a toddler.

I love how my bigness gets responses from my three-year-old. She reaches over and pats my tummy and says, "Baby, baby." She's also getting more excited, wanting to know where the new baby is going to sleep and asking, "Is the new baby going to sit in the high chair to eat?" When she was helping me get out some little baby clothes and baby shoes, she said, "These little shoes are so cute."

Stronger practice contractions. Your Braxton Hicks contractions may become more intense and feel like strong bands tightening across your abdomen. Use these prelabor contractions to practice the relaxation and natural pain-relieving techniques you are learning in childbirth class (see page 234). It is important to program your mind to relax your body, rather than tense up, as soon as you feel one of these contractions coming on. Chances are you're taking these in stride because you know you have only another month or two to deal with them.

Stronger kicks. While it's normal to feel fewer kicks in the final two months, they may feel stronger. Some kicks can be a real pain in the gut, ribs, bladder, groin — wherever your growing baby directs his energy. You may experience those nightly kick shows soon after you go to bed.

Martha notes: We loved playing family baby-kick games. I would place a piece of paper on the bulge and the kids would watch baby shake it off. We also played "guess the body part": Is it the heel of a foot or a bony little elbow?

Sleepless while pregnant. Neither pregnant women nor their babies kicking in the womb sleep through the night. If your enlarging uterus doesn't wake you up, its occupant probably will. (Read up on some sleep tips on page 82.)

CONCERNS YOU MAY HAVE

Managing Pain in Childbirth: Know Your Options

It's best to learn about natural and medical pain relief a couple of months before labor day. Don't wait for a crash course in pain management when the first contraction hits! Today's laboring mother has more options for pain relief in childbirth than ever before. Not only is there much more the laboring woman can do for natural pain relief, but medical pain relievers are now better and safer. Because there are so many analgesic options, today's mother needs to be well informed. Here's how you can use your mind and body to enhance the progress and ease the pain of labor.

Why childbirth hurts so much. It takes a lot of pushing and stretching to move a baby the size of a melon through a cervical opening the size of a kidney bean. Muscles don't work hard and tissues don't stretch without letting your body know it. Your uterus will be working very hard to accomplish the feat of childbirth. That's why it's called labor or, even better, hard labor. How much pain you experience depends upon the strength of your contractions; whether or not your contractions were augmented with Pitocin, which can cause more painful contractions; how big your baby is; and the baby's position. A face-down baby hurts less than a face-up baby. Besides those hardworking uterine and fast-stretching cervical muscles, there are a lot of pressure pains in surrounding tissues, such as bowels, bladder, backbones, and other nearby tissues, which also get squeezed and stretched as baby comes through.

Contrary to popular belief, it's usually not the contracting uterine muscles that produce the pain. Most childbirth pain originates in the dilating cervix and surrounding tissues as baby passes through. During the first stage of labor the uterus itself doesn't squeeze baby out; what really happens is that uterine contractions work to pull the cervical muscle up and out of the way so that the baby's head can then be pushed through. The muscles and ligaments in the pelvis are richly supplied with pressure receptors and pain receptors, so the pulling upward on the cervix, and then the baby being pushed through the birth canal, produces powerful pressure sensations with added pain sensations due to tension in the muscles. The more the tension, the more these powerful sensations morph into pain.

Like any muscle, uterine muscles hurt more if there is resistance to the work they need to do. When a muscle is taut, strained, and overly tired, the chemical and electrical activity within the muscle tissue gets out of balance. These physiological changes produce pain.

How you feel pain. Contractions begin, tissues get stretched, and the pain receptors in the nerves of these tissues get stimulated, sending lightning-fast impulses along the nerves to the spinal cord. In the spinal cord these impulses must pass through a system of gates that can stop some signals and allow others to pass through on the way to the brain, before they can be registered as pain. Therefore, the good news is that you can actually influence pain at three sites:

- Where it's produced in the laboring *tissues*

- At the *gate* in the spinal cord

- In the *brain* where the pain is perceived

In working out your own techniques for pain management, you will want to employ pain-relief measures that can manage pain at all three of these sites.

One way to understand this pain pathway is to picture pain impulses as miniature race cars. They speed from the stimulus site — the tense, strained tissues in the pelvis — to microscopic pain receptors, or parking spaces, located on the nerve cells of the spinal cord and brain. Blocking access to these pain-perception receptor sites is how pain-relieving drugs work.

You can influence the activity of these pain cars without drugs. First, you can limit the number of cars getting started in the first place. To do this, you can use relaxation techniques (described on page 298) to keep your muscles from getting tense and overtired. And you can use the positions for labor (see page 352) that keep your muscles working correctly and naturally. Next, you can close that gate in the spinal cord so that the pain cars can't all get through. A pleasant touch stimulus, such as massage, sends positive impulses that can at least partially block the transmission of pain impulses along the spinal cord. You can also cause gridlock at the gate by sending through a lot of competing vehicles, such as impulses from music (see page 298), positive mental imagery (see page 299), or counterpressure (see page 302). Finally, you can fill up the receptor sites in the brain with your natural pain-relieving neurohormones, such as endorphins (learn how on page 297), so that the pain cars have no place to park.

In addition to drugs (see page 307) and your body's own endorphins, distraction techniques can be used to fill up pain receptor sites in the brain and thus block the perception of pain. With the distraction method, you work to fill your brain with alternative imagery that is so captivating that your focus on it can overshadow your perception of pain. These techniques sound good in childbirth classes, and even seem to work when you are practicing simulated labor in your living room, but they can fail when the real labor begins. This kind of focus requires strong mental discipline, the kind that can even take years to acquire, so for many mothers the effort itself soon becomes mental strain, which tends to put the body on edge. In our experience, neither mind nor muscles relax when a mother tries too hard to concentrate on something else to escape from her labor. For some laboring mothers, though, distraction strategies do help.

PAIN HAS A PURPOSE

It's no surprise that so many women sign up for epidurals when they preregister at the hospital. Movies and television often portray labor as an emergency situation that must be treated with drugs while a woman lies on her back in bed. Childbirth educators, on the other hand, try not to even mention the P-word, substituting the more technical term "contractions" and analogous terms such as "surges" and "waves" for "pains."

Could it be that pain serves some useful purpose in childbirth? After experiencing the births of our own children, and watching thousands of women manage (or not manage) their labor pains, we have two conclusions about pain and childbirth:

1. Pain does serve a useful purpose.

2. Unmanageable pain is not normal, necessary, or healthy in childbirth.

In general, pain is the body's signal that a system is not working the way it is designed to, or that something is going wrong in the body and needs attention. If you are running a marathon and find that you are getting a sore knee or becoming painfully exhausted, you take this as a cue that you need some nourishment or liquid, or that you need to change your breathing technique or style of running. You make whatever changes are necessary to increase your energy and ease your pain, while still progressing toward your goal.

The same is true of birthing a baby. For example, if a mother feels sharp pain in her back, she can interpret this as a signal to keep changing her position until she feels relief. What's good for mother is good for baby: by changing her position, she allows baby to shift and find an easier — and less painful — way out. Pain, properly understood and wisely managed, is a valuable labor assistant. Listen to its signals.

Think of pain as the birth communicator: manageable pain means your cervix is doing its job, opening so you can push baby out; unmanageable pain means you need to change what you're doing. (Read Martha's water labor story, page 301, for another example of listening to pain.)

Ten Pain Management Strategies That Work

Even though no amount of reading or practicing can totally prepare you for what your labor is going to be like, odds are that the more informed and prepared you are, the less fearful you will be — and the less your labor will hurt. In showing you how to work out the right pain-management system for yourself, we will focus on ways to lessen both pain production and pain perception.

Pain tolerance is as individual as personalities. One woman's "intense sensation" is another woman's "Ow, that really hurts!" This is why no one pain-management program fits all pregnancies. Some mothers focus so much on "not having drugs" that they don't get in touch with their laboring body and relax into the hormonal symphony of labor. So, work toward a pain-relief balance. Unbearable pain can slow labor and be unhealthy for you and your baby. On the other hand, wrongly timed and wrongly dosed drugs can also slow labor. Appropriately used pain relief can speed labor and birth for a healthier mother and baby.

Martha notes: *Rather than striving for* control, *think* release, *which implies understanding your body's signals and working with them.*

1. Have a balanced mindset about pain relief. Some women enter labor absolutely opposed to taking medicines and willing to push their minds and bodies to the max; they regard anything less than an unmedicated birth as failure. Other women ask their doctors to "give me everything you've got" in their quest for a pain-free childbirth. Somewhere between these two extremes is the right balance. For most mothers, it's wisest to enter labor armed with all the natural pain-relieving tactics we describe *and* with an open mind regarding the options available for medical relief, should your labor or your individual obstetrical situation demand it. Birth is not a contest to see who can cross the finish line with the least medical assistance. It is your baby's entry into the world, and it is also a landmark in your life. The memories of this birth will last a lifetime. Whatever it takes to give birth to a healthy baby and help you feel good about the process is the right pain-management package for you.

Dr. BJ notes: *When you are laboring in a hospital, the nurses will likely ask you to rate your pain on a scale of 1 to 10. This ritual is a procedure that is mandated by the accrediting bodies for hospitals. While the rating scale has never been validated as a reliable indicator of pain in laboring women, it is still in widespread use. One of the concerns that I have with this is that it focuses the woman on "how bad her pain is" rather than how she is managing her pain. When a woman is repeatedly asked to rate her pain, it conveys to her that her pain must be worse than she may actually perceive it. I advise many women planning a hospital birth to ask the nurses not to use the pain scale. This can be done through your birth plan — a document, like an advance directive, that can be incorporated into the chart — so that the nurse is "off the hook." (Learn more about creating a birth plan on page 267.)*

2. Try to be less fearful. Fear enhances pain. The efficiency of the magnificent uterine musculature depends upon your hormonal, circulatory, and nervous systems all working together. Fear upsets these three systems:

- Fear and anxiety cause your body to produce excessive stress hormones, which counteract the helpful hormones your body produces to enhance the labor process and relieve discomfort. This results in a longer and more painful labor.

- Fear reduces blood flow and thus oxygen supply to the uterus. Oxygen-deprived muscles tire quickly, and a tired muscle is a hurting muscle.

- Fear produces muscle tension, and the last thing you want during labor is tight abdominal and pelvic muscles. Tense and tight muscles not only hurt, they also have a harder time working in harmony to dilate the cervix enough to allow you to push baby out. Normally, the muscles in the upper part of the uterus contract and pull up while the lower ones relax and open, allowing the cervix to dilate so that baby can pass through into the birth canal. Fear primarily affects those lower muscles, causing them to tighten instead of relax. As a result, the strong muscles of the upper uterus contract against the tight lower uterine muscles and cervix, producing much pain and little progress.

Some fear of labor is perfectly normal — it's only natural to be anxious about the unknown. However, unresolved anxiety and fears will impede your labor. Even though a fearless labor is as rare as a painless birth, you can work to resolve your fears before Birth-Day. What, specifically, do you fear about birth? Do you fear the pain, for example, having heard horror stories or having had negative experiences with pain in the past? Do you fear having a cesarean or needing an episiotomy? Are you afraid that you will lose control midway through labor? Do you have fears about problems with the baby? List all your fears, and next to each one, write what you can do to avoid having that fear come true. Realize, too, that some events and outcomes are beyond your control, and resolve not to worry about things you cannot change.

Surround yourself with fearless helpers. By now you've probably learned who among your friends and family sees birth as a horror story and who does not. Fear is contagious.

Be judicious about who you choose to be with you when you deliver your baby. Don't think that this is the time to finally prove something to your mother; if she has a fearful attitude about labor, it is better for her to watch your birth on video afterward than to be in the birthing room influencing you with her fears.

Avoid fearful replays. Don't carry scary baggage from your past into the birthing room. Labor has a way of stirring up uncomfortable memories of previous traumatic births. You may, at the height of an overwhelming contraction, automatically push "tense up" buttons in response to events long past.

Dr. Bill notes: Many fathers-to-be are afraid of birth. They don't understand childbirth pain, and they find it very upsetting when their mate hurts and they can't "fix" it. Even Mr. Sensitive-and-Fearless may become Mr. Frightened at the height of a particularly hard series of contractions, or in response to a sudden change in birth plan. It helps to inoculate your mate against fear so that he won't pass the bug on to you. Prepare your partner for the normal sights and sounds of labor. Tell him what may happen if events don't go as planned. And try not to share your own fears. If he sees that you seem not to be afraid, he is less likely to be so himself.

3. **Employ a professional labor coach.** An experienced woman who has gone through labor herself and who has made a profession of studying the normal sensations of labor and what to do about them is a valuable person to have at your side. This special woman will help you interpret your

TENS

Transcutaneous electrical nerve stimulation (TENS) is a pain-easing technique that is used in pain centers, mainly for postoperative pain. TENS is now being used in some birth centers to ease labor pain. It is most helpful with *continuous* pain, like that of back labor (see page 351), rather than the rhythmic pain of normal contractions, since they allow for rest in between. A TENS unit, about the size of a deck of cards, is held in the mother's hand. Wires from the unit are taped to areas of mother's skin, usually around the lower back. When mother senses a contraction or back pain coming on, she operates the electrical-current generator to send tingling sensations into the skin and muscle. Mother can adjust the level of electrical stimulation. Practitioners of both acupressure and TENS believe that pressure and electrical current interfere with pain signals and stimulate local endorphin release. These mechanisms are thought to decrease both the local sensation and the cerebral awareness of pain.

sensations during labor and offer suggestions for managing your pain. Specifically, your coach will show you how to cooperate with the forces of nature and progress less painfully. (See our tips on selecting a labor coach, page 260.)

4. Relax your birthing muscles. "Relax? Are you kidding? These contractions feel like a Mack truck plowing through my belly!" So said a mother we know to her coach midway through labor. "Relax" is more than just an empty word to throw at a mother who is experiencing the most intense physical work of her life. (A better term could be "release.") It is exactly what she needs to do in order to help the work progress. Relaxing all her other muscles so that her uterus can work unimpeded will help her cooperate with what her uterus is doing rather than resist it. Being able to relax and release is what will likely make the difference between a great birth experience you want to treasure in your memory and a not-so-great one you would just as soon forget.

Why relax? Relaxing all of your other muscles while only your uterus contracts eases the discomfort and speeds the progress of labor. If there is tension elsewhere in your body, especially in your face and neck, this tension will be communicated to the pelvic muscles that need to stay loose during a contraction. Tense muscles in labor hurt more than loose ones, and chemical changes within a tense muscle actually lower the muscle's pain threshold, causing you to hurt more than if the muscle were not opposing the work of labor. When tight muscles resist the relentless, involuntary contractions of your uterus, the result is pain. Tense, exhausted muscles soon lead to a tense, exhausted mind, which increases your awareness of pain and decreases your ability to cope with it. You lose your ability to explore options and make changes that would lessen your misery.

Laboring a baby out is hard and demanding, but it is done in spurts with periods of rest in between, a sort of "charge" and "recharge" cycle. Once a contraction is finished, you need to let go of it so you can totally rest. If you don't rest between contractions, you will not be able to recharge and welcome the next contraction with its good work. Labor becomes steadily more intense and energy-consuming as it progresses, so intermittent mindful rest is important for conserving energy for what's ahead — the pushing stage, when enormous energy will be needed for the hardest work you will ever do.

Relaxation also helps balance your hormones for birth. As we mentioned earlier, two sets of hormones help your labor. Adrenal hormones (also called stress hormones) give your body the extra power it needs in situations that call for tremendous effort, like labor and birth. The adrenal hormone epinephrine exerts a synergistic effect on the natural narcotics your body produces, adding more natural pain relief. During labor your body needs enough of these stress hormones to help you work hard, but not so many that your body becomes anxious and distressed, causing your mind and muscles to work against progress.

Another kind of hormone also works for you during labor — natural pain-relieving hormones, known as endorphins. (The word comes from *endo*genous, meaning "produced in the body," and m*orphine,* a chemical that blocks pain.) These are your body's natural narcotics, helping to relax you when you're stressed, and relieving pain when you're hurting. These physiological labor assistants are produced in the nerve cells. They attach themselves to pain receptor sites on the nerve cell, where they blunt the sensation of pain. Strenuous exercise increases endorphin levels, and endorphins enter your system automatically during the strenuous exercise of labor, as long as you don't tense up and block their release. Levels are high in the second stage of labor (pushing), when contractions are most intense. Like artificial narcotics, endorphins can work differently in women's bodies, which may explain why some women seem to feel more pain than others. Unimpeded endorphins are better for you than artificial narcotics. Instead of the periodic "blast" and subsequent groggy feeling you get with drugs, endorphins can provide a steady source of pain relief during labor and a feeling of mental well-being that laboring mothers often describe as "naturally drugged." Resting in between contractions will allow these natural pain relievers to work. Fear and anxiety increase your level of stress hormones and counteract the effects of endorphins. If your mind is less anxious, your body is less likely to hurt.

Endorphins also help you in the transition from birthing to mothering. Levels are highest just after birth and don't return to prelabor levels until two weeks postpartum. Endorphins stimulate the secretion of prolactin, the relaxing and "mothering" hormone that regulates milk production and gives you a psychological boost toward enjoyment of mothering. Endorphins also help you stay relaxed during pregnancy.

When you labor the way your mind and body were designed to do, your body produces just the right balance of stress hormones and endorphins. Fear and exhaustion drive these hormones out of balance. When you release during contractions and rest between contractions, you'll be amazed how your body can be under the control of your mind. You'll feel relief and your baby will be born more easily.

Spend as much time as possible practicing specific muscle release and total body relaxation. Here are some of the time-tested relaxation techniques that Martha and mothers we have counseled have used to break the "relaxation barrier."

Rest and release. Relax and rest *between* contractions and relax and release *during* a contraction. Keep these two words in mind during your labor. Condition yourself to think muscle-relaxing thoughts that help you surrender to the normal workings of your body. When you feel a contraction beginning, instead of bracing yourself and tensing your muscles for what's to come, take deep breaths, relax, and release. Practicing the "R&R" exercises below will condition you to say to yourself, "Contraction coming, breathe and release!" instead of "Oh no, not another contraction!" Use your imagination to see yourself tense up, and then respond to that by letting go. Then, when your pretend contraction is over, take a final deep breath and relax into rest.

The best time to practice these exercises is when you are having Braxton Hicks contractions — you will be rewarded with a lessening of tension-related pain. Collect a bunch of pillows and get comfortable. Practice over and over, with your partner, in various positions: standing and leaning against your partner, a wall, or a piece of furniture; sitting down; lying on your side; and even on all fours.

R&R Exercise 1: Check your whole body for muscle tension: a furrowed forehead, clenched fists, a tight mouth and clenched jaw, and raised shoulders are common hot spots. Then practice releasing each group of muscles from head to toe systematically, tensing then relaxing each muscle group to help you identify the two different states. When your partner cues you with

"contraction," think "relax and release." Then allow these tight muscles to loosen, and remember how that feels so that you can recall it during labor when the cue to release is easier said than done.

R&R Exercise 2: Practice "touch-relaxation" frequently, several times a day, throughout your final month of pregnancy. Touch-relaxation conditions you to expect pleasure rather than pain to follow tension. Find out which touches and what kinds of massage relax you best (see page 304). Do the head-to-toe progression described above. Tense each muscle group, then have your partner apply a warm, relaxed hand to that area as your cue to release the tension. This way you won't have to keep hearing the verbal cue "relax," which can eventually become irritating. You can also use this now to relax hurting muscles, by having your partner put just the right touch on that area. Practice: "I hurt here — you press, stroke, or touch here."

5. Play music to labor by. Enjoy your favorite lullabies of labor (see page 350). Music can be a wonderful relaxation aid. Carefully choose a medley to fit your taste and help you relax. Play this music during your practice R&R sessions at home so you are conditioned to relax when you hear these soothing sounds on labor day.

Why do you think dentists pipe in music for their patients? To occupy the mind while they work on the teeth. Music can actually ease bodily discomforts through a phenomenon called audioanalgesia. Studies show that mothers using music during labor require fewer pain-relieving drugs than mothers who do not listen to music, because music stimulates a mother's body to release endorphins, the natural pain-relieving and relaxing hormones. Music also fills the mind with pleasant sensations, leaving less room for painful ones. And music has a mellowing effect on birth attendants, too, reminding them to respect the peacefulness of this process.

Play a medley of already tested favorites, taking care to choose songs whose rhythms relax rather than stimulate or agitate your system. Many mothers make their own recordings using pieces that have previously helped them in times of stress. Music that triggers flashbacks of particularly pleasant events, such as the first time you danced together, is particularly appealing. Some moms report that environmental sounds (such as waterfalls, wind, and ocean waves) and soft instrumentals that ebb and flow are more soothing than vocal music. (Along with your favorite CDs or digital playlists, be sure to bring along a player and fresh batteries or the appropriate charger for your MP3 player.)

6. Practice mental imagery and visualization. A clear mind filled with soothing scenes relaxes a laboring body — at least between contractions. It also encourages the production of labor-enhancing endorphins. Sports psychologists use mental imagery to help athletes perform.

Determine now what thoughts and scenes you find most uplifting and relaxing and practice meditating on them frequently throughout the day, especially in the final month of pregnancy. In this way you'll bring to your labor a mental library of short features that you can click on for those moments of rest between contractions. Store up half a dozen images of your most pleasant memories: how the two of you met, a favorite date, or a special vacation.

Imagining my favorite sweet treat helped me relax. Our childbirth educator reminded us that "stressed" spelled backward is "desserts."

It helps to visualize what's happening during your labor. When a contraction begins, visualize your uterus "hugging" your baby and pulling up over his adorable little head. During the dilating stage, think of your cervix slowly getting thinner and more open with each contraction. Some mothers who have used visual imagery successfully during the pushing stage have visualized the birth canal slowly opening up like a flower. Change scenes from painful to productive. You can also try the strategy known as "packaging the pain." Grab the pain as if it were a big glob of modeling clay and soften it into a tiny ball; or wrap it up and tie it to a helium balloon and imagine it leaving your body and floating up into the sky. Do the same with distressing thoughts: put them into a thought bubble and let them float away. This exercise is especially helpful in conjunction with a cleansing breath as a contraction begins: breathe deeply, exhale, and either blow the pain part of it away or see it as a friend bringing your baby's birth one contraction closer.

Between and during the more difficult contractions, especially the ones right before you start pushing, imagine the finish line. When pushing starts, picture more and more of your baby's head showing (with all that hair!) — and soon, usually, you will be helped to see that little head and touch it. Picture yourself reaching down as your baby comes out, assisting your birth attendant in bringing your baby up onto your abdomen, and feeling that warm, wet little body.

Mental imagery is not a mind-over-body technique — it's mind helping body work more productively. Be sure to use mental imagery as a relaxing tool, not as a distraction. If you believe that you can put your mind on another planet to help you escape from what's going on in your body, you're probably in for a big surprise; contractions can be so overwhelming that efforts at mental escape will have little effect. It's more realistic to expect your mind to work with your labor rather than escape from it. That said, many unmedicated women say that when the mind gets so focused on the work the body is doing, they do "go to another planet" — not as an escape, but as

the result of literally blocking out everything else except that all-consuming task at hand: giving birth.

Martha notes: With my first few labors I tried distraction techniques, such as fixing my eyes, trance-like, on a focal point, breathing in patterns, and tapping out a tune with my fingers. But when my labors became so demanding that these techniques no longer worked, I intuitively began to do what did work: I let my body take over and do what it had to do. When I learned to release my body during labor rather than try to control it, I could relax my pelvic muscles.

PUTTING CHILDBIRTH PAIN IN PERSPECTIVE

After forty-five years of our own personal births and witnessing thousands of others, here's what we've learned about how veteran mothers view pain in childbirth. We realize that they have a whole different perspective on pain from that of first-time pregnant women. A first-timer may expect that the pain she will experience at childbirth will be the most awful pain in her life. She may enter labor with fear. The experienced childbirther sees that although labor could be "worse" than other pain, it's a different kind of pain. Realizing how it differs gets the experienced woman through labor in a much less painful way than a novice. A first-timer can listen, learn, and be encouraged by what experienced women tell her. When she hears "It feels like really severe wrap-around cramps," she has a frame of reference that can be useful.

She may be able to say to herself, "I can do this." Not so if she hears "Horrible!"

Ponder for a moment the worst pain you have ever suffered in your life, say, a really fierce toothache or migraine headache. It caught you by surprise; it went on for days. It started out severe and was unrelenting no matter what you did. It just wouldn't go away. You would have given anything for a few minutes of relief. Childbirth pain is different:

- This pain is *not* unrelenting. There are blissful (or, at least, very welcome) pauses between the contractions, and the pauses last a lot longer than the pains, at least before transition. Put this into perspective: each contraction is only sixty to ninety seconds long.

- It's predictable. You know that within, say, two or three minutes another contraction is going to come, and you can prepare mentally to accept it.

- After a while you will know what the next pain is going to feel like. It may be a bit more or less intense than the previous one, but it's going to feel similar.

- Childbirth pain builds slowly, giving you a chance to get accustomed to it and cope with it.

- It has an ongoing purpose, signaling you to make bodily adjustments for the benefit of baby.

- You know that it will end.

- When it ends, you get the world's most magnificent reward.

When you put the pains of childbirth in perspective, it's clear that labor is designed to be manageable. If it weren't, why would women continue to have babies?

7. Enjoy laboring in water. Oftentimes the simplest things in life — and labor — work the best. One of the most amazing labor-pain relievers also happens to be the least invasive and without side effects. The miracle? Water — not to drink, but to relax and "let go" in.

Martha notes: I personally experienced the benefits of water labor with the birth of our seventh baby, Stephen. After four hours of active labor managed by a lot of walking around and staying focused, I began to feel a much more intense pain low down in front. This was a strong signal to my body that something needed attention. So I got into a large tub filled with warm water.

After two more intense contractions, I was able to let my entire body relax. I experimented with different positions and found one that allowed me to "float" from my shoulders down so that my whole torso and pelvis could remain totally relaxed. At that point, the pain literally melted away — better than Demerol!

The experience of total release accompanied by nearly total relief was amazing. I stayed in the water for about an hour until I reached the pushing stage. Then I got out of the tub and gave birth to Stephen on our bed in a side-lying position. As the baby emerged, we discovered the reason I'd felt that much pain: his little hand was crowding in alongside his head,

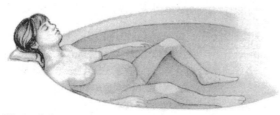

Water labor.

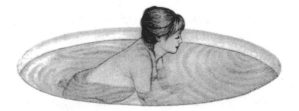

so two parts of him were needing to come through the cervix at once. That change in pain was the signal I needed to make a change: the water relaxation gave my pelvic muscles time to adjust.

Why water works. Remember your high school physics? Place an object in water, and the force of buoyancy equal to its weight lifts it up. To simplify Archimedes' principle, put it this way: water gives a laboring mother a lift. Buoyancy feels like weightlessness. With less weight to support, and less muscle tension, your body feels less pain and saves energy for where it is needed — your hardworking uterus.

Water relieves. Muscles that are weighed down less, tire and hurt less. Also, the supportive counterpressure from the water can ease the pain of sore muscles, especially during back labor. Recall our earlier discussion about relieving pain by filling the nervous system with pleasant sensations so there's less room for painful ones. Being in water is like a continuous body massage, stimulating all the touch receptors in the skin. It would take thousands of gentle fingertips to touch as many skin receptors as the water does when you soak in a warm bath.

Water relaxes. Immersing your body in a warm tub soothes your mind and body, reduces stress hormones, and allows your body's natural relaxing and pain-relieving hormones to take over.

Water releases. Changing positions to go with the flow of labor is the most important natural pain reliever and labor enhancer a woman can use. Being in water lets this happen more naturally and easily. Many women laboring on terra firma describe feeling rooted to one spot, afraid to move at all, lest it hurt more. A woman in water is free to float with her body supported as she finds a position that best eases her discomfort. Being in water also seems to free her mind, so that she can tap into her deepest instincts and let tension float away. Next time you're in a swimming pool, see if this doesn't ring true. Notice how you are free to move your body and clear your mind.

Water labor has been used in Russia and France for more than fifty years, but it's relatively new to North America. A study of eighteen hundred women who labored in Jacuzzi-type pools showed these encouraging results:

- The women had shorter labors.

- Cervical dilation was more efficient — 2.5 centimeters per hour compared with 1.25 centimeters per hour of active labor for mothers who did not take advantage of water.

- The descent of the babies was twice as fast.

- The women reported less pain.

- The cesarean section rate was one-third that of traditional hospital births.

- Mothers labeled "high-risk" because of high blood pressure showed a dramatic reduction in their blood pressure within minutes of immersion in the pool.

More gain with less pain — bring out the labor tubs!

Dr. BJ notes: *If the hospital that you plan to labor and birth in has tubs, be sure to* *ask how often they are used and what the policies or restrictions are related to water immersion in labor and birth. Many hospitals advertise tubs but because of restrictions they are rarely used.*

Using water for labor. Some hospital maternity units and many birth centers have Jacuzzi-size labor tubs. (If the hospital of your choice does not have them, voice your disappointment. This is just one more way in which women can influence how birth business is done.) An alternative is to rent a portable one; check with local midwives or childbirth organizations for information. (Of course, you will have to persuade your birth practitioner and the hospital to go along with this.) The tub should be large enough to bring out the mermaid in you — at least five and a half feet wide. Here are some ways to use water to your advantage during labor:

- Have the water at bath temperature, which is usually a little higher than body temperature.

- Enter the tub when the intensity of your contractions tells you that you need some relief. For most women the best time to take the plunge is between 5 and 8 centimeters dilation, when active labor is in full swing. You may find water labor especially comforting during transition — the most intense stage of labor. Lying in a labor tub can also be used to accelerate a slow labor. The splashing of water on your nipples can trigger the release of contraction-stimulating hormones. Water is also effective in easing a fast-and-heavy labor, where the contractions threaten to overwhelm you.

- Try lying on your back or side or kneeling forward on all fours, so the water covers your uterus, at least up to your breasts.

- If your labor stalls while you are comfortably floating in the water, get out and walk or squat on land to get your labor going again; reenter the tub once labor gets going.

- When you enter and exit the water, be sure to do so between contractions and with assistance, so you don't slip.

- When you feel the urge to push, it's time to get dry. (Babies have been born in the water when there was no time to exit or when a mother was so comfortable that she could not bring herself to leave the water. They do just fine as long as they are lifted up out of the water, and placed in mother's arms, without delay. This is so that they can take their first breath as soon as possible.

Unless your birth attendant advises you otherwise, it's safe to use water labor even after your membranes have ruptured. That's when contractions get more intense and you really need the relief of water. Maternity centers with experience in water labor (and water birth) report no increased rate of infection in women using water after their membranes have ruptured, as long as the mothers are in active labor and proper infection-control hygiene is followed.

It is usually not necessary to leave the water for routine procedures. If you have an IV in place, a saline lock can be used in the veins of your hand, covered with a waterproof plastic bag sealed with a rubber band. If intermittent fetal monitoring is necessary, it can be done on a part of your abdomen that you can lift above the water; and a plastic bag can be slipped over the handheld monitor if not using a special monitor designed for underwater use.

If your hospital or birth center does not offer a labor tub and you're unable to rent one, at least try sitting in a regular tub or standing in a shower. A jet of warm water is often especially effective in easing back labor. And, in addition to the feel of water, the soothing sounds of the shower running or the tub filling are welcome during labor.

Don't expect all the pain of labor to magically float away into the water. Our personal experience, however, and that of other women who have used labor pools, suggests that water is one of the most wonderful laborsaving devices available.

8. Enjoy the right touches. A soothing massage, a caring caress, a passionate kiss, even a simple foot rub can be blissful relief to a laboring mother. (See more on page 363.) By stroking the receptor-rich skin and kneading the pressure receptors beneath the skin, you bombard the brain with pleasant stimuli.

You won't know exactly where or how you will want to be touched until labor is under way. But in the final months some practice rubdowns to relieve backache, or touches to help you relax during Braxton Hicks contractions, will prepare you for labor, when the right touch really counts. A lot of prenatal practice encourages your husband to use these techniques during labor once he sees how helpful they are ahead of the big day.

Using pure vegetable oil or massage lotion, try different strokes on different areas of your body. Firm caressing with fingertips is preferred on the face and scalp. Deep pressure and kneading is welcome for large muscles, such as the shoulders, thighs, buttocks, calves, and feet. Ask your partner to try counterpressure with the heel of his hand for easing the pain in lower back muscles. Using scented oils — especially lavender, rose, or myrrh — can also enhance the relaxation. Peppermint-scented oil can help if you feel nauseated.

Find out ahead of time which massage strokes you like, and which you don't. For example, stroking downward in the direction of body hair growth is pleasant, whereas stroking upward, against the hair shaft, can irritate a laboring woman. Help your partner learn the intensity and rhythm of the pressure you enjoy. Take turns — when you massage him, show him what you like.

My first labor was slow and I got the best, most relaxing foot rubs. My second was fast and furious and my husband rubbed my legs hard and fast. Somehow he knew instinctively that only something intense could compete with the pain of passing a cantaloupe!

A tip for the masseur: don't take criticism of your massages personally. Expect your partner to be touchy during late pregnancy and irritable during labor. Rubs that she used to love may get you a curt "Stop that!" or "Don't touch!" on labor day, as you discover the "hot spots" that annoy rather than relax her. During your childbirth class you may practice with massage tools such as tennis balls or paint rollers, but be prepared to improvise. Experiment with many different touches in different places throughout different stages of labor. Just be quick to switch gears if she doesn't like what you're doing, and be patient. She'll try to let you know what she wants, but she'll be too preoccupied for politeness. Rest assured, she'll appreciate your efforts immensely.

9. Breathe right for birthing. Every exercise has its optimal breathing pattern, and this is especially true of labor. Forget those old birth videos that show laboring women panting robotically at the first uterine twitch. The theory, as Martha remembers from forty years ago, is that by keeping the breathing high in the chest the diaphragm would not push against the contracting uterus. To do this the breathing had to be fast to keep enough oxygen coming. Most women found themselves getting light-headed and tense, the very thing you don't want.

My husband and I practiced our patterned breathing every night, but once I was in the grip of an overwhelming contraction, I forgot how I was supposed to breathe.

When breathing patterns are intended as a distraction, the true purpose and role of breathing in the body's physiology can be sabotaged. Breathing that is slow and deep has a relaxing effect and supplies the blood with plenty of oxygen. Fast, shallow breathing can easily do the opposite. If you find yourself breathing fast during a contraction, it's probably because you are in panic mode. Slow down your breathing, and you will automatically feel calmer. For this you don't really need patterns — slow, deep abdominal breathing is intuitive for mindful release of tension.

As a labor and delivery nurse for ten years and now a professional labor coach, I have been involved in more than a thousand births and rarely have I seen couples use rehearsed patterned-breathing techniques successfully during labor. Most women become so frustrated with the concentration it takes that they find it confuses and stresses them rather than relaxes them. Patterned breathing, meant to distract, simply isn't sufficient to distract from the intensity of contractions, especially during later labor and transition. I have noticed that at this point most mothers switch intuitively to an internal focus, and to consistent, deeper, slower breathing that relaxes and tunes them in to the workings of their own bodies.

The right breathing technique is the one that works for you: it will be the style of breathing that delivers the most oxygen to you and your baby with the least amount of effort. Try these do's and don'ts.
Do:

• When a contraction begins, inhale deeply through your nose, then slowly exhale through your mouth in a long, steady stream. As you breathe out, focus on letting your facial muscles relax and your limbs go limp (imagine tension leaving your body). Your exhalations signal release, and you can sense that release especially in your pelvic muscles.

• As the contraction peaks, remind yourself to continue to breathe at a relaxed, comfortable rate. Your husband and your labor coach can help you with this pacing if you start breathing too fast in response to an intense contraction.

• If you still find yourself breathing too fast, refocus by taking a deeper breath, followed by a long, drawn-out blow, as if you are blowing off steam.

• Breathe naturally to rest between contractions, as you do when you are falling asleep. Visualize oxygen flowing into your baby.

• For the labor coach and/or partner: Watch the mother's breathing patterns for cues as to how she is coping. Slow, deep, rhythmic breathing shows that she is handling her contractions well. Fast, spasmodic breathing communicates tension and anxiety. Use massage, model proper breathing, or suggest a change of position.

Don't:

• Don't pant. Panting is not natural for humans. (Dogs and cats in labor pant because they don't sweat. It's their way of releasing body heat.) Panting not only exhausts you, it can lead to hyperventilation.

• Don't hyperventilate. Breathing too fast and too heavily blows off too much carbon dioxide, causing you to feel light-headed and to have tingling sensations in your fingers, toes, and face. Some women tend to hyperventilate during the height of intense contractions and need caring reminders to relax and slow their breathing. If you start to hyperventilate, breathe deeply in through your nose and out through your mouth, as slowly as you can.

• Don't hold your breath. Even during the strain of pushing, the blue-in-the-face, blood-vessel-popping, breath-holding, and bearing down you see in movies is not only exhausting, but can also deprive you and your baby of much-needed oxygen.

• Don't worry too much about how you will breathe during labor. If you keep your wits about you, you will naturally breathe in a way that's best for you and your baby.

HYPNOBIRTHING

Hypnobirthing, the use of hypnosis as a labor-easing and labor-speeding tool, has become increasingly popular, especially among the drug-free childbirth set. English obstetrician Dr. Grantly Dick-Read, author of *Childbirth without Fear,* proposed that hypnosis could ease the fear-tension-pain cycle that plagues so many women and increases the pain and length of labor. The less fear a mother has, the less tense her body becomes, and consequently the more relaxed her birthing muscles are and the quicker and less painful the birth. Fear suppresses endorphins, the body's natural anesthetics. Lessening fear enables mother to take advantage of her own natural pain-relieving internal medicines.

Hypnosis enables the laboring woman to program her mind to trust her body and give birth the way nature intended. By attending classes and listening to audiotapes at home, mother practices self-hypnosis. When labor day arrives, she uses these now-familiar hypnosis techniques to calm her mind, which relaxes her birth muscles for a calmer, quicker birth. Those mothers who have a natural knack for using their minds to control their bodies can benefit from hypnobirthing. Even though hypnosis does not always result in a natural and drug-free birth, it's simply one more tool to help increase the chance of having a more relaxed and less painful birth. And it works! Hypnobirthing statistics show a reduction in epidural use from a national average of 71 percent to 23 percent in hypnobirthing-prepared students, and a lower surgical birth rate of 17 percent compared with the national average of 32 percent.

Dr. BJ notes: I tell the moms who want to use hypnosis as a labor tool that the process of labor and birth is enhanced when the "controlling" part of the mind is out of the way so that the body can work uninhibited. We grew up to believe that controlling what happens is important and, while that philosophy works for many aspects of life, it doesn't usually work for childbirth. Hypnosis was a strategy that was very powerful during my birth. Not only did it help with labor and birth but has been an ongoing life tool during times of stress to help me balance.

For more information about the use of hypnosis during labor, visit hypnobirthing .com and hypnobabies.com.

10. Know about medical pain relief. All drugs have a risk/benefit ratio that a patient, in partnership with her doctor/midwife, should know. Here we give you tools to empower you to develop your own pain-management program during labor. Study your options now before you need them. When you're at the height of an uncomfortable labor pain and feel like shouting "Just give me something — now!" is not when you will be in a state of mind or body to "study your options." Complete pain relief without risk is a promise on which no doctor can deliver. While today's analgesics and anesthetics are better and safer than ever, there is no such thing as a perfect pain reliever, that is, one that works completely *and* is perfectly safe for mother and baby. By understanding what obstetrical drugs are available, what benefits and risks they carry, and how to use them wisely, you will be able to decide which of them, if any, you want to use. Medical pain relief can be a welcome addition to — but not a substitute

for — the natural self-help practices we've described. Remember, studies show that mothers who take natural childbirth classes and learn ways to manage their own pain require much less pain-relieving medication during their labors than uninformed mothers do.

Narcotic pain relievers. If only there were a perfect analgesic that acted on just the pain pathways in mother and didn't cross over the placenta to baby. Unfortunately, there is no such panacea. While narcotics relieve mother's body of pain, they also affect baby. An additional concern about narcotics is their effect on the mind, since they can impair one's ability to focus. When combined with natural pain relievers, however, properly used narcotic medications can get a struggling woman enough relief to allow her to rest and recharge, to help get her back on track. Here is what every mother-to-be should know about choosing and using narcotic pain relievers.

How narcotics work for mother. Narcotic analgesics relieve pain by blocking the pain receptors in the brain. Analgesics affect different persons differently. Not only does the degree of pain relief narcotics provide vary from woman to woman, but so do the mental and emotional side effects:

- Some mothers feel a lot of relief within twenty minutes of the shot, while others report only partial relief ("It took the edge off the pain so I could manage it better").

- Some people find that the foggy mind they get on narcotics is worse than a hurting body.

- Some women enjoy the euphoria that narcotics induce, a floaty feeling that helps take their mind off their labor. Other mothers find that narcotics compromise their ability to make decisions that benefit their labor progress. If a mother's mind is too muddled to participate in managing labor with movement and changes of position, her labor may be prolonged, along with her pain.

- Narcotics can also make you feel sleepy, so much so that you sleep between contractions and come to only as each one peaks, unable to focus and stay "on top of" the contractions; you can wind up feeling overtaken by the pains.

If this is your first pregnancy or your first use of a narcotic analgesic, you don't know how you might react. While you may tolerate these drugs well and experience pain relief without a lot of undesirable side effects, be prepared for the possibility of nausea, vomiting, dizziness, and the above-mentioned spaced-out feeling. If you used narcotic analgesics to your advantage in a previous labor, chances are they will work for you again, though there is no guarantee.

How to use narcotics wisely during your labor. You may enter the labor room having studied up on drugs, armed with all the natural alternatives, and at some point conclude, with your birth attendants, that it would be in the best interest of you, your baby, and the progress of your labor to get some medical pain relief. Here are the safest and most effective ways to use analgesics during your labor:

Select the right drug. Discuss with your doctor or anesthesiologist which drug is best for your particular labor situation. Which one is likely to give you the quickest, most effective pain relief with minimal effects on your baby? In our experience, Nubain is the most effective in taking the edge off the pain and has the fewest side effects. We have also found that it is not readily available in some hospitals because of cost. A popular analgesic used today is Fentanyl, as it is fast-acting and quickly eliminated. There has also been a resurgence in the use of nitrous oxide (laughing gas) in labor.

It's important to avoid becoming exhausted during your labor. Sometimes it's sleep a mother needs more than pain relief. Instead of suggesting a narcotic during early labor, your doctor may advise taking a sedative or sleeping medication to help you sleep for a bit so that you can enter active labor with more energy reserves.

Select the right time. Analgesics given too early can slow the progress of labor. In the early stages of labor, narcotics are known to decrease the strength of contractions and slow dilation of the cervix. If given too late, too close to birth, they can depress baby's breathing. The best time to administer narcotics is when your labor is very active (6 to 8 centimeters), just before you enter transition, or if your contractions become so overwhelming that you feel you are losing control. Because the effect of narcotics on a newborn's nervous and respiratory system peaks around two hours after they are given, doctors prefer not to give these drugs within two hours of when they expect you to give birth. They want to give the drug time to wear off, at least to the point that it will not compromise baby's ability to breathe after birth. Thus, physicians do not feel it is safe to give narcotics once the pushing stage has begun. Fortunately, once you have the urge to push, your need for medical pain relief will be greatly diminished. Don't worry, however, if a situation arises in which you *must* have a narcotic pain reliever during the pushing stage; baby can be given an injection of a narcotic blocker (Narcan) immediately after birth, which reverses the effect of the drug on baby's ability to breathe.

Select the right route. Getting the drug intravenously gives you relief more quickly than an intramuscular injection. Intravenous drugs also wear off faster. After an intravenous injection a mother usually feels some relief within five to ten minutes; this relief may last around an hour. Intramuscular injections, on the other hand, typically take half an hour to an hour to reach full effect, but the relief may last three to four hours. In either case, some mothers notice that the second dose is not as effective as the first. Most women choose the intravenous route. If labor pain is overwhelming enough to

require medical relief, you want it to happen fast. When you get medication intravenously you are also getting extra fluids, which your body needs during labor. You can request a *heparin lock,* an intravenous catheter allowing administration of medication that is not hooked up to an intravenous bottle; this allows you to adjust positions more easily.

As in so many aspects of pregnancy, birth, and parenthood, using medical pain relief is a judgment call of both mother and doctor. Make these decisions carefully. The progress of your labor and the health of your baby depend on it.

As a childbirth educator, I meet many moms who understand the physical effects of interventions and surgery, but they don't understand the after-birth impact. They don't understand that a certain medication can affect breastfeeding for weeks (or even months) after the birth, or the psychological impact of having an epidural and not being able to feel the baby come out.

Martha's note: *For our first baby, born in 1967, we were young and naive, willing to take the advice of our obstetrician, whose standard practice was to administer a spinal anesthetic and assist the delivery with forceps. (A spinal removes all sensation and all movement, including the ability of the mother to push her baby out.) I still remember the feeling of total numbness as the baby was pulled from my body, and the disconnect when the nurse showed me our baby. My body had no memory of giving birth, so my mind could not grasp that he'd been born. It was not a good feeling then, and the memory still bothers me.*

Epidural anesthesia. Many women want to hug their doctors for giving them an epidural during labor. *Epi* is a Greek word meaning "upon," and *dura* is the sheath that surrounds the spinal cord. (A "spinal" refers to an anesthetic injected into the space enclosed within the dura. This space contains the spinal cord, spinal nerves, and cerebral spinal fluids.) In an epidural, the pain-relieving drugs are injected into the space outside the dura. In a spinal, they are injected into the space around the spinal cord. The epidural has done away with the belief that you must experience pain to birth a baby. Yet before you grab this magic medicine, learn about its benefits and risks. There are different types of epidurals, different times during labor to get one, and trade-offs you should know about.

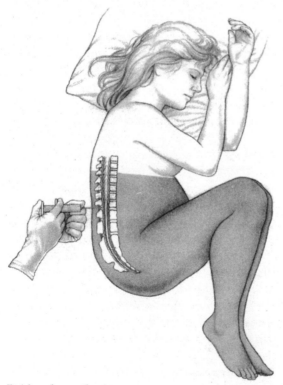

Epidural anesthesia.

How epidurals are given — what you may feel. Before you receive an epidural, you will get a liter of intravenous fluids to build up your blood volume and prevent the decrease in blood pressure that sometimes accompanies an epidural. Your doctor or anesthesiologist will then ask you to sit up, or lie on your side, and curl into the knee-chest position to round your lower back. This widens the space between the vertebrae, making it easier to find the right area for injection. As your doctor or nurse scrubs your lower back with an antiseptic solution, it will feel cold. Next, you will feel a slight stinging sensation as some local anesthetic is injected under your skin to numb the area. When the area is sufficiently numb, he or she will insert a larger needle into the epidural space and inject a test dose to determine whether the needle is in the right place. Once the needle is properly inserted, the anesthesiologist threads a catheter through the needle into the epidural space and removes the needle, leaving this flexible catheter in place. The pain reliever will then be injected into the catheter. A few minutes later you may feel a shooting sensation, like an electric shock, down one leg. Within five minutes you are likely to begin to feel numb from your navel down, or you may notice that your legs are feeling warm and/or tingly. Within ten to twenty minutes the lower half of your body may feel heavy, or numb, depending on the type of medicine used, and the pain of contractions will subside. The exact level of decreased sensation cannot be predicted precisely. The current generation of epidurals are more weighted toward sensory block, not motor block, so most women are able to move around (but not out of bed) and feel pressure sensations but little pain. The anesthesiologist has several ways to adjust the block, using different anesthetics, analgesics, and positioning.

This is the point at which most women sing the praises of the epidural, but this is also the instant at which a woman becomes more of a patient than a participant. Yes, once the pain is relieved, you can rest and recoup your energy. But because the lower half of your body feels heavy, you will need assistance changing positions. Since the sensation to empty your bladder is impaired, a nurse will insert a urinary catheter. Because of the possibility of the epidural lowering your blood pressure, the nurse may monitor your blood pressure every two to five minutes until it is stable, and every fifteen minutes thereafter. To keep the pain relief even on both sides of your body, the nurse may turn you from side to side. To be sure baby is handling the epidural well, you will be hooked up to an electronic fetal monitor. You will also notice that the doctor or nurse periodically rubs the skin of your abdomen, checking to see if you can feel it, to be sure the drug is giving you sufficient pain relief but not ascending high enough to interfere with your breathing. Now comes the juggling act of getting you just enough anesthetic to give you pain relief and help you manage your labor but not so much that it slows down your labor. As you will see from these stories, laboring mothers view epidurals differently.

I had a horrendous labor with my first baby and, quite honestly, wasn't sure I ever wanted to go through that again. But labor memories do fade and I got pregnant again. This time I opted for an epidural, and I'm glad I did. Even before my labor started, the fact that I knew I was going to have an epidural took a lot of the fear and dread out of labor. I actually loved the experience of birthing a baby without so much pain. I don't feel guilty or less of a woman because I opted for an epidural. For me, this was the right decision. My epidural was marvelous. I can't wait to have another baby.

I felt like a beached whale. My legs felt like a sack of potatoes. I couldn't move. Everyone had to help me, and the nurse even had to tell me when I was having a contraction. Sure it didn't hurt, but I felt out of touch with what was going on in my body. For my next birth, I may rethink the whole epidural question.

With my epidural I felt my body and I were out of sync. My urge to push was obliterated. I needed the nurse to put her hand on my uterus and tell me when to push. I felt like a bystander at my baby's birth.

Types of epidurals. Not only are epidurals getting better and safer each year, but there are more kinds of them available, allowing laboring women and their doctors to choose the one that best fits an individual labor. Here is the menu of epidurals that may be available at your hospital:

A *continuous epidural* means that a bedside pump continuously infuses your epidural space with pain-relieving medication. The continuous epidural is the most common epidural used because it offers constant pain relief. Unlike with an intermittent epidural (see next option), blood pressure is more stable and overall a lower dose of medication is needed.

With an *intermittent epidural* the medicine is injected periodically as needed, allowing mothers to juggle the level of pain they can tolerate with the degree of movement they desire. Some mothers do not like the roller-coaster effect of intermittent injections.

EPI-LITE

Another pain reliever in the anesthesiologist's medicine bag is a low dose of narcotics, or a combination of narcotic and anesthetic medicines, in the epidural. This lower dose allows a woman to maintain sensation, the feeling of pressure, and movement without so much pain, thus allowing her to manage her labor without fear. In blocking all of the sensations of labor, epidurals can mask unusual pain that can signal that something is not going right and that can prompt mother and those helping her to make adjustments. Critics also believe that since some epidurals greatly diminish a mother's awareness of what's going on in her body, she becomes detached from her labor. Father becomes equally detached because he doesn't have to be involved. Epi-lite may be the answer to these concerns and a more beneficial and safer compromise.

With an epi-lite, mother can still feel when she's having a contraction. While the dose is high enough to relieve a certain level of pain, it does not mask major pain that could be the body's signal a problem exists that needs attention — from mother and doctor. A low-dose epidural can relieve just enough pain of labor so that an exhausted mother can relax and get a second wind for pushing. It allows mother to be able to at least sit upright in a rocking chair — a "rocking epidural." Even if she can't walk, at least she can rock. In a further improvement, the anesthesiologist uses a combined spinal and epidural. A small dose injected into the spinal space takes effect immediately and lasts only two hours, but the continuous epidural remains in place, allowing longer pain relief.

Epi-lite allows a woman to maintain sensation, giving her the best of both worlds — feeling without hurting.

Patient-controlled epidural anesthesia (PCEA) gives the woman control to self-regulate the amount of relief she receives by pressing a button that allows a preset computer-controlled amount of medication to be injected into the epidural tubing. With PCEA, some women use less medicine, some more, but at least you have a choice.

New epidurals. Both mothers and doctors have long dreamed of an anesthetic that would allow women to enjoy sensation and movement during labor, but without the pain. With newer epidurals this dream has almost come true. Anesthesiologists are experimenting with combinations of narcotic analgesics and anesthetics, or with analgesics only, in hopes of blocking the pain nerves while sparing the motor nerves. Dubbed "walking epidurals," these types of analgesia allow the mother to stand, kneel, squat, and maybe even walk with support. They are even "lighter" than the usual epi-lite. Studies show that epidurals that allow mothers to walk or at least be upright during labor are associated with more efficient labor and healthier babies than epidurals that take away a mother's mobility and ability to labor upright.

The "walking epidural" is actually a spinal and epidural administered together. A small amount of narcotic is injected directly into the spinal space (not the surrounding dura) in a small enough dose to ease the pain of labor but not block movement. Mothers can walk with assistance, shower, sit, stand, or squat. This type of anesthesia is particularly useful in cases where mother is experiencing unbearable contractions, and her pain and exhaustion are preventing her labor from progressing. An epidural given too early (before 5 or 6 centimeters) can slow the progress of labor, but spinal analgesia may bring just enough pain relief to allow mother to rest and recharge before she enters the next, more strenuous, stage of labor.

You should be aware that "epidural" can mean many things. Ask what your options are. Discuss them ahead of time with your doctor and have some idea of your preferences. Discuss your options again with the anesthesiologist, whom you may not meet until you are in active labor. Be sure to tell your practitioners that you are open to change should your labor situation change. You will not know before labor day what your contractions are going to feel like and how you will want to manage them. Being informed about your options will help you make the best choice.

The timing of epidurals. When to get an epidural is as important a decision as which type to get. Getting an epidural too early in labor will limit your mobility and is simply unnecessary. Getting an epidural at the very end of labor defeats the purpose of the epidural, and can simply impede the pushing phase. How an epidural affects a mother's labor is highly individual, so it is difficult to come up with absolute "shoulds" and "should nots" in obstetrical anesthesia. But there are some general guidelines.

Your obstetrician/midwife and anesthesiologist are likely to recommend waiting to administer an epidural until they are satisfied that your labor is active, you are having regular contractions, and your cervix is dilating progressively. Different women reach this point at different times, but typically this will be when your cervix is dilated around 5 centimeters and you're definitely into the active phase of labor. Because you have to get "halfway there" before you are at the stage of labor where an epidural is safest and most effective, it is important to develop a pain-management system (as previously discussed) even if you know ahead of time you will want an epidural. An epidural might be recommended earlier if you are becoming exhausted or if there is some obstetrical or health reason the obstetrician or anesthesiologist would like an epidural placed. For example, with twins the possibility of having to do maneuvers on your abdomen or even an emergency cesarean to deliver the second baby would make having an epidural catheter in place a good idea.

Some mothers and their birth attendants adopt a "wait and see" attitude about epidurals. If your own pain-management system is working, you are not overly tired, and your contractions are bearable, you may want to delay the magic stick in the back. But remember that the decision-to-effect time (the time between deciding on an epidural and it being in place and relieving pain) can be at least thirty minutes. Waiting too long may mean you won't be able to get the relief you need.

I was coping just fine until the contractions came on like gangbusters and I begged for an epidural. The doctor checked me and said I was already beginning transition, so it was too late to get one. It would have been difficult for both the doctor and me to try to do an epidural during the height of these contractions, and besides, by the time the epidural took effect the worst would be over and I probably wouldn't need it. So, I toughed it out. But next time I won't wait so long to cry uncle.

When to ask for the epidural to be turned down or off is also an important decision. It's best to think about this one hour ahead of time, too. Many mothers and physicians prefer to stop the infusion early enough to allow the effects of the epidural to wear off just as the pushing stage begins. This enables mother to move around and adjust her body to the most comfortable position for pushing. If you wait until your cervix is completely dilated to turn off the epidural, you won't have the urge to push and won't be able to push effectively for about an hour. The pushing stage could last as long as three hours — one hour of ineffective pushing, followed by two hours of real pushing. Many obstetrical units recommend not starting pushing until the mother really feels the urge, avoiding pushing efforts, and instead using time and uterine pushing alone to bring the baby farther down the birth canal. Your labor attendants can give you advice here — some women push very effectively with an epidural in place and there is no need to let it wear off; other women benefit from having the epidural turned down or off so that they can really feel the urge to push and can push more effectively.

Dr. BJ notes: *In general, the data has shown that turning an epidural down or*

off does not make a difference unless the epidural is "dense," meaning that the mother cannot move her legs. The problem with turning it down or off is that the rebound pain will seem worse, and the mother may be unable to manage it and therefore unable to push effectively.

Questions You May Have about the Safety of Epidurals

Is an epidural safe for our baby? The truth is that doctors do not know for sure whether epidurals are completely safe for babies, although our opinion is that they are probably safe enough. Even the U.S. Food and Drug Administration labels epidural anesthesia "generally regarded as safe" (GRAS). This is a hedge, meaning that the FDA is not certain either. There is no such thing as a risk-free pain reliever. Small amounts of the narcotics and anesthetics used in epidurals do cross the placenta into baby's bloodstream within minutes. Some babies show changes in fetal heart patterns following an epidural, though these changes have been judged to be not harmful. Some observers have noted that newborns whose mothers had epidurals are more likely to show feeding difficulties in the weeks after birth. When compared with newborns of unmedicated mothers, newborns of medicated mothers do not search for the breast as vigorously when placed on their mother's abdomen immediately after birth. For unknown reasons, some mothers develop fevers following an epidural, and as many as 5 percent of babies of mothers receiving epidurals may also have fevers. It is difficult for the doctor caring for the baby to decide whether this fever is simply a side effect of the drug or whether it signals a newborn infection. To be on the safe side, sometimes a doctor will have to order a series of tests to rule out infant infection.

When we were investigating the various obstetrical anesthetics, we found it very difficult to evaluate them in terms of efficacy and safety. The field of obstetrical anesthesia is improving so fast that on one occasion when we asked an anesthesiologist to comment on a fairly recent study, his reply was, "Oh, we don't use that drug anymore." Much of what you do read and hear about the potential problems associated with epidural anesthesia is indeed out of date. With improved needles and better drugs used in lower doses, today's epidurals are safer for baby and have fewer annoying side effects for mother. It's important to discuss the safety issue with your anesthesiologist. Sometimes a mother's epidural actually benefits the baby; it's not good for baby if mother suffers through a prolonged, exhausting labor in which the blood flow to the uterus is compromised. An epidural can support both mother and baby.

The problem with epidurals is they are used for a large percentage of women who could do without that level of pain relief and instead could be motivated to use natural approaches. Too many women decide to get an epidural too early in their birth. There is an imbalance in the risk/benefit ratio — and the number of babies affected by the side effects is too large. It's hard to study the long-term effects.

Is having an epidural safe for me? As with any drug, a few women may experience unpleasant side effects: a drop in blood pressure, shivering, nausea and vomiting, generalized itching, difficulty urinating, spinal headaches, and even seizures if the epidural "goes spinal," that is, enters the spinal cord and travels up the spinal canal. Some women who receive epidurals also report long-term backaches. While these side effects are merely uncomfortable and temporary, they may be enough to make you stop and think about whether you really want an epidural. Most women, however, breeze through their epidurals with few unpleasant side effects and carry home healthy babies and pleasant memories of their birth.

Might an epidural interfere with my progress in labor? An epidural can help or hinder the progress of labor. We have been present at births where a well-timed epidural actually moved labor along, and we have observed births where a poorly timed or poorly chosen epidural interfered with labor. Like the studies on the safety of epidurals, the studies on their labor-prolonging effects reveal mixed results. In general, epidurals do seem to have a tendency to prolong the second stage of labor (pushing), especially for first-time mothers. The newer low-dose epidurals, however, do not generally prolong labor. Here are two examples of how epidurals can affect labor:

Jan and Tony were first-time parents who wanted to birth their baby "right." They attended two separate series of childbirth classes, took great care in choosing their birth attendants, hired a labor support person, and did all their homework, as befitting the importance of this event. They entered the birthing room well informed about all their options and well practiced in all the natural pain-relieving tools that they had learned about.

Jan's personal pain-management system seemed to be working for her until midway through her labor, when contractions got increasingly intense. Jan and Tony realized the natural way wasn't working anymore. Even though Jan walked, knelt, soaked, and squatted; even though Tony rubbed, supported, and coached; and even though the obstetrician and labor support person did everything they were supposed to do, Jan's progress was slowing. She had used up all of her resources on coping with the pain and was now becoming increasingly exhausted. Her labor stalled: lots of pain, no gain. Together with her husband and her birth attendants, Jan made the decision to avail herself of whatever medical intervention was appropriate so that she could achieve her goal of a gratifying birth experience. She opted for an epidural, which allowed her to rest, regain her strength, and go on with the labor. Jan felt a twinge of "I couldn't do it naturally" remorse, but she knew when to say when, and she felt good about her decision. After about three hours of relief from the epidural, Jan asked that the epidural be stopped and allowed to wear off. Most of its effects had indeed worn off by the time she entered the pushing stage, and she was able to squat to push out her healthy 9-pound baby.

In this case, the wise use of an epidural helped Jan's labor by allowing her time to get her energy back. Jan and Tony viewed the use of epidural anesthesia not as a failure of their resources, but as one more tool available to them in their quest for a safe and satisfying birth.

First-time parents John and Susan had a crowd of friends who praised the virtues of epidurals and wondered why any woman would want to go through the ordeal of labor without this "godsend." John and Susan attended the childbirth class at their hospital but concluded that, since Susan was going to have an epidural anyway, there was no reason to take time to practice relaxation, breathing, and position changes that they wouldn't need to use. Susan got her epidural as soon as the contractions began to intensify. After it was administered, however, and she was confined to bed, her labor slowed. To get her labor going again, her doctor administered Pitocin, a synthetic version of the contraction-stimulating hormone oxytocin. The nurse who was caring for Susan couldn't help thinking, "First, she had a drug that weakened her contractions, then another one to make them stronger. Can two wrongs make a right?" Her labor stalled: "failure to progress." She gave birth by cesarean section.

This is the downward spiral of one intervention necessitating another. If this mother had become informed and empowered how to also make her own pain-easing medicines and then used the epidural in addition to and not instead of medical pain relievers, her birth experience might have been more satisfying.

It's important to understand how any medication in childbirth, especially an epidural, can affect a mother's natural birthing hormones. Levels of oxytocin have been found to be higher during the second stage of labor in mothers who do not have epidurals. Studies also show that mothers having epidural anesthesia tend to have lower endorphin levels. In unmedicated labors, mothers get some degree of natural pain relief from endorphins; these endorphins are also thought to be responsible for the "high" of childbirth most unmedicated women report. Thus, epidurals take away some of the pleasure of birth, as well as the pain. Of course, sometimes epidurals are the best thing for a mother's hormones — for example, when a mother who is overwhelmed by the intensity of contractions is becoming increasingly exhausted. As her stress hormones rise, uterine contractions become weaker and blood flow to the placenta decreases — neither of which is good for mother or baby. For these mothers, epidural anesthesia helps reduce the level of stress hormones, enabling uterine contractions to become stronger and more productive.

Am I more likely to have a cesarean section if I choose to have an epidural? Because there are so many reasons that a woman may need a cesarean, it is difficult to answer this question. Many of the studies that are inconclusive are based on older anesthetics and higher doses than are commonly used today. The newer lower-dose epidurals do not seem to increase the cesarean rate. For a moment, though, forget the studies and employ common sense. As we've discussed, in order to help baby progress down the birth passage, mother must be able to move and adjust her positions according to the sensations she feels. A regular epidural prevents mother from moving, so she cannot take advantage of a valuable labor assistant — gravity. When she has no sensation, there are no cues telling her when or how to move or change position. An epidural also requires fetal monitoring, which can produce false alarms, leading to surgical intervention. And a mother having an epidural often requires Pitocin, which requires still more fetal monitoring. This technological spiral often continues all the way to the operating room, as you read in the birth story of John and Susan.

As in the story of Jan and Tony above, an epidural can, in some instances, help a mother avoid surgical birth by preventing or relieving exhaustion. We have, at times, witnessed this birth scenario: A mother is "failing to progress," so the doctor advises a cesarean. In preparation for the cesarean, mother has an epidural, which relaxes and recharges her, and while the operating team is preparing for the surgery, to everyone's surprise, mother pushes out her baby.

Sometimes, choosing one intervention can prevent another more serious one. The use of an epidural in some medical conditions, such as high blood pressure during labor, may reduce a woman's risk of needing a cesarean birth.

After a long, drawn-out labor, I had had enough of doing it "on my own." After two days of long, close contractions with very little to show for it, I had an epidural and Pitocin to dilate me to 10 centimeters. Then I had them turn off the epidural for pushing. When it finally wore off, it was great to feel the urge to push rather than just being told "Here's a contraction, now push."

Ultimately, a satisfying birth experience does not depend on massage, music, or medication. It depends on making informed choices that you are comfortable with. Your doctor's goal is the same as yours — maximum comfort with minimum risk. Realistically, few women can have it all: medication brings risks, but no medication means discomfort/pain and effort. By understanding the options before you, your individual preferences, and your unique birthing circumstances, you will be able to make choices wisely and have a birth that is safe and satisfying for you and your baby.

MY PREGNANCY JOURNAL: EIGHTH MONTH

Emotionally I feel:

_____

_____

_____

_____

Physically I feel:

_____

_____

_____

_____

My thoughts about you:

_____

_____

_____

_____

My dreams about you:

_____

_____

_____

_____

What I imagine you look like:

_____

_____

_____

_____

_____

My top concerns:

_____

_____

_____

_____

_____

My best joys:

_____

_____

_____

_____

Visit to My Healthcare Provider

Questions I had; answers I got:

_____

_____

_____

_____

Tests and results; my reaction:

_____

_____

_____

_____

Updated due date: _____

My weight: _____

My blood pressure: _____

Feeling my uterus; my reaction:

_____

_____

_____

_____

How I feel when I feel you kick:

_____

_____

_____

What Dad feels when he feels you kick:

_____

_____

_____

What I bought when I went shopping:

_____

_____

_____

_____

Reactions of your brothers or sisters when they feel you move:

_____

_____

_____

_____

How I feel when I think about the pain of labor:

_____

_____

_____

_____

I'm going to try these ways to ease the pain:

_____

_____

_____

Things I'll try with this birth that I didn't try with my last birth:

_____

_____

_____

Photo of me in full bloom:

Comments:

_____

_____

_____

_____

_____

_____

_____

_____

_____

_____

_____

_____

_____

The Hormonal Symphony of Birth

EXPECTANT MOMS AND DADS, READ THE FOLLOWING SECTION

To deeply appreciate the wonderful workings inside a laboring mother's body, read this next section, periodically pausing to imagine a mother soon conducting the greatest masterpiece a woman can create — birthing a little human being.

Mothers, during your pregnancy hundreds of hormones have played in harmony with one another to grow your baby. Now it's time for the finale!

When you can listen to your internal hormonal signals and respond as you would when you are deeply moved by beautiful music, powerful in its crescendos and quiet in its lulls, you can be in tune and in sync with the work of the composer. And in the "opus" of laboring and giving birth,

the composer is none other than the magnificent design built into the biology of your body.

Let's spend some more time with the primary players in your hormonal symphony orchestra, the Symphonic 7:

- Estrogen
- Progesterone
- Oxytocin
- Endorphins
- Adrenaline
- Cortisol
- Prolactin

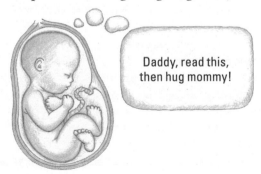

Daddy, read this, then hug mommy!

Grow-and-Prepare Hormones

Featuring estrogen and progesterone.
Throughout pregnancy your placenta produces

primarily two baby-growing hormones, progesterone and estrogen, both of which increase more than ten times over pre-pregnant levels. That's why you feel more feminine. In the final month the concert is coming to a close. Your hormonal changes prepare the birth canal to push your little passenger through. What triggers labor still remains a mystery, but here's what is known. Up until Birth-Day these two pregnancy hormones are in balance: progesterone relaxes uterine muscle and protects it from contracting too much; estrogen, on the other hand, tones the uterine muscle for the homestretch. When labor begins, estrogen surges while progesterone plummets. While your labor may seem anything but musical, there really is a magnificent symphony playing inside your body.

To appreciate this magical design, let's peer into the muscle cells of the uterus to see how these hormones work. Hormones attach themselves to sites on cell membranes called receptors, sort of like doors that the hormones push and say "let me in." The more receptors, the greater the hormonal effect. During the later weeks of pregnancy,

estrogen prepares the uterus for the oxytocin effect. By wiring the uterine muscles with more oxytocin receptors, estrogen primes the uterine muscles for its birthing buddy, oxytocin, to increase the strength of contractions, more appropriately called "forces" or "waves" rather than pains.

The two labor-preparing hormones, estrogen and progesterone, open up natural pain-lessening pathways, called opiate pathways, between the brain and contracting uterine muscles, as if prompting your body to work harder but still somehow feel better. Now that the uterus is primed for work, the birth orchestra is ready for "opening night" — or day. Let the symphony of birth begin!

Power-and-Progress Hormones

Enter oxytocin. You may not have realized it, but you have already been enjoying the oxytocin effect: you get a bit of an oxy-spike during lovemaking and orgasm. The most heard — or felt — hormonal player in the symphony of birth, oxytocin is like the percussion section of a well-tuned orchestra, knowing when to be loud, enabling labor to progress, and when to ease off and let mother enjoy an interlude of rest. Oxytocin has been rehearsing its part since you first felt those Braxton Hicks contractions. When true labor starts, oxytocin's moment of stardom begins.

Oxytocin comes from the Greek, meaning "hastening birth," and that's exactly what it does. Just as the drums reach a crescendo — at the maximum-force peak of a contraction — and mother is ready to say "enough already!," another prime player, this

---

THE BEAUTIFUL BALANCE OF BIRTHING HORMONES

Moms, appreciate the pregnancy perk of biochemical balance. Birth hormones can be perceived as your own internal birth "medicines," where the unpleasant side effects of one hormone (which can be perceived as "pain") are balanced by the effects of another hormone, a natural pain-reliever.

time an enzyme, enters. The placenta secretes oxytocinase, which temporarily dials down the intensity of the contraction forces.

The drums temporarily quiet, allowing the two stars — mother and baby — to rest and recharge for the next crescendo three to five minutes later. Each crescendo is likely to be stronger than, and closer to, the one before. Another welcome player, serotonin, also sounds a few notes at the time of peak contraction pressure to calm anxiety and help ease the sharp sensations. These welcome mini-intermissions are just what the hardworking mother needs.

Ideally mother is supported by wise, knowledgeable, and patient attendants who allow the oxytocin effect to continue. As baby's head descends lower, the cervix is being drawn up and out of the way and the vagina gradually opens to accommodate the little passenger. Receptors in these tissues trigger more uterine muscle–contracting hormones, especially more oxytocin, enabling descent to progress. This vaginal squeeze is like a huge therapeutic hug that better prepares baby for a more physiologically stable adjustment to life outside the womb.

Relieve-and-Relax Hormones

Beta-endorphins are "don't worry" hormones of birth. Mother makes her own pain-easing medicines, called beta-endorphins, or simply endorphins. Appropriately labeled the "reward-and-reinforce hormones," these physiological opiates are released in increasing spurts with increasing intensity of contractions, reaching their highest dose during those final forceful pushes. These neurochemicals peak at birth and remain in mother's brain and bloodstream during the first few days afterward to reinforce her mothering. They are also secreted into the colostrum of her milk. After birth, endorphins behave like biochemical facilitators, helping mother and baby get to know each other. Not only does mother make her own medicines for reward and pleasure during birth, baby makes hormones from his own pituitary gland.

Endorphin levels gradually rise in mother's blood during pregnancy, and studies have found an increase in pain tolerance toward the end of pregnancy. Endorphins also activate dopamine, which is associated with pleasure and euphoria.

Moms, if we seem unapologetically passionate about informing and empowering you to make your own birth medicines, it's because we wish you to have the healthiest birth you can have.

Synchronous symphony. Endorphins go up as the strength of contractions goes up. Oxytocin and endorphins play together in labor-progressing and pain-easing synchrony. Just as oxytocin starts to play "too loud," meaning that the contractions are getting too strong, endorphins tamp down the pain and bring calmness and relief. Endorphins, especially when combined with oxytocin, account for that euphoria and "on another planet" experience mothers report during pushing.

Labor is good for baby's genes. The new science of epigenetics (the developmental origins of health and disease) is beginning to prove what mothers and many birthcare providers have long suspected: the hormonal orchestra of birth switches on certain genes that better prepare baby for life outside the womb and better equip mother to take care of her baby. Though the science of epigenetics is still in its infancy, research suggests that the hormonal harmony of pregnancy and birth may induce "hormonal imprinting," meaning the baby will be born with an increased number of receptor sites, those microscopic doors on the target cells throughout the body, allowing more healthy hormones to selectively enter. This birth experience can influence baby's later tendencies to many illnesses, such as diabetes and cardiovascular disease; and it can influence baby's brain wiring for emotional health. To give your baby a head start, play the best hormonal symphony you can.

Relaxing "music." The ovaries secrete the hormone relaxin, which softens and relaxes the previously tight cervical muscle, enabling it to dilate. When the push-and-contract hormones work in harmony with the relax-and-dilate hormones, progressive music occurs and the symphony of labor is shorter and more productive.

Physiological birth is better for mother and baby than a pharmacological birth. The difference between these mother-made medicines and the ones from the hospital pharmacy is that the natural medicines talk to one another because they share the same neurochemical language. This hormonal harmony programs mother and baby to birth and bond.

Performance-Enhancing Hormones

Enter the energy hormones. Another section in the birth orchestra is for epinephrine (also known as adrenaline) and norepinephrine players, collectively called catecholamines. Remember those "fight or flight" hormones, neither of which you plan to do during birth? Yet, to have a healthy labor and birth a healthy baby, you need these internal medicines to be dispensed into your bloodstream at the right time and in the right dose during labor. Like all other smart hormonal players, they have their place, knowing when to shout their instructions and when to be still. Catecholamines gradually increase during labor, becoming loudest around transition, when mom needs a boost of energy and alertness. Baby also has a catecholamine rush at birth, which helps shift blood to the central organs of the brain and heart, better preparing her for a healthy life outside the womb.

However, unresolved stress, especially fear, enables catecholamines to make too much noise too early in labor and birth, which may slow rather than speed labor. This is the biochemical basis for the dysfunctional fear-tension-pain cycle, which causes the hardworking mother to use up too much birth energy too soon and consequently wear out before she can play her full score.

Adrenaline and cortisol. During the crescendo of delivery, another player enters the orchestra with adrenaline: cortisol. Just as a marathon runner needs an "adrenaline rush" to labor toward the finish line, so your body gets an adrenaline surge to push the baby out. Adrenaline also calls upon its buddy hormone, cortisol, to add fuel to the sprinting body. The good news is that these two hormones, and all the others, work in concert to mobilize fuel to the hardest-working muscles and ready them for baby passage. The uncomfortable news is that they also have quirky behaviors that account for the laboring mother acting in ways she never even thought she could. (Birth attendants take note: mentally plug your ears and smile. The concert, even the parts that are not so melodic or repeatable, will soon be over, and the encore will be indescribably beautiful.)

Dr. BJ notes: *I love to hear a laboring woman say, "I can't do this!" It's like the marathon runner who "hits the wall." This is my cue to get prepared because the baby is coming! This is when close support is needed to help her let go of her baby.*

To prepare baby for a healthy transition from placenta-dependent life to life outside the protective womb, he must also make his own medicines for health. A newly delivered baby enjoys a high dose of catecholamines that help stabilize his biochemistry, especially blood sugar, body temperature, heart rate, blood pressure, and breathing. They also help baby maintain adequate glucose and other essential nutrients, like free fatty acids. Catecholamines even enhance baby's sense of smell, further attracting him to his source of warmth and food — mother's breasts.

Ever marvel why some babies are so alert, wide-eyed, and eager to connect with mom (physiologically called the state of quiet alertness, the optimal neurological state for bonding), especially when immediately placed on nature's best "incubator," mom's chest? Credit the catecholamines for prompting babies to do this for their own well-being at birth.

Music for both mother and baby. Birth is a symphony in motion, called the movements of birth. As the pair choreograph birth, mother moves, baby moves. Her changing positions prompt baby to change position to navigate through the birth passage. This happens best in minimally medicated or nonmedicated births.

Produce-Milk and Bond-with-Baby Hormones

Prolactin plays its music. Another helpful hormone in the orchestra is prolactin, which, as the name describes, "promotes milk." But this hormone doesn't only help make milk; it also plays nicely in mother's brain. Prolactin rises during pregnancy, takes a dip during labor, then plays even louder, when its melody is most needed, in that first hour after birth, acting as a neurochemical facilitator to help activate lactation and connect mother and baby.

When mother gives baby her breast, baby's suckling and skin-to-skin contact give back to mother the calming, anti-stress feelings of prolactin and oxytocin. By suckling, baby stimulates mother's brain to produce more prolactin and oxytocin, which help her sleep better, reduce mommy stress, and have other physiological effects that make her more maternal. This is a smart mother-baby cycle: mother is neurochemically programmed to breastfeed baby, and baby's suckling makes mommy more maternal. New fathers also enjoy higher prolactin levels, which prompt them to be more paternal. Finally, prolactin is credited with enhancing baby's brain development and may be one of the many reasons why breastfed babies tend to grow up to be smarter kids.

Biochemically speaking, neuroscientists believe prolactin triggers a "positive addiction" between mother and baby and a "brain-based reward" for the labor of birth. Another marvel of birth: the hormonal harmony of labor increases what we call attachment hormones in mother and baby to draw them closer to each other.

THE NEXT MOVEMENT OF LABOR: BABY MEETS MOMMY

When the birth attendant wisely and quickly moves baby to where he instinctively wants to be, placed in skin-to-skin contact onto mother's bare abdomen, amazing things happen as baby and mother perform their first after-birth dance together. When baby is placed tummy-to-tummy on mom's soft, warm, newly softened belly, all of baby's senses and reflexes are activated. Baby can rest and get oriented to his new space, but soon (often within minutes) pheromones exuding from the glands on mother's areola, which act as a biochemical magnet, draw baby toward the nipple. Appropriately called the "birth crawl," this has been beautifully described and scientifically validated by Nils and Jill Bergman in their must-read book, *Hold Your Premie* (New Voices Publishing, 2010), and described on the website BirthCrawl.org. Baby's strong legs and feet, in what's called the step reflex, propel him in the right direction so that he can connect with his source of safety and survival — the nipple.

Martha notes: These strong pushes on mama's belly even have a purpose: the kneading effect actually stimulates the newly emptied uterus to begin the process of contracting to close off uterine blood vessels.

Additional stimulation comes when baby grasps and mouths the skin on mother's chest, then the breast. His eyes lock on to the dark-colored areola surrounding his target,

and his nose locks on to mother's scent. Left to himself to locate the nipple as he eagerly explores, he will find it and latch on and start sucking, as we say, "for dear life," exactly what he is hormonally primed to do. Baby's sucking triggers another surge of oxytocin in the mother, stimulating the newly emptied uterus to continue contracting and squeezing the leftover vessels in the placenta, protecting her from excessive postpartum bleeding. The interplay between mother's musical hormones of birth and baby's musical hormones prepare baby for life outside the womb.

THE ENCORE: BIRTH BONDING

Sucking, touching, and eye contact are all part of the music nature writes for baby to begin life outside the womb, and now baby steps in as the guest conductor. When baby is placed in that place of safety close to mother, another movement unfolds — mutual giving. As you learned earlier, baby's sucking gives mommy an extra burst of hormones that help push out the placenta. When baby and mother are tummy to tummy right at birth, mother gives baby warmth because her breasts are natural warmers. The temperature of her entire chest area increases by three degrees to welcome and warm her baby. More mutual giving: mother warms her baby, baby warms mother's heart.

The scent, the warmth, and the skin-to-skin contact actually work on the emotional center of the baby's brain, the amygdala, firing neurons that cause baby to believe, "I feel safe!" Too often well-meaning attendants rush in with their tools to "stabilize" baby. Yet it's usually better, for baby and mother, to realize that mother's soft, warm abdomen

THE TOP TWO MINUTES IN A BABY'S LIFE

The time between birthing of baby and clamping of the cord is vital to baby's health. During those magic two minutes baby has important physiological transitions to make. The medical term for this is stabilization. Here's how to help your baby make the healthiest transition from placental "breathing" to lung breathing:

Have a physiological birth. The hormonal harmony of birth translates into more stabilizing and attachment hormones that flow from mother into baby's most important adaptive organs: brain, heart, and lungs.

Hold the cord cutting. When possible, delay cord clamping for several minutes to give baby a "final squirt" of healthful blood.

Give baby skin-to-skin contact. Mother is the most physiological "incubator" for keeping baby warm. Hold the procedures (eyedrops, injections, weighing baby, etc.) until later. Even if oxygen is needed, baby can usually remain on mother's abdomen, and most procedures can simply be done there so as not to interrupt baby's safe and secure place.

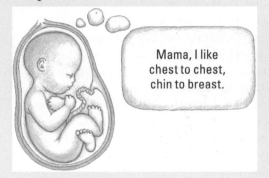

Mama, I like chest to chest, chin to breast.

and breasts are better baby stabilizers, and wise birthcare providers should enable this to happen. This early bonding, in effect, stabilizes baby's unsettled post-birth vital signs, especially body temperature, heart rate, blood pressure, and breathing. If you put yourself behind the eyes of your baby, where would you like to be when you are introduced to the big, wide, scary world? On mama, or in a plastic box? As Nils Bergman, says, "Mother is the best incubator."

Birth meeting continues. What else is going on in there? While it's natural (and necessary) to just gaze at your beautiful suckling baby, there are still a lot of healthy hormonal happenings going on. As you begin your birth-bonding dance together, you are

both rewarded with hormonal surges that prompt the dance to continue. Blood levels of oxytocin — the hormone of love and the "cuddle chemical" — are highest in the first hour after birth, just when mother and baby are most open to falling deeply in love. Oxytocin also calms the pair at the very hour when the newness of motherhood and life outside the womb makes them *need* calming. Even in the "babymoon" weeks after birth the continued high levels of birth hormones account for new mothers feeling, "I'll just sit in my rocking chair and nurse my baby, and I don't care what a mess my house is."

We are going into these biochemical details to underscore the magnificence and power of a mother's body giving birth. Although the mindset in many maternity settings is one of mother as a passive patient with birthcare providers as the conductors, in the natural birth symphony she is always the star conductor of the performance. The obstetrician, midwife, doula, nurses, and friends support the stage and periodically even remain backstage, offering their skills at the right time, in the right amount, but only to help mother make more melodious music.

Enter the birthcare providers. Sometimes mom loses confidence in her ability to make her own birth medicines. She becomes uncertain what her body's signals mean. A midwife or doula, an attendant experienced in reading these signals, can help. Sensing that mom is about to play off-key or even give up her baton, this person gives mom a cue to help her symphony stay on track. "Try changing your position," "Focus on letting go." No one intrudes, everyone supports, and mother gets her tempo back.

SUPPORTIVE BIRTHCARE PROVIDERS

The midwife's music. The midwife acts like a co-conductor. She draws upon her personal and professional experience to intuitively observe when the mother forgets her score, doesn't know her score, or loses confidence in her score, and starts playing off-key. The co-conductor doesn't "intervene," but rather supports. She observes the mother's body language and intuitively helps her get back on key, perhaps with a change in position, a word of encouragement, a bit of emotional and physical nourishment, or a change of scenery like dimming the lights or changing the music. According to a midwife's training, mindset, and experience, birth is a normal, healthy,

harmonious process. Midwives also have the wisdom and experience to know when to call in medical assistance, when mother may need technology and pharmacology, and sometimes surgery, to give the blessing of birth the best ending: a healthy mother and a healthy baby.

The obstetrical section of the orchestra. The symphony of birth is so intricate that sometimes mother's hormones or anatomy or baby's position will not follow the physiological script — for example, in the case of placenta previa, breech presentation, and premature labor. For the best health of mother and baby, other players must be called in: obstetricians, anesthesiologists, and so on, as well as whatever technology and pharmacology players are necessary. But the central theme remains: mother continues to make her own birth medicines, with the help of others who complement hers. As a result of "technological births" women have become afraid of the workings of their own wombs, and even at some point believe that it's safer to have a doctor cut through their abdomen and womb to pull baby out than to enable baby to safely navigate through the normal passageways to the outside world. Billions of births over millennia have fine-tuned the birth symphony. To quote Nils Bergman again, "Humanity first, technology second."

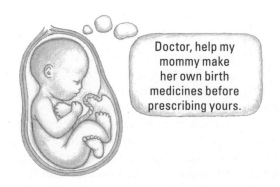

Doctor, help my mommy make her own birth medicines before prescribing yours.

Family and friends. It's important for mom to have people around her who appreciate the birth symphony. Only positive people with relaxed attitudes, please.

DADS AT DELIVERIES

Dads often feel helpless in this obviously female-centered performance. You might ask, "What can I do?" Love your wife. That's what you can do better than anyone else on this stage. You might be relieved you don't have to remember all those quickly forgotten breathing exercises that were presented during childbirth classes. You can play beautiful music at birth, too, by tuning into your own hormones to "love the mother."

Dr. Linda notes: Men also produce oxytocin, which helps them better bond with their mate and their baby. It's an equal-opportunity hormone.

THE LESS-SYNCHRONOUS SYMPHONY OF A PHARMA-TECH BIRTH

The physiological birth is a hormonal harmony perfected over the course of human history. Yet in the past century, modern medicine has attempted to improve on nature's design. In a small percentage of births, around 10 or 15 percent, modern obstetrical medicine has to complement mother's music, for the best health of mother and baby. The advances in obstetrical care of challenging pregnancies and newborn intensive care of compromised babies has

enabled more mothers and babies to enjoy a successful symphony of birth. Appropriate interventions can benefit mother and baby, but the further mother departs from a physiological birth, the greater the likelihood her hormonal symphony will be disrupted.

Pharmacological versus physiological birth. What happens when outside "players" are invited to join mother's orchestra — say, a synthetic hormone like Pitocin or Syntocinon, a technological player like electronic fetal monitoring, or a pharmacological pain reliever like an epidural? The entire orchestra runs the risk of being out of sync.

Enter the hormone disrupters. "You haven't dilated much . . . you're failing to progress." The word "fail" causes the baton to fall out of mother-conductor's hand. When disturbing notes sound, there can be an unnatural break in the action of birth, and fear can set in, prompting the players to be off-key: oxytocin decreases, contractions slow, and the orchestra is out of sync. Outside medicines can interfere with mommy-made medicines. Pharmaceuticals are meant to complement, not replace, and only after mommy-made physiological medicines have been supported.

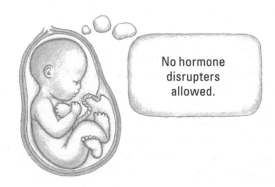

No hormone disrupters allowed.

TERMS OF ENDEARMENT

Fearful language disables a laboring mother. Words are seeds. Don't plant fearful words that sprout fearful thoughts. Birthcare providers, always use encouraging words:

Say this:	*Not that:*
Do	Try
Temporary pause	Stuck
Enable	Allow
Babies don't know how to tell time	Failure to progress, overdue
Decline	Refuse
Holding for now at 5 centimeters	Still only at 5 centimeters
Support	Intervene

How Pitocin performs. Custom-made for baby and mother, oxytocin comes in bursts and pauses, automatically released into mom's bloodstream at the right dose, at the right time. Natural oxytocin contractions are not only easier on mommy but safer for baby. Your mommy-made oxytocin arrives at your hormonally primed uterus in pulses, telling the receptors when you need more and when you need less. The intravenous "pit drip" doesn't have that pulse effect; it doesn't automatically know when to dial up and when to dial down.

Dr. Linda notes: *Pitocin, synthetic oxytocin, nicknamed "pit," is chemically the same but the dosing is not. A "pitocin drip" is administered by medical protocol and dialed upward until the contractions are "adequate" by obstetrical standards. This can be a good thing, and when used appropriately Pitocin can speed up an abnormally long labor. This can help avoid a surgical birth, or a vacuum or forceps delivery, and give women a little extra "oomph" when the pushing efforts of mom are exhausted. Be sure you and your caregivers have gotten as much mileage as possible out of your mommy-made oxytocin, and that you are only calling in the orchestra understudies when absolutely needed. If a well-meaning birthcare provider recommends Pitocin, make sure it is absolutely necessary, and other available alternatives have been tried first. Birth doesn't always follow the desired musical score. When possible, stick to the script of the great classical masterpiece of birth, knowing there are times to improvise, which, too, can lead to great moments.*

Some obstetrical neuroscientists are concerned that the pit drip can lead to receptor insensitivity, meaning that higher doses of Pitocin (and more painful contractions) are needed to force the receptors open. The emerging science of psychoneuroendocrinology suggests that the brain may not recognize the synthetic pharmaceuticals as the real thing because synthetic oxytocin may not cross the blood-brain barrier and actually register its effects there. So although mama-made oxytocin acts on the uterus (contractions) and the brain (analgesia and calmness), synthetic oxytocin may act only on the uterus.

Labor-inducing drugs have a tendency to

produce longer, stronger, and closer-spaced contractions than those a mother would experience with her natural hormones. It's thus possible that the synthetic labor-stimulating hormones might compromise the blood and oxygen supply from the placenta because the placenta, and baby, have less time to refuel and re-oxygenate between contractions. The synthetic contractions are usually more painful for mother and cause her to be out of sync with her own pain-relieving hormones, oxytocin and beta-endorphin, necessitating more pain relief and epidurals, which can lead to more complications.

Pharmacological pain-relievers, especially epidurals, may also "relieve" mother of her own natural birth and attachment hormones, and therefore blunt the euphoria mommy enjoys from these birthing neurochemicals.

One of my birth attendants said to me: "You might need a pit drip to jumpstart your stalled labor!" I felt like saying, "I'm a mom, not a car battery."

Painful "music." When your contraction-producing hormones are in disharmony, the cervical hormones don't relax when the pushing hormones tell them to, causing harder uterine contractions to push against tightly closed cervical muscles — ouch! More painful labor results, which is why we emphasize the hormonal harmony of labor. Your body knows how much oxytocin to drip into your system and when to release it better than the IV machine at your bedside. Furthermore, you often have to lie in bed while getting a "pit drip," and this position can slow your labor progress. In laboring

mother lingo: "Pit contractions are too strong, too long!"

Enter epidurals. Epidural analgesics, if timed appropriately, can help the concert to continue. They enable the exhausted conductor to rest, recharge, and resume her symphony. But if given too early they can delay the finale of birth. Inappropriate use of pharmacological analgesics can blunt the pain-relieving and labor-progressing effects of mother's physiological hormones.

Possible Pitocin effects on baby. Some birth scientists are concerned that the "too long–too strong" effects of Pitocin may also compromise placental blood flow to baby, which is why, for safety's sake, electronic fetal monitoring (EFM) is required while synthetic oxytocin is given.

Enter technology: electronic fetal monitoring (EFM). While sometimes lifesaving, our love of technology has allowed it to infect birth. The electronic fetal monitors may pick up confusing wiggly lines of possible disharmony, often leading to premature canceling of the whole performance and redirecting the orchestra

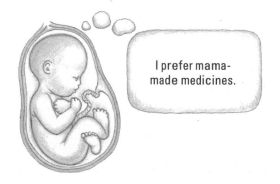

I prefer mama-made medicines.

offstage into the operating room, which now occurs in more than 30 percent of births.

One intervention, such as synthetic Pitocin, often requires another, such as electronic fetal monitoring, which requires more lying on the back, which causes unbearable pain, requiring epidural or prescription analgesia. If these interventions are untimely, they may upset the hormonal harmony of birth and downgrade mother from conductor to a more subservient role. When mother and her birthcare providers work in harmony, in the final moments of the concert all the hormones work together in a powerful crescendo to birth baby.

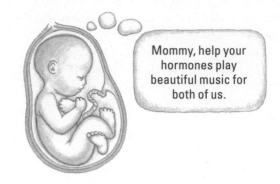

Mommy, help your hormones play beautiful music for both of us.

MOMMY-MADE VERSUS FACTORY-MADE OXYTOCIN: PHYSIOLOGICAL VERSUS PHARMACOLOGICAL BIRTH		
Oxytocin Effect on...	*Physiological*	*Pharmacological*
Brain	Calming and pain-relieving.	May act only on the uterus and not get into the brain.
Contraction intensity	Arrives in pulses, allowing painless pauses.	Too strong, too long, too painful.
Synchrony with oxytocin receptors in the uterus	Oxytocin released when receptors are ready and most sensitive, allowing receptors to remain sensitive.	Oxytocin release and receptor sensitivity may be out of sync, leading to receptor insensitivity.
Dosage	Naturally matched to mother's need and receptor sensitivity.	May not match mother's need and receptor sensitivity.
Contractions affecting baby	Contractions less intense and shorter. Relaxes placental blood vessels longer, restoring healthy blood flow to baby.	Contractions more intense and longer. May squeeze placental blood vessels; shorter relaxation phase, possibly compromising blood flow to baby.

Cervix	Match cervical ripening and readiness, enhances progress.	Stronger contractions may occur before cervix is ready, increasing pain and decreasing progress.
Pain relief	As oxytocin increases, endorphins also increase as a balancing analgesic.	May not enjoy the natural endorphin analgesic effect.
Method of delivery	More likely to have vaginal birth.	Increased chance of having surgical birth.
Maternal blood levels of birthing and mothering hormones	Higher levels of oxytocin and endorphins.	Lower levels of natural oxytocin and endorphins.
Newborn	Birthing hormones higher in cord blood; bonding hormones higher. Oxytocin and its buddy hormones benefit baby.	Bonding hormones lower.
Breastfeeding success	Higher milk-making hormones; feeding more pleasurable.	Lower milk-making hormones; breastfeeding less successful.

AN EXPERT'S FINALE OF BIRTH MUSIC

A few months before this book was "delivered," Martha and I had the privilege to be speakers at "Turning the Tide," an Australian conference on the latest advances in maternal-fetal medicine. We, along with some of the world's experts in physiological births — obstetricians, midwives, university professors, and neonatal intensive care nurses — all gathered along with four hundred other birthcare providers with a single purpose: to inform and empower the modern mother on how to increase her chances of having the healthiest pregnancy and birth she can have. At the meeting we asked two of the speakers, Dr. Nils and Jill Bergman, perinatal medicine specialists and concert lovers, to summarize our hormonal harmony analogy. Here's what they told us:

There is a hormonal harmony at a natural birth that is like a classical symphony. Like any good symphony this comes in four movements.

Mother conducts the first movement (allegro), which reaches a crescendo at birth itself. The baby then conducts the second (adagio), which starts very softly and quietly, with many individual instruments playing their own tunes. In the third movement (scherzo) they play together, and then in the fourth (finale), all the instruments play in harmony to create full symphonic sound. The "instruments" in this symphony are hormones that play healthful music in mother's and baby's brains and bodies.

The first movement starts with the beginning of labor and sets the tune. Oxytocin is released in pulses to contract the uterus and open the birth canal. This canal opening makes even higher levels of oxytocin in mother's brain, preparing her for bonding.

As a counterpoint, labor increases adrenaline and cortisol in the baby. These stress hormones provide intense stimulation to the baby's brain and lungs. The squeezing of the lungs as baby passes through the birth canal tunes them to be ready to breathe. The baby in the womb has spent most of her time sleeping, but now baby needs to be awake, ready to conduct the next movement.

The stress hormones in mother and baby at birth are higher than they will ever be again, a real crescendo to end the movement.

At birth the baby draws a first breath. Crying is not necessary for this. While high-stress hormones were needed at birth, they must now be rapidly lowered. And so, baby conducts the second movement: the adagio is slow and gentle, and needs to be in a safe place. Skin-to-skin contact with mother provides warmth from her body to stabilize baby's heart and breathing, and provides a familiar smell for the feeling of safety. The main instrument playing in the baby now is oxytocin, which lowers stress. This also starts a set sequence of behaviors, like a tune where each note must follow the last in the right order. Baby now becomes the active one, as mother lies back. The baby's sense of smell guides him to her nipple. Baby may touch and taste it along the way to sucking. Baby knows where to go — his life depends on mother's life-giving colostrum and milk. Without any help, he will latch on to the nipple and start to suckle. Baby then locates mother's face, making eye contact, even while continuing to suckle.

This starts a number of new instruments! Prolactin is released, and this activates the glands in the breasts that will make milk. Breastfeeding also activates dopamine, the pleasure hormone, making mother feel emotionally content. This hormonal harmony makes caring for her baby feel very rewarding, almost addictively so. Another surge of oxytocin begins to act on different parts of mother's brain. One action is to make her fiercely protective; another activates her emotional capacity to bond with baby. Later, oxytocin will stimulate milk-ejection reflexes, each of which reinforce protection and bonding.

Suckling is pleasurable for the baby also, as well as soothing for pain relief. The baby will decide how long this movement should be, and the movement ends with the baby falling asleep on mother. Smell tells the baby that mother is present (so it is safe to sleep), which allows the brain to cycle through different levels of sleep, necessary for wiring of baby's brain growth. This sleep should not be disturbed.

Procedures should be clustered when baby is awake.

The third movement, like the scherzo, is a dance with mother and baby. It begins when baby wakes from his first sleep, perhaps after one or a few hours. He wants eye contact and bonding time, and more time at the breast. Then another cycle of sleeping, playing, and feeding. As this continues during the first few cycles, mother *has the opportunity to wire her brain to her baby's, sleeping when her baby sleeps, and waking with her baby. The first 1,000 minutes (about 16 hours) is the sensitive time when mother and baby are learning to dance together.*

(See resources, page 429, for books and DVDs by the Bergmans.)

NINTH-MONTH VISIT TO YOUR HEALTHCARE PROVIDER
(34–40 WEEKS)

The frequency and content of healthcare provider visits during the final month depend greatly on your particular obstetrical situation. Your provider may wish to see you weekly. During this month's visit you may have:

- An examination of the size and height of your uterus

- A palpation of your uterus to determine position of your baby

- An internal exam, if indicated

- A weight and blood pressure check

- An ultrasound exam to determine the size and position of your baby, if indicated

- Vaginal culture for Group B strep colonization

- An opportunity to discuss when to call your practitioner if labor begins

- An opportunity to discuss the difference between Braxton Hicks contractions and the "real" ones

- An opportunity to discuss signs that labor has begun

- An opportunity to discuss when to go to the hospital or birth center

- An opportunity to discuss your birth plan, including labor assistants, avoiding an episiotomy, or special birth requests

- An opportunity to discuss your feelings and concerns

Your healthcare provider may discuss what to do when you're "overdue." You may have weekly ultrasound examinations to assess the volume of the amniotic fluid, or discuss possible induction of labor at some point. If you are overdue, your healthcare provider will counsel you on worrisome signs to watch for.

19

Ninth Month: This Is It!

Now that baby's birth is near, excitement is building: you are more eager than ever to meet your baby. You may also be tired of hearing "What? You're *still* pregnant?" At least now you can say, "Not much longer!" For many women, month nine is the longest month of the pregnancy. So many times mothers have told us they wished they could just fast-forward to the Big Day. If you haven't already, you might want to start saying how far along you are in terms of weeks, e.g., "I'm thirty-six weeks' pregnant — only two more weeks to go!"

It's more obstetrically correct to talk of "labor month" rather than "labor day," since you will actually spend a good part of your ninth month "in labor." Of course, this extended labor will be nowhere near as powerful as what you will experience on the day or so leading up to your baby's birth. Throughout the weeks prior to delivery, your mind and body will get ready for one of the most memorable events in your life.

HOW YOUR BABY IS GROWING, 34–40 WEEKS

You will feel bigger because your baby nearly doubles his weight in one month, going from less than 4 pounds to about 7½ pounds, and may now be nearly 21 inches long. During this "finishing" stage, baby gains a tremendous amount of subcutaneous fat, filling him out for birth. His lanugo hair has disappeared, along with some of the vernix caseosa — just enough of this cheesy substance remains to lubricate him for a smoother passage during birth. By this time, your baby has pretty much run out of room and is tucked up like a little ball in position for birth. During the final weeks inside the womb with less room to exercise, baby makes stepping movements, turns his head, blinks, sucks his thumb, grasps with his hands, practicing all the movements he will need after he makes his appearance in the world. For months now, baby has been swallowing and peeing amniotic fluid. The air sacs of his lungs are now well lined with surfactant, which will help keep the lungs expanded after birth with each breath of air, enabling nearly all babies born at this month to breathe on their own outside the womb.

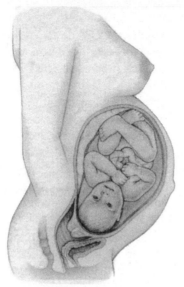

Baby at 34–40 weeks.

HOW YOU MAY FEEL

Ready! "I'm so ready!" is how most nine-monthers greet their healthcare providers during their now weekly checkups. Naturally, most moms are eager and ready before baby is. This is a good time to take a deep breath and call up a healthy dose of patience. Martha recalls vividly how she felt at the end of the ninth month with our third child. Our first two had been born several weeks early, so having to be patient was new to us. Our doctor told us, based on Martha's eagerness to give birth, "We'll see how things look at your next visit." We had a strong hunch that if she had given him the green light he would have been happy to give things a pharmaceutical "nudge." As it turned out, Martha went into labor later that week. She needed patience, not drugs.

HOW LABOR HORMONES WORK

Remember our description of your hormones being like a symphony orchestra (reread "Listening to Your Hormonal Symphony Orchestra" on page 152)? In the final month the concert is coming to a close. Your hormonal harmony changes to prepare the birth canal for passage and to push your little passenger through. While what triggers labor still remains a mystery, here's what is known. Up until Birth-Day your pregnancy hormones are in a fine balance: Progesterone relaxes uterine muscle and protects it from contracting too much. Estrogen, on the other hand, tones the uterine muscle for the homestretch. As you near the finish line, the progesterone effect will be dialed down and the estrogen effect dialed up. More and more estrogen will stimulate the uterine muscle toward the crescendo of increasingly stronger Braxton Hicks contractions to the point where the practice contractions morph into actual labor. As your estrogen hormones trigger increasingly stronger and more painful contractions, this considerate hormone signals the brain to secrete its buddy hormone, serotonin, which calms your anxiety and somewhat eases the pain. While you may view labor as anything but musical, there really is a magnificent hormonal harmony playing inside your body.

I hope to be able to convey the same attitude toward birth to my daughter that my mother conveyed to me. Since I was an older sibling, I got to watch what a joy being pregnant and giving birth were to my mother. So, when my daughter comes to me and asks, "What's it like?" or "Is it scary?" I will tell her that pregnancy is the most special thing her body is designed to do.

Wanting to get back to "normal." Yes, you're eager to hold your baby. Maybe you can't wait to be done with pregnancy and get your body back. You're probably even looking forward to lying on your stomach! Yet, you could also be feeling fleeting pangs of regret over having to give up the specialness of being pregnant. You have a unique and special closeness with your baby now, an intimate experience with baby that no one else shares, and it may feel hard to let go. The good news is that this intimacy will soon evolve into something even more incredible. You'll be amazed at how quickly you forget both the pains and the pleasures of pregnancy once you hold your precious baby in your arms.

I found myself dwelling on kicks, talking to my baby, and hugging my tummy during the last month, trying to imprint these very special feelings on my brain. But once the baby came, I realized that while pregnancy was beautiful and I loved sharing my body with my son, having him as a separate person was even more fulfilling. Being pregnant was amazing, but being a mom really blew me away!

More need to rest and nest. While you won't become a recluse, most women in their final month turn their hearts toward home. You may become more meditative. Your desire and ability to entertain dwindles and social activities don't seem so important. You might discover you couldn't care less about world events. You may find yourself becoming very protective of your peace. This is nature's way of guarding you from outside influences, which can distract you from the highest priority event in your future. You now have the best excuse (and will have for months to come) for saying no to any requests for your time and energy that would take you away from your nest. Don't be surprised if you feel a sudden, compelling urge to clean the house or undertake a big project, such as putting ten years' worth of loose photos in albums or organizing them on the computer. Dr. Linda cleaned the basement while waiting for baby number one. The basement didn't get cleaned for another two decades. By baby number three there was no burst of energy whatsoever.

I decided as I entered my ninth month to cultivate the quiet and rest my mind and body needed. I wanted to be both fit and rested for labor. I saw from watching my friends how exhausting that would be. So I knew this would be my only chance to stockpile energy. Yet, two weeks before delivery day I started washing walls. I never wash walls.

There may be a well-timed shift to high gear to go along with the urge to prepare your home for the important newcomer. A day or two of yielding to this energy spurt can provide you with a healthy diversion from the tedium of these seemingly endless last weeks and maybe give you an added sense of accomplishment. But don't overdo it. Even though the nesting instinct is common among females across the animal kingdom, human mothers don't need such a spotless and sanitized nest. You don't have to have everything perfectly decorated and in place before baby is born. Many well-appointed nurseries go unused for the first few months (or years!). These things can be done by someone else or done gradually after Birth-Day, with baby snuggled in a sling, sleeping peacefully. This is not the time to use up energy. Even though you may think that labor day is still two or three weeks away, don't count on it. During the ninth month, rest as if the next day could be "it."

Baby dropping, feeling better—sort of. Sometime during the final few weeks you may notice that your baby bulge has moved lower down. You may even get comments that your side profile has changed. Most first-timers notice their babies dropping within two weeks of delivery, though some babies drop as many as four weeks before. Many second-time mothers find that their babies do not drop until labor begins because their pelvic muscles have already given birth, and no warm-up is needed. Baby's head settling into the pelvis is also called "lightening" (because the lower-riding load seems smaller and lighter) or "engagement" (since baby's head engages the pelvic opening). Whether baby "drops," "lightens," or "engages," you will feel and look different. One thing you'll probably notice is that your breasts no longer touch the top of your abdomen.

Two of the more common annoyances of the eighth month, breathlessness and heartburn, usually ease during the ninth month. When baby descends lower into your pelvis, your diaphragm has more room to do its job, which helps you breathe more easily. And now that your stomach is less squished,

you may feel less heartburn. Of course, while the discomfort at the top end of the uterus may improve, common discomforts reappear at the bottom — you'll need to urinate more frequently again as baby's head begins to press more on your bladder. And while the upper digestive tract may feel better, the crowded lower tract may once again feel constipated and bloated. Hemorrhoids may enlarge, too.

More pelvic pressures. As your baby descends into your pelvic cavity, you may find yourself prone to sharp, stabbing pains at the base of your spine or in the middle of your pubic bone, making it uncomfortable to walk. Some women get uncomfortable twinges or "pins and needles" in the cervix itself. You may feel pressure or even a sharp pain in your pelvic area whenever you try to lift up your leg to put on your underwear or get out of bed. Sometimes these pains can radiate around to your back or down your thighs. The increased pelvic aches and pains of the ninth month are most likely due to the relaxation and stretching of your pelvic ligaments in preparation for the job to come. You can ease these discomforts by moving into different positions. It helps to continue to exercise gently every day — take long, slow walks.

Baby's head pressing against the nerves and blood vessels in your pelvis can also cause cramps in your thighs. As with pelvic aches and pains, these changes are due to the influence of pregnancy hormones on the ligaments of all of your joints. The overall loosening of ligaments has been known to cause the knees and wrists to feel weak, too, making even light lifting tricky. However, movement keeps your body tuned up. Don't become a couch potato or your muscular, cardiovascular, respiratory, and digestive systems will lose tone. Toned body muscles are important during your birth time to provide support for you so the strong uterine muscle can be most efficient. Most moms in their ninth month find swimming to be the most relaxing and comfortable exercise.

Dr. Linda notes: I remember watching pregnant women "waddle" with a wide gait and thought I'd never get that out of shape. I didn't realize it was due to loose pelvic ligaments — and yes, I did get the waddle!

One benefit of having some aches and pains in late pregnancy is the opportunity this presents for you to practice the deep breathing you've learned in childbirth class. Often couples don't take this practice seriously and don't get around to working it into their day. It can seem weird to practice having a contraction when there's nothing to work with. But, when you have an actual ache, a stabbing pain, or a strong Braxton Hicks contraction, put it to good use: Go into your relax mode, however you've been taught, and deep breathe. Take a minute or two and imagine this is a real "labor pain." Watch and see how the thing changes as you stop bracing against it and just let it happen.

Feeling different kicks. Babies move even less in the ninth month than they did in the eighth, but what these movements lack in frequency they make up for in power. You may feel hard kicks in your ribs and punches in your pelvis. Sometimes it may even feel as though baby is moving into your vagina — a very odd sensation.

When baby is kicking you in an awkward position, try moving your body to get her to move. This is a mini-rehearsal for changing

your body positions during delivery to help baby navigate through the winding passage.

Feeling bigger and off-balance. Now you are big — really big. You may find that the muscles in your abdomen hurt from working so hard to support your belly, or that your crotch and your thigh bones ache when you walk. Bigness becomes an all-over feeling. Even your legs feel heavy. You may wonder how you are going to lug yourself around for another month, especially up and down stairs. Even getting up off the sofa will begin to take some planning.

CONCERNS YOU MAY HAVE

Continuing to work. If you work outside the home, you will need to decide when to stop working. While some mothers say, "I want to work until the day I begin labor," we caution you regarding this approach. This is a time when your body is undergoing as many physiological changes as it did when you were first pregnant. At that time you "gave in" to the process and allowed your body to rest because of the overwhelming fatigue you felt. The process of preparing for birth is energy intensive for both the mind and body, and giving in to the process is again required. Setting too many deadlines or pressuring yourself to keep on working can keep your body from relaxing and allowing nature to take its course. Women who continue working up until the time of labor can experience conflict within themselves and "hold in" their baby as there are other things that must get done first. The last month is truly a time to let go of everything else so that you can ease into your birth time and new motherhood, rested in mind, body, and spirit. If possible, start your maternity leave a week or two early to give yourself the time to rest and replenish your reserves. Studies have shown that the more rest and sleep that women have prior to their birth time, the easier their labor is — something all women want!

PACKING AND PREPARING FOR BIRTH

In the last few weeks before Birth-Day, you will have many things to do and people to call. Here are some tips to jog your memory:

☐ Arrange care for your other children.

☐ Tie up loose ends at work.

☐ Preregister at hospital or birth center.

☐ Tour birth place.

☐ Compose birth plan and discuss with healthcare provider.

☐ Send copy of birth plan to hospital.

☐ Remind labor assistants of due date and update them if it seems that you might go early.

☐ Stock up on nonperishable groceries and freeze some dinners ahead.

☐ Pay bills.

☐ Be sure you understand when to call your healthcare provider and when to go to the hospital.

☐ Finish outfitting baby's layette.

☐ Buy last-minute comfortable clothing: gowns and nursing bras.

☐ Buy baby's car seat and have it installed correctly — some police departments offer this service.

Pack your bag a few weeks before your due date. Put as many things as you think you'll need into your case and leave it open for last-minute additions. When the moment hits, you won't have time to run around grabbing — and forgetting — items you are likely to need or want.

Here are items to pack for the birth:

Laborsaving devices

☐ Your favorite pillows (in colored cases, to keep track of them)

☐ Your favorite music on an MP3 player, plus extra batteries or a charger

☐ Unscented massage lotion or oil

☐ Your favorite snacks (e.g., trail mix, fresh fruit, juice), plus sandwiches for dad

☐ Hot water bottle or rice pack

☐ Special aids that you have been using during your labor practices, such as a birth ball, tennis ball, knee pads (for all-fours position)

☐ Clothes to wear in labor (bathing suit top if you plan to use tub for labor immersion) and to wear home after baby is born — don't forget bathrobe and slippers

(continued)

Toiletries

- ☐ Hairbrush, dryer, hairbands or elastics

- ☐ Soap, deodorant, shampoo, conditioner (avoid perfumes that may upset baby)

- ☐ Maternity-size sanitary napkins (also supplied by hospital)

- ☐ Toothbrush, toothpaste, lip balm

- ☐ Glasses or contact lenses (or both — you may not feel like dealing with contacts in labor)

- ☐ Cosmetics

Homecoming clothes for baby

- ☐ Socks or booties

- ☐ Undershirt

- ☐ Sleeper with legs (to fit into car seat)

- ☐ Receiving blanket

- ☐ Bunting with legs and heavy blanket if you'll deliver in cold weather

- ☐ Cap (usually supplied at birth place)

- ☐ Diapers (usually supplied at birth place)

Other items

- ☐ Hospital preadmittance forms

- ☐ One or more copies of your birth plan

- ☐ Insurance forms

- ☐ Cameras (video and still)

- ☐ Cell phone and charger

- ☐ "Birth-Day" gift(s) for baby's sibling(s)

- ☐ Favorite book and magazines

- ☐ List of family and friends' telephone numbers

Sleepless in the homestretch. Most moms-to-be admit frustration this month over not being able to get enough sleep; no matter how tired they are, they don't sleep well and never feel fully rested. This can be because of the physical and emotional drain of the ninth month, or from an overactive mind finding things to worry about. Either way, you now have another chance to practice relaxation and deep breathing. When you see how you can relieve tension, store that thought away for use during labor.

First-time moms will now be getting used to a light sleep pattern they've never experienced before. This becomes, and

remains, a familiar and practical mode for mothers at night. Nursing the baby, seeing that older children are covered with blankets, comforting them after nightmares, sitting up through their illnesses, reassuring a wakeful one — all these things dictate light sleeping for a number of years.

Small changes in weight. Even though your baby will gain several pounds during this month, your weight may increase only slightly, stay the same, or actually drop a pound or two. Weight loss in the final month is usually due to a decrease in the amount of amniotic fluid, as hormones begin shifting fluid around in your body. You produce less amniotic fluid, and the increased frequency of urination may lead to an overall drop in total body water, and therefore a decrease in your weight. It's just your body letting go of fluid it no longer needs.

WHAT TO DO WHEN YOU'RE "OVERDUE"

Why you should not worry. Don't worry if your due date has arrived but baby hasn't. Even though you're ready, clearly baby isn't. In fact, most babies labeled "overdue" aren't. While the normal range of maturity is between thirty-eight and forty weeks, your estimated due date can be off by a week or two (see page 125). With modern ultrasound dating, fewer than 4 percent of babies who go beyond forty-two weeks are actually overdue. Perhaps your due date wasn't that accurate after all; even ultrasound dating is not infallible. Babies are labeled "overdue" more often if your menstrual periods were irregular and you started out with a highly uncertain due date. First pregnancies tend to last a bit longer, as the body has never done birth before. In any event, worry won't prompt delivery and, as you've already learned, stress just increases the risk of complications.

Why your healthcare provider may worry. You and your healthcare provider could simply watch and wait. But babies who overstay their welcome in the womb (after forty-two weeks) do have a statistically higher incidence of some problems. These include:

- Baby outgrows the placenta, causing baby to be undernourished, which happens in only about 10 percent of babies who go beyond forty-two weeks.

- More commonly, an overdue baby is born too big, leading to a more difficult birth.

- The level of amniotic fluid may decrease to a concerning level, adding to birth complications. Since amniotic fluid helps to cushion the umbilical cord during labor, overdue babies have more trouble tolerating labor due to umbilical cord compression; the heart rate may go down during labor, possibly resulting in a cesarean section.

- A post-term baby is more likely to inhale meconium (intestinal material), which can get stuck in baby's breathing passages, leading to temporary breathing problems after birth.

- Blood sugar instabilities are higher in post-term babies.

Your doctor or midwife will monitor your baby's amniotic fluid level twice a week to be sure it's not decreasing too much. Usually between forty-one and forty-two weeks your doctor or midwife will begin the extra monitoring of the pregnancy and, if your baby is not born by forty-two weeks, then an induction may be scheduled.

(continued)

Induce your labor? Because the risk of the above complications goes up after baby is truly "overdue," your healthcare provider is likely to intervene. For the health of your baby, she may not want to take any chances, even though it's uncommon (less than 1 percent) for babies to reach forty-three weeks, the time at which the risk of complications greatly increases. Babies who have gone beyond forty-two weeks may not tolerate labor as well, mostly because the placenta is aging and cannot provide the same reserve during labor. Labor requires both the ripening (softening) of the cervix and having regular, coordinated contractions of the uterus. So, if warranted, your healthcare provider could induce labor in these ways:

- By applying a prostaglandin gel (misoprostol) to your cervix to ripen it and stimulate labor.

- By placing an inflated Foley bulb in the cervix overnight to promote gentle softening and effacing of the cervix.

- By artificially rupturing your membranes if baby has descended low enough to make this a safe procedure.

- By "sweeping" your membranes: During a vaginal exam, your healthcare provider inserts a finger into your cervix to stretch it a bit, and then makes circular "sweeping" movements to separate the membranes from the cervix. This may stimulate the labor-starting hormones, prostaglandins.

- By inducing labor with Pitocin. This has to be done very carefully if baby hasn't yet descended enough.

- By suggesting "do-it-yourself" options, such as sexual intercourse and nipple stimulation, to get labor started.

Of course, walking around upright is the safest and most sensible way to prompt baby to descend a bit, and may just be the labor prompt you need. Take long walks around the block or go out into the countryside to enjoy nature.

FROM LABOR TO BIRTH

Thirteen Ways to Help Your Labor Progress

You've spent the last nine months growing a baby and quite a few weeks learning about the art and science of giving birth. Now comes the event you've been waiting — and training — for.

You can help your labor progress and avoid what we call the "cycle of discouragement." Imagine this scenario: You've been having contractions for a while at home, you've been admitted (meaning you *are* in labor), and after a few hours your birth attendant checks you again and announces, "Nothing's really happening." You become discouraged and anxious, making your progress slow even more, and you face a long, drawn-out labor. For some women, slow, steady progress is their healthy norm, but there are ways for nearly all women to get their bodies working more efficiently — and less painfully.

1. Be informed. During your childbirth classes you've been learning a lot about the anatomy and physiology of labor, especially about how the uterus contracts, the cervix gradually dilates, and your baby turns and bends as he navigates the winding road of your pelvic passages. You've come to understand the importance of relaxation, the labor-stalling effects of fear, how your birth hormones work, and what you can do to help them work better.

Review all you have about the wise use of technology and medications:

- A well-timed epidural, as discussed on page 313, can help an exhausted mother rest and get a second wind, possibly accelerating labor in the long run.

- On the other hand, the wrong medication or the right one given at the wrong time can interfere with the progress of labor (see page 308).

- Using technology that requires you to stay in bed will slow down labor. If you need an IV, request a heparin/saline lock, which will allow you to be mobile rather than tethered to a bedside IV pole. If you need electronic fetal monitoring, ask to have it done intermittently.

- If for medical reasons you need continuous electronic fetal monitoring, request telemetry (a wireless method), which keeps you mobile.

Dr. Linda notes: If you plan to use a labor tub, inquire about a waterproof monitor.

2. Be rested. The harder a job is, the more breaks you need to take. Fortunately, labor provides two breaks: the first is during early labor, when contractions are typically not so difficult to deal with; the second is between each contraction. Except during transition, when labor is at its most intense, there is always time to take a rest between the end of one contraction and the beginning of the next. (During transition, some women have back-to-back contractions.)

A common mistake first-time laborers make is not resting during early labor. You may reason, "These contractions aren't so bad. I can handle them. Now is the time to vacuum or address birth announcements before the real work starts." Wrong! The real work will be much more difficult to manage if you are not rested physically and mentally. While you are still laboring at home, retreat into a quiet place. Turn off your cell phone and go to sleep, or at least get some rest. Do not dwell on your to-do list.

Remember to rest between contractions, even early in labor, when these breaks last five minutes or more. Use the relaxation techniques you have rehearsed. We have seen veteran mothers use their relaxation techniques so effectively that they are able to momentarily zone out, even during active labor. Don't spend your time between contractions worrying about what the next one will feel like; remember, you handled this one, you can handle the next! Between contractions think R-R-R: rest, relax, rejoice.

3. Be nourished. A hardworking uterus needs a lot of energy from food and hydration from fluids. Doctors used to discourage eating or drinking during labor in case the mother needed a general anesthetic for a cesarean delivery, relying instead on intravenous fluids to hydrate and provide energy. Since most mothers who need a surgical birth can now use an epidural or spinal anesthetic, keeping the stomach empty during labor is not as important as it once was. General anesthesia, which might still be needed for emergency delivery, can cause you to vomit while you are unconscious and then inhale your stomach contents into your lungs. For this reason, laboring women should ingest only small amounts of quickly digestible foods. Eating heavily is likely to make you uncomfortable and nauseated. Here's how to stay well nourished during labor:

Eat early. Eat early in labor to store energy; when labor gets more intense, your stomach may not cooperate.

Eat often. As you learned early in your pregnancy, grazing is much friendlier to squeamish tummies than eating big meals.

Eat foods that are stomach-friendly. Some mothers experience nausea during labor and find it difficult to eat and drink. Nevertheless, you need to eat. Bring along food and drinks that were easy on your stomach during the early, nauseous months of your pregnancy. The foods you tolerated then are the ones you are most likely to be able to tolerate now. Avoid fatty and fried foods, gassy foods, and carbonated beverages — if you are nauseated, flat ginger ale helps.

Drink to your body's content. Avoid becoming dehydrated, which depletes your energy, upsets your body's physiology, and slows your labor. Hydrate yourself with at least 8 ounces of water per hour in early labor, and sip between contractions. Be sure

to bring to the hospital at least two water bottles filled with your favorite healthy fluids to have in addition to water, such as juices or smoothies. Consider bringing an electrolyte solution such as coconut water, as muscles need salts as well as water. Many mothers get so involved in their labor that they neglect to quench their bodies' thirst. One of the jobs of the birth partner is Chief Water-Bottle Pusher.

LOVE YOUR LABORADE

Take along your previously tummy-tested smoothie to your birth place. Labor day is not the time to experiment with some new potion. (See our recipe on page 24.)

Intravenous feedings. If you are too nauseated to eat or drink, and your practitioner feels that you are becoming dehydrated, she may recommend giving you intravenous fluids. This can perk up a stalled labor or an exhausted mom. An additional benefit: more fluids means more trips to the bathroom, which, because of the walking and squatting, are themselves labor stimulators.

4. Be quiet. Design a peaceful birthing environment for yourself. Birth attendants (husband, friend, nurses) need to respect your privacy during contractions so you can concentrate on your work, and between contractions so you can rest. This is where your mate comes in. Give him the job of peacekeeper, pledged to banish chattering, noisy, or interfering people from your labor room and to protect the privacy and dignity of this event. Keeping the lights dimmed can set the mood for peace, along with quiet, relaxing music.

Dr. BJ notes: Be wary of calling friends and family as your birth time begins — it will make it difficult for you and your partner to maintain a peaceful environment. Everyone will want to get frequent updates or to come to visit. I recommend that you identify one person as your main contact. Once you are well into labor (6 centimeters or so), let your go-to person know, and she can keep everyone updated on your progress. That way you and your partner can avoid unnecessary distractions and focus on the task at hand.

5. Be funny. Laughter is good for labor. It increases the level of endorphins and decreases stress hormones. Try watching a funny movie on the TV in your room or on your computer, particularly one that you already know you love. Some mothers listen to books on tape in early labor, choosing their favorite authors. Keep your mood light. Try joking around with the nurses and other workers. When the time comes to get serious, your light mood will have kept you relaxed and more able to go where your body takes you next.

6. Be romantic. Love makes the world go 'round, and it helps babies come out, too. The same hormones released during lovemaking also enhance labor. Nipple stimulation, by the mother herself, by her mate, or by water splashing on her nipples during a soak in the tub, releases the contraction-intensifying hormone oxytocin. Kisses, a caressing cuddle, a sensual massage can all get your birthing hormones working for you. These hormones also counteract anxiety, which, as we have said, can cause your labor to slow rather than progress.

For me, giving birth is the ultimate expression of my sexuality and my femininity. So, the setting was very important for me. I wanted soft music, dim lights, and a private atmosphere. The right environment for birth is similar to the environment you would want for lovemaking.

7. Be positive. A negative birth environment is no help to a laboring mother. Banish negative people from the birth room. You don't want to hear someone else's war stories, comments about how they couldn't progress, or their labor-strategy comparisons in which you are the clear loser. Invite only positive people to your birth. If the number of people with you becomes a problem as labor intensifies, their presence will become a negative. Let them know ahead of time that at some point you will want to have only your mate and your labor coach with you. Your mate and your coach need to be aware of how the mood in the room can affect you, so they can make adjustments. And, you certainly need them to stay positive, too. (See whom to invite to your birth, page 331.)

8. Be comfortable. Pamper yourself with as many labor-enhancing amenities as you can think of (and that will fit in your bags). Bring along your favorite music. Bring some kneepads in case being on your hands and knees turns out to be your most comfortable position. Take a shower, soak in the tub, nibble on healthy delicacies, keep your masseur busy, prop yourself up with pillows — do whatever you need for your peace and comfort. If for medical reasons you will need to spend a lot of time in bed, bring a foam-rubber pad contoured like an egg carton. (Check ahead of time to see whether your hospital provides one; if not, purchase one in the bedding department of a discount or department store.) These pads soothe the skin and muscles.

9. Be equipped. The more labor tools you bring to your birth, the better progress you are likely to make. If your hospital lags behind in labor-assisting devices, bring your own. Along with a professional labor coach (see "Choosing a Professional Labor Coach," page 260), bring your MP3 player or your own collection of index cards with encouraging quotes to relax and empower you. If you like this idea, collect memorable lines from birth books, verses from poems or scriptures, or humorous limericks. You may want to read these yourself or let your birth partner read them to you. Hearing a poem read by your lover may be just what you need to help you relax between contractions. Hearing a strengthening scripture passage can renew your focus. For other labor aids, see page 355.

I sang psalms during my contractions. Really helped!

10. Be vocal. Reserve your etiquette for dinner parties; you needn't be embarrassed about the sounds you make in labor. After all, you are not laboring in a library or church! When asked how a laboring woman should act, veteran birth attendants — especially those who have birthed babies themselves — respond, "Any way she wants." Many women find power and comfort in letting go with a yell, prolonged moan, or gutsy grunt when the going gets tough. These (sometimes involuntary) sounds vocalize your release of tension and are a powerful way to muster up inner energy to get through a really tough contraction. They are similar to the sounds athletes make during particularly grueling events or those that require tremendous concentration. Some sounds hinder labor. Low-pitched, long groans (called "sounding") are releasing and energizing. High-pitched, sharp, sudden screams are body tensing and frightening (to you and to the woman laboring in the next room). Be sure to let your husband know that you are likely to let loose with strange sounds; otherwise, he may misinterpret these scary noises as a sign that you are losing control and will want to do something to quiet you down, or he may worry that something is wrong.

I'm a trained singer, and I found singing sounds to be a great release during labor. I bundled up the pain of the contraction and let it go in the sounds I made.

11. Be mobile. Included in every laboring mother's Bill of Rights are the freedom to move about during labor and the freedom to improvise whatever birthing positions work best for her. In order to take advantage of your body's natural ability to guide you to the best positions for labor and birth, however, you may have to first go through a bit of cultural deprogramming. Scratch from your memory the on-your-back scenes from the movies. Studies show that women who are not culturally locked into the horizontal birthing mindset tend to assume any of eight different positions during the course of their labor, and most of these are upright, semi-upright, and moving. (Read more about the best positions for birth on page 353.) Walking is especially helpful in labor, both to ease discomfort and to speed progress.

My otherwise wonderful nurses were stuck in recommending the old back and stirrups position.

12. Be upright. Research has shown that laboring upright increases uterine efficiency, shortens labor, and opens the cervix better. It also widens the pelvic passage, giving baby an easier way out. When you are upright, your pelvic joints, relaxed by the hormones of pregnancy, are better able to shift and accommodate a baby with a large head and broad shoulders. Being upright also allows a more natural stretching of the birth-canal tissues, making tears less likely.

Upright laboring does not mean that you are standing, leaning, walking, or squatting nonstop. Here are the two top position-changing guidelines for helping your labor progress:

- Labor upright *during* contractions
- Lean or recline and rest *between* contractions

With my first son I dilated to 10 centimeters, but because of intervention too soon, my son was never given the chance to descend into the birth canal, and therefore I never developed the urge to push. I ended up with

a C-section. When I became pregnant with my second, my husband and I made plans to do things differently. I was determined to push my own baby out. For the entire nine months of pregnancy I visualized my baby descending and pushing him out. My mantra from early on was, "Down and crown." I visualized the physical feeling, the emotional feeling, and how I would deal with it all. When the time came, my labor progressed beautifully. During labor I repeated my mantra, "Down and crown." It progressed exactly as I visualized, except for the fact that it went so much faster than I anticipated. Before I knew it, my midwife told my husband it was time to move me to the birthing pool. I assumed the position that I visualized giving birth in. After about an hour, I had my moment of victory. The baby crowned and the head slipped out! My two pieces of advice are to have a supportive and encouraging doula and attendant, and to visualize the birth, both the physical process and the emotional process, and how you are going to handle it.

13. Be wet. Birthing tubs should be a birthright. Most laboring mothers have an innate desire to get into water. (See why on page 302.)

HOW FAR ALONG AM I?

It helps to understand the terminology that your birth attendants use and how this translates into what's happening in your body. Your birthcare providers will gauge your progress by three measurements: effacement, dilation, and descent.

Effacement (or "being effaced") is a measurement of how much your cervix has thinned as it changes from a thick-walled cone to a thin, wide cup under baby's head. During an internal exam your birthcare provider measures how effaced you are.

(continued)

- 0 percent effaced: your cervix has not yet started thinning.

- 50 percent effaced: your cervix is halfway there.

- 100 percent effaced: your cervix is totally thinned out and ready for the opening to fully expand (dilate) so you can start pushing.

The cervix of a first-time mother may need to be completely effaced before it begins dilating. With subsequent pregnancies, effacement and dilation can occur together. During an internal exam close to your due date, you may hear your healthcare provider announce that your cervix is "ripe," which means that it is soft enough to begin effacing and dilating.

Dilation refers to how far open, or dilated, your cervix is. During an internal exam, your birthcare provider inserts her first and second fingers into your vagina to estimate your degree of dilation in centimeters. In the prelabor stage or very early in labor, you may be 1 or 2 centimeters dilated; as labor intensifies, you will dilate from 3 to 9 centimeters, and during transition you gain the last 1 or 2 centimeters. When your birth attendant gives you the good news that you are 10 centimeters dilated, your cervix is completely open. Obstetrically speaking, being "in labor" means your cervix is progressively dilating.

Descent describes how far down baby's presenting part (usually the head) is in the pelvis. During an internal exam, your birth attendant will determine to what "station" baby has descended. Station zero is the middle of the pelvis. Each centimeter above or below station zero marks another station. The highest station is "floating," meaning that the baby's head is above the pelvic inlet and not yet engaged. If your attendant announces, "Your baby is at minus four," that means that he is floating four centimeters above station zero. If your birthcare provider announces, "Your baby is at plus four," your baby's head has descended all the way through the pelvis and your attendant can get a glimpse of it.

Besides effacement, dilation, and descent, another factor in labor progress is baby's changing position. Baby not only has to come down the birth canal; his body has to turn to navigate the path of least resistance through the pelvis. Sometimes during labor the degree of dilation and descent stays the same for an hour (or more) while your baby and your body work to change baby's position, affording him an easier way out. Although this change won't be charted on your dilation and descent notes, it is progress all the same.

Don't be discouraged if your birth attendant announces, "You're still 4 centimeters." Obstetricians generally regard "normal" progress in active labor as a rate of 1-centimeter dilation per hour and 1-centimeter descent per hour (1.5 for subsequent pregnancies), but these are only rough rules of thumb. They may not necessarily be the rules followed by your uterus. A labor that progresses more slowly than usual is not necessarily abnormal. Recent research shows that a dilation rate of 1 centimeter every four hours can be considered a normal pattern. Not every birth goes by the book.

Working Out Your Best Birthing Positions

I realized that if I was lying in bed when my obstetrician came to visit, she perceived me as a patient. But when she saw me walking around my room, strolling in the halls, or laboring in the arms of my husband, she perceived that I was managing nicely, and there was no need to intervene. Lying in bed, I was clearly a target for intervention. I guess being in bed made me seem dependent and sick, and the doctor felt obliged to do something.

Just as there is no single right position for making love, there is no one "best" position for pushing out a baby. It is important to know what positions to try and to have the freedom to experiment. Midwives are very comfortable with birthing in different positions and will suggest them during pushing and birth. Try these labor-tested favorites:

You should have seen the look on my obstetrician's face when I asked her to kneel and catch the baby from below while I pushed in the squatting position with my husband supporting me from behind. But it worked great, and the next time someone asks, I bet she'll be ready — with kneepads!

Squatting. Squatting benefits mother and baby. It widens the pelvic opening, relieves back pain, speeds the progress of labor, relaxes perineal muscles so that they are less likely to tear, improves oxygen supply to the baby, and even facilitates delivery of the placenta. If you have practiced squatting during pregnancy, it will be easier during labor. You can be supported in your squatting if you need help with balance. Squatting makes contractions more intense because it positions baby's head to put pressure against the cervix — that's why squatting accelerates your progress. If you find it makes your contractions overwhelming, you can modify your squats.

Here are some tips for squatting:

- Unless it helps your earlier labor progress, reserve squatting for the second stage of labor, when your cervix is fully dilated and you can start pushing. Squatting is seldom necessary during the first stage of labor unless it is a comfortable position for you to manage your contractions. It's better to avoid tiring your legs until your contractions really get serious, and best reserved for the pushing stage.

- The urge to push is your signal to squat. When a contraction begins, get or be helped into a squatting position. If you are in bed, ask for a squat bar, which attaches to the bed, or use someone's neck for support (see the illustrations on pages 356–57).

- To avoid tiring and losing your balance, place your feet at least shoulder-width apart and squat gradually. Don't bounce, as this strains your knees.

- As you squat, release your abdominal muscles so that you look as though you are eleven months pregnant. Tensing your abdominal muscles is likely to increase your pain.

- The "dangling squat" (see the illustration on page 356) is a natural releasing position, reminding your body to let go, release the tension, and birth the baby. Positioning your body this way will also send your mind messages to surrender.

Kneeling. Kneeling is helpful in easing overwhelming contractions, relieving back pain, or turning a posterior baby. It also helps you improvise: try lowering onto your heels into a kneel-squat, or getting on all fours.

Sitting. Sitting upright with your legs spread widens the pelvis, but not as much as squatting does. One of the most labor-efficient positions is sit-squatting on a low stool. Alternatives are to sit astride a toilet seat, a chair, or a birth ball. If you must stay in bed because you've had pain medication, sit astride the corner of the bed.

Standing and leaning. Since your labor is likely to progress more quickly and efficiently if you walk a lot, you may find yourself upright during an intense contraction. Stop where you are and lean against the wall or your birth partner, or rest your head against pillows on a counter or high table as an alternative to going into a squat.

Side-lying. Even though being upright helps your labor progress, it is not practical or even possible to be upright during your whole labor. Your hardworking body will need some rest, and if you don't get it, it may stop doing its job so well. Side-lying is a better alternative to lying on your back. It's best to lie on your left side as shown in the illustration on page 85. Be sure to place one or two pillows between your legs to help keep the pelvis open.

How often and how much you remain on your side depends upon your labor. If you want to ease a hard and fast labor, use the side-lying position, especially during a strong contraction. If you want to speed up a dragging labor or increase the efficiency of contractions, kneel or squat during the contractions and then return to side-lying between them.

Some mothers feel so comfortable lying on their side that they deliver their babies in this position. If you wish to use this position, one of your birth attendants will need to hold up your top leg to widen your pelvis.

HAVE A BALL!

One of our top picks for laborsaving devices is the birth ball. In our living room sits a 28-inch "physioball" (available in birthing supply catalogs and sporting goods stores) that our grandchildren play on. Each time a pregnant woman visits our home, she gravitates toward it. "My, how relaxing to just perch on this ball" is a common response. One friend asked to borrow it for labor. She spent more time sitting on this ball than in her bed during labor. This makes sense because sitting on the ball naturally relaxes the pelvic muscles.

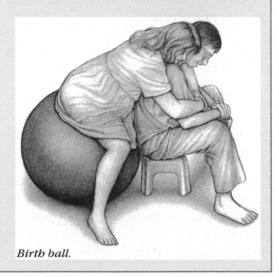

Birth ball.

Be sure to rehearse these positions during your childbirth classes and at home. Remember to think "upright" during contractions and "rest" between them. In labor, keep experimenting until you find the positions that help you manage your discomfort and help your labor progress.

Now that you are empowered with self-help labor-progressing tools and information, here is a description of the usual stages of labor most women experience.

Stages of Labor and Birth

During your ninth month your eagerness for Birth-Day can make you think that every twinge in your uterus is "it." It usually isn't "it," and days or weeks will likely pass before you'll be able to meet your baby. Some mothers start their labor with a bang — suddenly, unquestionably,

powerfully — and progress fast. Others ease into labor slowly, sometimes unconvincingly. Some tired moms will have a labor that starts, stops, goes in spurts and pauses, and drags on for days. It's easy to be confused by all the terms: "prelabor," "false labor," "early labor," "real labor," "active labor"; the list goes on. While every mother's labor and delivery are as individual as her pregnancy, there are typical stages most women go through as "it" approaches.

Prelabor: What You May Experience

Consider most of your final month of pregnancy as prelabor. When your birth hormones relax your pelvic ligaments, they cause your vaginal tissues to become more stretchable, and soften your cervix to get it "ripe" and ready to dilate. Many things

---

BEST LABORSAVING IDEAS AND DEVICES

Gathered from our own twelve births and the thousands we have attended, here are our top picks for a less painful and more efficient labor. You may wish to bring along this checklist to remind yourself and your birth attendants:

☐ Choose the right coach (see page 260).

☐ Hydrate yourself (see page 348).

☐ Nourish yourself (see page 347).

☐ Rest between contractions (see page 373).

☐ Ask for quiet between contractions (see page 348).

☐ Laugh (see page 349).

☐ Listen to music (see page 77).

☐ Move more, sit less (see page 350).

☐ Labor upright (see page 351).

☐ Enjoy a birth ball (see page 354).

☐ Ask for a massage or touch counterpressure (see page 304).

☐ Try tennis balls or a paint roller for back pain (see page 304).

☐ Apply hot and cold packs (see page 223).

☐ Breathe (see page 305).

☐ Enjoy water labor (see page 301).

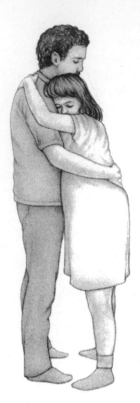
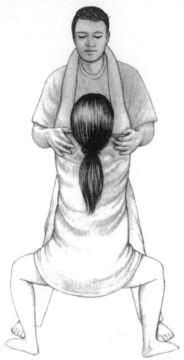
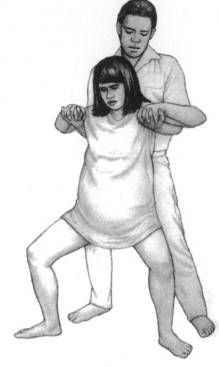

"Slow dancing."　　　　*Dangling squat.*　　　　*Supported squat.*

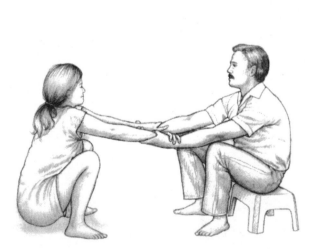
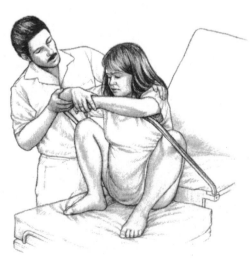

Supported squat.　　　　*Using a squat bar.*

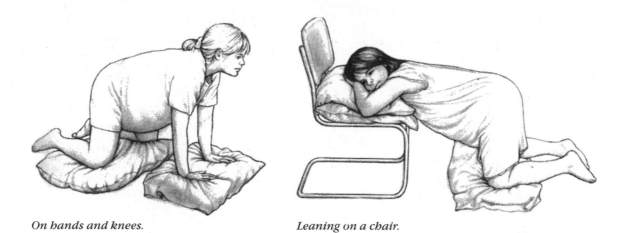

On hands and knees.

Leaning on a chair.

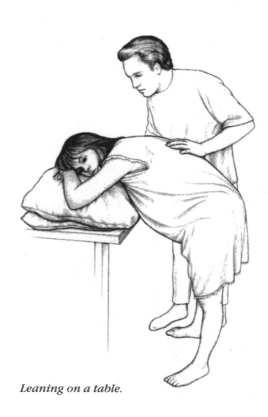

Leaning on a table.

happen to get your body ready to give birth. Here are clues that labor is near:

Feel baby dropping. Toward the end of the eighth month or early in the ninth month (for a first-time pregnancy), baby settles downward into your pelvis. Many second-time mothers find that their babies don't drop until a week or less before labor begins.

Frequent urination. Now that baby's head lies closer to your bladder, you may be going to the bathroom a lot more often.

Low backache. As baby gets heavier and drops, count on some aches or pains in your lower back and pelvis as your uterine and pelvic ligaments stretch even more.

Stronger Braxton Hicks contractions. You may notice that your warm-up contractions become painful rather than just uncomfortable, like menstrual cramps. Even though these prelabor contractions are not as strong as labor contractions, they are strong enough to be starting the work of effacing your cervix from a thick-walled cone to a thin-walled cup. These contractions, which get even stronger just prior to labor, can continue, on and off, for a week or two before labor starts. They become less intense when you change position or start walking. Remember to practice your relaxation techniques. (Read about the differences between prelabor and labor contractions on page 359.)

I felt as though I had a belt inside my abdomen that suddenly tightened and released and then tightened again. This went on for two weeks before my "real" contractions began.

Diarrhea. Birth hormones acting on your intestines may cause abdominal cramps and loose, frequent bowel movements — nature's enema, emptying your intestines to make more room for baby's passage. Those same hormones can also make you feel nauseated.

Increased vaginal discharge. You may notice more egg-white or pink-tinged vaginal discharge. This differs from the "bloody show" described below.

"Bloody show." The combination of baby's head descending into the pelvic cavity and the prelabor contractions thinning the cervix can "uncork" the mucus plug that seals the cervix. The consistency of this mucus varies from stringy to thick and gooey. Some women notice the one-time passing of an obvious mucus plug; others simply notice increased blood-tinged vaginal discharge. Some of the tiny blood vessels in your cervix break as your cervix thins, so you may see anything from a pink-tinged to a brownish-red-tinged teaspoon of bloody mucus. If your discharge shows more blood than mucus — like a menstrual period — or a lot of bright red blood, report this to your practitioner immediately.

Once you notice a "bloody show," you are likely to begin labor within three days, although some mothers hang on for another week or two.

Water breaks. Only one in ten mothers experiences her bag of waters breaking prior to labor. For most mothers this doesn't happen until they are well into labor. If your water breaks before labor has started, plan on your labor starting more intensely within the next few minutes or hours, or at least within the next twenty-four hours. Labors are usually less intense if the water breaks later in labor. Be sure you have discussed with your doctor or midwife what to do if your water breaks. She may recommend inducing labor, especially if you have tested positive for beta strep (see page 412). There are pros and cons to simply awaiting labor or inducing labor, but your caregiver will probably want to be notified of leaking fluid.

The signs listed above tell you that labor is coming, but not necessarily when. Some women experience some or all of the signs within a few days of giving birth; others notice them a week or two before. When these cues occur, and to what degree, varies from woman to woman. Many women are not aware of these changes as they happen. If you experience several of these signs, it's best to get some rest, because chances are great that you will be giving birth within a few days.

Labor Begins: How to Tell

You're officially in *active labor* when your cervix is 5 centimeters dilated. (See page 360 for a description of the phases.) Some women can stay just shy of this stage of dilation for days or a week or two before they experience consistently regular, hard contractions. Your labor has begun when your contractions become regular and increasingly intense. When this happens you are likely to see your baby within a day.

We find it helpful to divide contractions into prelabor contractions, which prepare the passage for baby, and labor contractions, which deliver the baby. Many women, especially first-timers, can't pinpoint the exact moment that labor contractions begin. After the fact, of course, mothers can look

back and say, "Oh, yes, that was when they started." Here's how to tell the difference.

Prelabor contractions (also known as "false" contractions):

- Are irregular, following no discernible pattern for more than a few hours.

- Are nonprogressive; they don't become stronger, longer, or more frequent.

- Are felt most in front, in the lower abdomen.

- Vary from painless to moderately uncomfortable; they feel more like pressure than like pain.

- Become less intense and less uncomfortable if you change position or walk, lie down, or take a hot bath or shower.

- Make your uterus feel like a hard ball.

Labor contractions (also known as "real" or "true" contractions):

- Follow a regular pattern (though timing is seldom precise to the minute).

- Are progressive; they become stronger, longer, and more frequent, with shorter intervals between them.

- Are felt in the lower abdomen and also radiate around to the lower back.

- Vary from uncomfortable pressure to a grabbing, pulling, cramping pain that can usually be managed, even lessened, by a conscious release of tension in your body.

- Don't change if you lie down or change position; walking may even make them more intense.

- Are usually accompanied by a "bloody show" (see page 358).

- Make your uterus become rock hard; you have to stop everything you are doing to focus on getting through each contraction.

Unless you are experiencing danger signs (see page 364), there's no need to call your healthcare provider unless it's during regular office hours and your curiosity just won't let you wait. Your practitioner can do an internal exam to tell whether you are in prelabor or early labor. If your cervix is softening, thinning, effacing, and possibly dilating, you will feel encouraged.

Once you (and perhaps your healthcare provider) have determined that this is the real thing, it's time to look for the signs of each phase of labor. Everyone's labor is different; nevertheless, labors have certain stages and phases in common.

First stage of labor

- Early or latent phase: 1 to 4 centimeters dilated

- Active phase: 5 to 8 centimeters dilated

- Transition phase: 9 to 10 centimeters dilated

Second stage of labor

- Resting and pushing phase

- Crowning and delivery phase

Third stage of labor

- Delivering the placenta

For some women the phases of the first stage are distinct; for others they blend together. Bear in mind, too, that the length and intensity of these phases vary tremendously from woman to woman and from labor to labor in the same mother. The descriptions that follow contain general guidelines; your labor will have its own unique duration, timing, and intensity.

The First Stage of Labor: Early Phase

What you may feel. For most women the early or latent phase of labor is the easiest part; it's also the longest. Some women may not even realize they are in labor or may think they're just experiencing stronger Braxton Hicks contractions. In this early phase, contractions can range from five to thirty minutes apart and last from thirty to forty-five seconds. They are not usually strong enough to prevent you from moving around your home doing business as usual, and most women feel calm and in control. You may feel like chatting, enjoying company, or taking a walk. You may be excited that the time is really here, yet apprehensive about what labor will be like and how you will cope. You may have an attack of the nesting instinct, and you may experience several of the bodily signs discussed in the section on prelabor above (diarrhea, low backache, increased vaginal discharge, menstrual-like cramps, "bloody show," frequent urination). During this phase some mothers may leak amniotic fluid or the membranes may rupture, although this usually does not happen until the next stage, the active phase of labor. The early phase of labor lasts an average of eight hours for first-timers, but it can vary from a few hours to a few days. Some women sleep through this phase if it occurs at night.

What's happening in your body. During early labor your cervix thins out, becoming nearly completely effaced. It also dilates, reaching 4 to 5 centimeters by the end of early labor.

What you can do. Your body can play tricks on you in this phase of labor. You may feel euphoric and chatty, or get a sudden burst of energy and want to keep busy. You may not feel the desire to retreat into a quiet place and rest yet, but you *must*. Many first-timers waste so much energy during this early phase of labor that they are tired by the time the harder work begins. Although you need to rest, mental excitement and mild bodily discomfort can make you restless. Ask your husband for a relaxing back rub, take a warm bath or shower, read, or watch television. Try to sleep, especially if it's nighttime. Do whatever you can to conserve your energy for the work to come: put your relaxation strategies to good use. If you simply cannot stay still, take a leisurely walk. The upright position and gentle movement will allow gravity to help baby descend into your pelvis and will keep your contractions progressing.

Be careful not to go into fear mode. This can happen if you had a difficult labor previously or if you distrust your body. Fear can cause you to resist your labor mentally and physically. If you feel yourself becoming anxious, try to talk it out with someone who can help you manage, for example, your labor support person or an experienced friend.

It is important to assess where your thoughts are taking you. Anxiety and fear are about what might happen next or has happened in the past. If your mind stays in the past or in the future, you can't focus on what your body needs *now*. Though these early contractions may not hurt, try those natural pain-relief techniques you've been practicing, deep breathing and relaxing.

As your contractions get stronger, use these techniques and experiment with different positions. Try resting in the side-lying position between contractions. If a backache becomes more intense, try spending some of your resting moments in the all-fours position. As latent labor becomes active and intense, you may find yourself spending part of your contraction time leaning against someone or something for support.

Most women spend this early phase of labor in the comfort of their homes. (Some hospitals have a policy that states you must be in active labor to be admitted to labor and delivery.) Be sure to eat frequently to store up energy. Keep your bladder empty, as this helps your labor progress. Above all, keep your mind and body relaxed so you can stay peaceful and conserve your energy.

Your mind or your body will tell you when you are nearing the end of the latent phase; your contractions will increase in frequency (to around five minutes apart) and intensity. One common sign of the onset of active labor is that you come down from your euphoria and become introspective, wanting to tune out what's going on around you and retreat into a quiet place. This emotional change is often a clue that it's time to contact your healthcare provider.

Tips for dad during the early phase.
Encourage your wife to sleep if it's nighttime
and to rest if it's daytime. (If she agrees, you
should do the same! After all, you have a
busy day ahead of you, too.) Offer massages
and back rubs and whatever physical and
emotional support you think she'd like. Ask
her what she needs. Remind her to eat and
drink.

This can be a scary time for you. You may
have a preconceived notion about "dangerous"
labors in which women scream in pain and
men pace about frantically outside the
delivery room. This may have conditioned
your mind to click into fear mode. You may be
flooded with irrational thoughts — for
example, you are suddenly afraid that your
lovemaking nine months ago has put your
beloved in danger. You may begin to feel
responsible for her increasing discomfort and
powerless to alleviate her distress. Other
in-the-future fears can crop up: worries about
what life will be like after the baby comes,
whether your wife will ever enjoy romantic
evenings again, whether you can make
enough money to meet the medical and
educational needs of your new child, whether
you'll be a good father, and on and on.

If you are one of the many men who don't
do well with hospitals, pain management, or
blood, the next forty-eight hours may be
difficult for you, despite careful preparation.
Be brave. You can do it. Your love and
concern for your partner will carry you
through. What she needs most is for you
simply to stand by her and share the hours
ahead. Sure, this can be a stressful time, but
you will be so thrilled and proud when you
hold your new baby that you will forget the
fear and worry. This little person and his
mom will be dependent on your steady, calm,
supportive presence in the days, weeks, and
months to come. Your life will be enriched
beyond measure by the most important gift
your wife will ever give you — your child.

The First Stage of Labor: Active Phase

What you may feel. As a general guide,
once your contractions are intense enough to
stop you in mid-sentence — you can't casually
talk through them — you are in active labor.
During the early phase of labor you may have
been lulled into thinking, "These aren't so
bad. I can handle this." Now, as your
contractions come on harder and faster, last
longer, and demand your total attention, you
may change your tune: "Wow! This is tough!"
Typically, contractions in the active phase
occur every three to five minutes and last
forty-five to sixty seconds. You may be
walking along and find that a contraction
stops you in your tracks, all but taking your
breath away. You can no longer manage by
distraction only; you need to call on your
previously rehearsed relaxation and pain-
relieving techniques. Remember, you must
take your contractions one at a time and rest
completely, mentally and physically, in
between each. Try not to worry about the
next contraction. In fact, don't even think
that far ahead, let alone worry.

Women often describe active labor
contractions as waves starting at the top of
the uterus and going to the bottom, or from
the back radiating around to the front. These
waves reach peak intensity midway through
a contraction, then gradually ease off. In
active labor your whole body seems to be
engaged in the contractions. You may feel
intense pulling and stretching right above
your pubic bone, along with a deep backache

or pelvic pressure. This is the phase of labor when your membranes are most likely to rupture and produce a gush of fluid. (For more about when your water breaks, see page 359.) Waterproof your mattress!

You may find your emotions changing even before your body tells you that you are in active labor. Just prior to or at the onset of active labor, many mothers instinctively seek out a more peaceful environment. Husbands and other caretakers should recognize this signal and adjust their routines accordingly.

This active phase of the first stage of labor lasts an average of four hours, but your uterus has its own timetable. Many women experience active labor in bursts and pauses; labor is intense for a while, a lull follows, and then contractions intensify again.

I woke up soaked. I thought I had peed in my sleep. So I got up, changed my bed and had a shower. After the shower I could still feel liquid running down my leg. I then thought to myself, "OMG, my water broke!" I started packing to go to the hospital.

What's happening in your body. During this active phase, your cervix completely effaces, and you dilate from 4 to 8 centimeters. Baby's head descends lower into your pelvis, which often breaks the membranes and releases the amniotic fluid with a gush. Your brain responds to your increased discomfort by releasing endorphins. Try to avoid the fear-tension-pain cycle. Now is when you want your labor hormones working for you, not your "fight or flight" stress hormones. You may notice that you begin to shiver but are not cold; in fact you are usually hot during this time. Shivering, a sign that you are in active labor, is how all of the other muscles that are

supporting your labor reenergize and keep from cramping up. A warm bath or shower helps reenergize the muscles.

What you can do. Employ your relaxation and pain-relieving techniques (see page 300). Early in the active phase of labor is the time when many women opt for medical pain relief (read more about having a balanced mindset about pain relief on page 293). Remember these important keys to easing the discomfort and enhancing the progress of labor:

- Rest between contractions to recharge your body.

- Relax and release during a contraction. Take a deep breath as it begins. Breathe slowly and rhythmically in through your nose and out through your mouth. Once it's over, take another deep breath to let go of any tension that may have built up.

- Change positions frequently. Improvise; do whatever works for you.

- Drink a glass of water every hour.

- Empty your bladder every hour.

- Consider immersing yourself in water.

During this phase there may be periods when your mind seems to escape to another world. You may feel this zoning-out sensation during or between contractions. Don't be afraid. Your body is doing just the right thing to help you handle your pain.

Tips for dads during the active phase. It's important for everyone on the labor scene to respect the mother's desire for calm by

WHEN TO GO TO THE HOSPITAL OR BIRTH CENTER

You may picture yourself rushing frantically to the hospital or birth center, only to deliver your baby in the backseat. Maybe you worry that your mate-turned-midwife will have to do an emergency bedroom delivery because you waited too long. Despite what you see in the movies, this rarely happens. With a little coaching from their birth attendant, most mothers-to-be time their hospital or birth center arrival just fine. During one of your last prenatal visits or an earlier phone call to your healthcare provider, you will receive instructions on when to go to the hospital. (If you have a specific obstetrical problem and are told to go early, do it.) Here are some general guidelines:

- A rule of thumb that works for most first-time mothers is to go to the hospital when you reach 4-1-1: contractions 4 minutes apart, lasting 1 minute each, and occurring consistently for 1 hour or more.

- Leave for the hospital if contractions are strong enough to stop you in your tracks, prevent you from speaking, or require you to muster up serious comfort techniques.

- Follow your inner voice. If it says, "It's time to go *now*," go.

Unless your practitioner instructs you otherwise, be sure your labor is well established before going to the hospital. Try to labor in the comfort of your own home for as long as possible. Arriving too early into the strange environment of the hospital can cause your labor to stall.

Don't worry about what the birth attendants at the hospital or birth center will think if your arrival is a false alarm. They are used to this. They won't patronize you, snicker, or embarrass you with questions like, "What are you doing here so soon?"(If someone says that, ignore it!) If this is your first baby, you are not expected to know what labor is like, nor can you check your own cervix to determine how far along you are. If this is not your first time, you have every reason to believe that labor will happen faster.

Get some notes on "when to call" from your caregiver. Typical instructions would include:

- Regular, painful contractions lasting more than an hour. This may be modified based on whether you have already been dilated, have had fast labors in the past, or live very close or very far from the delivery site.

- Bag of waters breaking. Usually labor will start on its own if you are not already in labor; but if there are concerns about strep or the baby's position (the cord is vulnerable to prolapse if the head isn't against the cervix), your doctor or midwife may want you at the hospital.

If you experience the following, call immediately:

- Active vaginal bleeding in the form of clots or bright red bleeding. This can result from normal stretching of the cervix, but it can also indicate a problem with the placenta.

- Sudden onset of severe headache and upper abdominal pain can be a sign of preeclampsia.

addition, baby's head squeezing through the cervix puts tremendous pressure on your rectum and pelvic bones, accounting for the overpowering sensations you feel. Fortunately, your brain also recognizes the intensity of transition and continues to release endorphins.

What you can do. Because transition is so strenuous, you will need to muster all the relaxation and pain-relieving tools you brought to this birth.

- Change positions to find what works: kneeling, sitting, on all fours, side-lying, squatting. Your body will tell you when it's time to shift position.

- Stay off your back.

- Use a labor tub or shower to regain your relax-and-release mode.

- Rest completely between contractions; don't think of the last one or the next one.

- Focus on releasing; visualize your opening cervix as it is pulled up over your baby's head.

- Overcome any urge to push by blowing out air over and over. If you allow yourself to bear down a lot before your cervix is fully dilated, you can cause your cervix to swell, and it will take longer to be pulled up over baby's head. Resisting the urge to push too soon is very hard to do. Let your birth attendant know if you feel an urge to push so that she can check your cervix and give you the green light if it's time.

Dr. BJ notes: Your body may just take over and make it difficult not to bear down.

Listen to your body. When you begin to make the noises that are recognized as "pushing," you will be evaluated to make sure your baby's head has slipped through the cervix. If your cervix is not completely opened, you will be coached to hold off pushing.

Mothers who have chosen not to have an epidural often change their minds and request one during transition. Don't feel disappointed if your birth attendant tells you that it is too late; by the time the epidural is placed and takes effect, transition is likely to be over.

Tips for dads during the transition phase. Remember, there are no rules for how a laboring woman is supposed to act. Transition is not a romantic time; your loving sweetheart may turn on you and her other helpers and become unintentionally hostile. She will probably be unable to tell you how you can help. She will be too preoccupied to think of anything you might do to make things better; she will also be too impatient and exhausted to explain her needs. Don't be hurt if she yells, "Don't do that!" or "Stop that!" Certain touches can be distracting in this phase. If she snaps at you to "get away," back off but stay with her. Reassure her, praise her, and try to keep her breathing on track by just breathing slowly and deeply with her. If you are under the care of a midwife or using a doula or labor support person, this will be the time when you will be glad to lean on her experience. The mom-to-be will need both of you.

When your wife is at her worst, you need to be at your best. Be a tower for her to lean on, an anchor to steady her. You don't have to fix anything — just be there. Love her. She'll appreciate it more than you know, but don't expect her thanks until later.

The Second Stage of Labor: Pushing Baby Out

What you may feel. The two most welcome features of the pushing stage are that it's usually much less difficult than transition, and that it ends with the birth of your baby. Your contractions will now be less intense, less painful, and farther apart, around three to five minutes from the beginning of one to the beginning of the next, and lasting only a minute each.

A blissful rest. Between transition and the beginning of the urge to push, many women get a ten- or twenty-minute lull in their labor called the "time of peace" by childbirth educator Helen Wessel, or the "rest and be thankful" phase by childbirth educator Sheila Kitzinger. If you have this brief break in the action, *rest.* Most women also experience a burst of energy, a sort of second wind for the pushing stage.

The urge to push! Once your cervix is fully dilated, baby's head begins to descend into the birth canal. You will feel an uncontrollable urge to bear down.

This was an irresistible, overpowering feeling, almost like having the most intense bowel movement of my life (but then again, not at all like that). It was the most earthy feeling I've ever experienced, and it felt wonderful compared to transition.

As you push your baby through the birth canal you may feel an alarming sensation of burning as your perineal tissues stretch to accommodate baby's head. Remember, the perineum is designed for this stretching. In minutes the pressure of baby's head against the perineum will numb these sensations. During pushing some women feel as though they're having a bowel movement, and some women, in fact, do. It's nothing to be embarrassed about.

Some lucky moms deliver their baby with a few hard pushes; others labor strenuously for a couple of hours. The average length of the pushing stage is from one to one and a half hours in most first-time moms. (Second-pregnancy pushing usually goes much faster.) As with most of labor, there is wide variation in the length of the pushing stage, and it may be longer than nature intended if an epidural anesthetic lessens your urge and ability to push. This is why many women and their birth attendants decide to turn the epidural down or off during transition, allowing the mother to participate fully in the pushing phase. Depending on the strength of the medication, it may take up to an hour for the drug to wear off completely.

What's happening in your body. Your cervix, fully dilated after transition, allows baby's head (or buttocks, if breech — see page 272) to enter the birth canal. In the previous stage your uterus did all of the work; now it's up to your abdominal and pelvic muscles to help finish the job. As baby's head stretches the vaginal and pelvic-floor muscles, microscopic receptors in these tissues trigger the urge to bear down, called the Ferguson reflex. This reflex also signals your system to release more oxytocin, the hormone that stimulates uterine contractions. These two natural stimulants work together to push baby out. One tells you to push with your whole body, while the other tells your uterus to contract and help push baby down. When you push, your abdominal muscles and diaphragm push against the top of the uterus, helping your powerful uterine muscles move baby steadily down and out.

What you can do. Knowing when and how to push will help you get to hold your baby sooner and with less work. Here are some pushing pointers we have learned from our own births and from veteran mothers.

Use self-regulated pushing. For unmedicated births, or if your medication has worn off sufficiently, you can bear down when your body tells you to, not when someone else yells, "Push!" As soon as you have the overwhelming urge to push, bear down. This urge may come at the beginning of a contraction or well into a contraction. You may feel one long, continuous urge during the contraction or several pushing urges per contraction.

Dr. BJ notes: *Curl around your baby by putting your chin to your chest and focusing the push as if you were doing a crunch, with the pressure on the top of the abdomen. Avoid pushing in your throat!*

Avoid staff-directed pushing. Birthcare providers are like fans cheering a runner at the end of a race, urging the mother on with encouraging words during the pushing stage. This cheerleading can be done in a way that is peaceful and supportive. Inform any overbearing "coaches" that they are disturbing your inner rhythm by urging you, "Bear down harder!" "Hold your breath!" "You can do it — try harder!" "Push! Push!"

This directed pushing is a carryover from the days when mothers were so medicated and immobile that they could neither feel when to push nor push efficiently when they tried.

Dr. BJ notes: *Be sure to let any birth attendants know that you do not use the "count to 10" method to time your pushing. That way there will be no pressure to push longer with each push or more often than your body is telling you to.*

If you can't feel the urge to push because of medication, you will need coaching on when and how to push. The labor and delivery nurse or your labor support person can let you know when to push. Also, you can place your hand on your uterus so you can sense the coming contraction. When the contraction begins, your director may offer instructions: "Take a deep breath in, blow it out, take in another deep breath, round (don't arch) your back, and bear down. (See the related section on the timing of epidurals, page 310.)

Push properly. Erase from your memory any movie scene in which a purple-faced mother is lying flat on her back pushing until her eyes practically pop out. Unlike the physiological pushing we described above, "purple pushing," urged on by a loud and anxious cheering squad, is usually not helpful for mother and can be harmful for baby. After all, this is not an Olympic weight-lifting contest. When a mother bears down, holding her breath for a long time, pressure within her chest increases. This slows blood return to her heart, drops her blood pressure, and can slow blood supply to her hardworking uterus. The longer the breath holding and the bearing down, the more likely it is these circulatory disturbances will happen. Studies link prolonged breath holding and bearing down for more than six seconds at a time to changes in the fetal heart rate, suggesting that baby may not get enough oxygen.

Research validates what many mothers do instinctively: short, frequent pushes conserve your energy, preserve blood vessels in your face, deliver more blood to your uterus, enhance contractions, and deliver more oxygen to baby. In fact, studies show that most mothers push properly without anyone telling them how. Besides being healthier for

baby and less exhausting for mother, proper pushing also decreases the likelihood of perineal tissues tearing and decreases the chances of having to have an episiotomy.

So what's the best way to push? Push with as much effort as you can without overdoing it. Short (five to six seconds) and frequent (three to four per contraction) pushes will not tire you out and will keep the oxygen level in your blood constant. After five or six seconds of bearing down to your maximum intensity, blow the air completely out of your lungs. Then inhale quickly, filling your lungs with enough new air for the next push.

SCIENCE SAYS: MOST MOTHERS DON'T NEED AN EPISIOTOMY

Obstetrical surgeons used to favor episiotomy for these reasons: They felt it was easier to repair than the tear that results when episiotomy is not used. They thought it might preempt a bigger tear. And they believed it might increase the speed of delivery, or aid in the use of forceps or vacuum extraction. For an episiotomy, the doctor or midwife, using a local anesthetic to numb the tissue, makes an incision into the skin and muscles of your perineum and vaginal canal just before your baby crowns in order to make the opening larger.

Routine episiotomy is a holdover from birthing's past, when medicated women delivered on their backs with their legs up in stirrups, a position that tenses perineal muscles and makes them more likely to tear during delivery. Forceps were used to get babies out. Women now birth their babies differently, leaving many mothers, midwives, and obstetricians to conclude that routine

episiotomy is not advisable and should be limited to "restricted use," meaning to "avoid episiotomy unless indicated for fetal well-being." Modern episiotomy research has clarified many myths:

Myth 1: A straight cut made by scissors heals better than a natural tear. *False.* Research shows that a few little tears, which may involve only the skin layer, heal better than one big incision, which goes through all the layers of skin and muscle. What nature separates, nature heals.

Myth 2: Natural tears during delivery are likely to extend into and damage the rectum. *False.* Research shows that episiotomy incisions are more likely to extend themselves and tear into the rectum, causing more long-term problems. Women in the "restricted use" group (receiving episiotomy only when deemed medically necessary) showed less tearing and were more likely to have intact perineal muscles than those given routine episiotomy. And fewer women needed suturing after delivery than those in the routine group. Hold a thin piece of cloth by the edges and try to tear it. Then make a tiny cut in the cloth and try to tear it. The cloth tears easily where it has already been cut.

Myth 3: An episiotomy shortens the second stage of labor and is therefore healthier for baby. *True and false.* Episiotomies may occasionally shorten the second stage of labor, but studies have shown that this makes no difference to the health of the baby, except in emergencies.

Myth 4: A woman is less likely to suffer long-term pelvic floor–muscle problems, such as bladder incontinence, if she has an episiotomy. *False.* Research suggests just the opposite: women who do not have an episiotomy tend to have stronger perineal muscles postpartum. Episiotomy does not help prevent pelvic floor–muscle dysfunction, such as later prolapse.

Myth 5: An episiotomy keeps your vagina from stretching out of shape. *False.* Nonsense. Your vaginal canal will already be stretched to its max, and it is unlikely that cutting a few minutes off the total stretching time will make any difference long term. No surgical procedure can return the vagina to its "like new" stage.

Myth 6: Episiotomy allows quicker return to sexual function. *False.* Research confirms that women who give birth

without an episiotomy are able to resume sex more quickly, experience less pain during sex, and report greater sexual satisfaction. (Vaginal tightness is determined more by the strength of your pelvic-floor muscles than anything else, so do those Kegel exercises!)

Not only does new research show that routine episiotomy is unwise and unnecessary, it may even be risky. Tearing is not inevitable at birth, and episiotomies are often done when no tear (or a minimal tear) would have occurred. An episiotomy opens you up (literally) to problems: the perineum is an area of the body that often does not heal easily, and it is also likely to become infected. Many women experience months of discomfort from their episiotomy.

The episiotomy was worse than the birth. I couldn't sit for two weeks. Then I had to drag around my rubber doughnut every place I went.

There are a few obstetrical circumstances that can necessitate an episiotomy:

- Fetal distress — when it's necessary to get the baby out quickly

- Shoulder dystocia — when baby's shoulder is stuck

- Vaginal breech delivery

- Forceps or vacuum delivery

Researchers believe that by following these guidelines, fewer than 10 percent of mothers may need an episiotomy.

What you can do to avoid "needing" an episiotomy and minimize tearing. Here are ways that you can lower your chances of tearing a lot or having this unkind and often unnecessary cut:

Practice your Kegel exercises (see page 68) at least a hundred times a day for the last six months of pregnancy. Also, don't forget to practice the *release* mode of this exercise. Relaxed tissues are more likely to stretch and less likely to tear.

Avoid the back-lying, feet-up-in-stirrups position for delivery. This position not only narrows your pelvic outlet, but it tenses your perineal muscles, making them more likely to tear or invite an episiotomy. Studies have shown that mothers who push in the squatting or side-lying position are much less likely to tear or get an episiotomy. Mothers who have epidurals and labor on their backs are more likely to get their perineum cut.

Control your pushing. Pushing too hard and birthing too fast is likely to tear your perineum or get you an episiotomy. If the birth attendant sees that the perineum is not being allowed to stretch gradually, he may cut to avoid a tear. Pushing gently with your body's natural urges stretches the vaginal and perineal muscles slowly, making them more likely to open without tearing. Childbirth educators teach the coat-sleeve analogy: If you try to shove your arm quickly through the long, tight sleeve of a sheer blouse, you are likely to twist things up. If you persist forcefully, you could tear the fabric. So, you move slowly to gradually widen the sleeve, smooth the fabric, and ease your hand through gently.

Perineal support helps. Using perineal massage technique, your birth attendant can gently smooth out the tissues of your perineum as baby's head stretches them. She can also support your perineal tissues with a warm compress while baby's head is crowning. You can do your own perineal massage with oil to increase elasticity of the vaginal opening. (See Resources, page 431, for perineal massage instructions.)

Ease into the crowning stage of delivery. Once you feel the burning sensation that goes along with the stretching of your perineal tissues as baby's head crowns, you need to let up on your bearing down. This will not be easy, because the urge to bear down doesn't let up. As your birth attendant supports the perineal tissue, your job is to ease baby out by blowing away your breath rather than holding your breath to push. You can't keep blowing your breath away and also bear down at the same time — try it now and you'll see the effect. Called "breathing baby out," this is a good technique to practice with your other daily exercises. Your attendant may still need some pushing from you, and will let you know when.

When your baby is crowning is not the time to initiate a dialogue with your obstetrician about the benefits of a no-episiotomy birth. Discuss the subject of episiotomy during one of your eighth-month or ninth-month visits. Let your preferences be known to your doctor or midwife: unless it's absolutely necessary for the health of your baby or yourself, you wish to avoid this surgical procedure. Be sure your wishes are recorded in your birth plan.

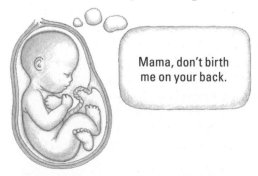

Mama, don't birth me on your back.

Assume the best position for pushing. Lying on your back is the worst position for pushing; upright squatting is best. If you are lying on your back, you will be trying to push your baby uphill, the least efficient route. If you are perched on your lower backbone (your coccyx), you will probably prevent it from flexing outward as baby passes through, slowing the progress and increasing pain. Squatting widens your pelvis and takes advantage of gravity so baby can move down and out faster. There are various ways to get the effect of squatting, one of which is a semi-reclined position that gets the pelvis widened by having your legs pulled back as you push. However, this arrangement takes advantage of gravity to a lesser degree than more upright squatting.

If your baby is coming down too fast, you can use the side-lying position with a birth attendant or labor support person supporting your perineum with a warm compress. You will need someone to hold up your top leg.

Take your time. Often mothers and birth attendants want to speed up the pushing stage of labor. You will be eager to get labor over with and to hold your baby. The "medical urge" to push babies out quickly is based upon an outdated belief that the longer baby is squeezed in the birth canal, the more she risks being deprived of oxygen. Current research shows that a long second stage, properly managed and properly monitored, does not adversely affect baby. New studies suggest that it is intense and prolonged bearing down during the pushing stage that can deprive baby of oxygen, not the length of the second stage itself. Don't be alarmed if you hear the beeps on the electronic fetal monitor slow down during your contractions, as long as they bounce back to normal after the contraction is over;

baby's heart rate normally slows down during contractions and recovers between them. If these beeps worry or bother you, ask to have the sound turned off. One of your birth attendants can keep an eye on the monitor.

Rest between pushes. As much as childbirth educators and veteran mothers offer this advice, many first-timers do not take advantage of the downtimes in their labor. When your pushing contraction is over, ease into a position that lets you rest. Suck on some ice chips, listen to soft music, keep your room and attendants quiet, and use whatever relaxation techniques you need to drift into your own calm world. Visualize "opening" and "releasing" scenes between contractions, as well as during them. Imagine the graceful unfolding of a tulip as a way to encourage your mind and body to open and bring forth baby.

Relax your perineum. The first few strong urges to push may take you by surprise, prompting you to tense instead of relax your pelvic-floor muscles. Here's where your Kegel and relaxation exercises really pay off.

Tips for dads during the second stage. Remind your partner to relax and help her do so. Support her desired labor position, wipe her forehead with a cool cloth, offer ice chips, offer to massage or give counterpressure where she needs it, stroke her arms and legs. Remind her to breathe in deeply and let go. Keep the birth room quiet and peaceful; banish disturbing influences and people. Encourage her progress even though she thinks it's slow ("Great job!"). Remind her how strong she is. And don't forget the well-timed kiss.

Crowning: baby's head appears. After you push for a while, your labia and perineum will begin to bulge — visible results of your work. Soon your birth attendant can see a puckered little scalp with dark hair appearing as you bear down, then retreating when the contraction stops, to reappear with the next one. When your birth attendant announces, "Baby's starting to crown," your perineum gradually begins stretching until eventually your vaginal opening fits like a crown around baby's head. This gradual back-and-forth descent slowly eases the vaginal tissue open. Once baby's head rounds the corner and ducks under your pelvic bone, it won't be able to slip back after a contraction anymore. (You can reach down and touch baby's head at this point to direct your pushing effort better.) As your labia and perineum stretch, you will feel a stinging, burning sensation called a "ring of fire." (Grab the corners of your mouth and pull. Notice the stretching and burning sensation. Magnify this for birth.) This stinging feeling is your body's signal to stop pushing for the moment. In a matter of minutes the pressure of baby's head naturally numbs the nerves in the skin, and the burning sensation will stop.

Once baby crowns, your birthcare provider will at times advise you not to push — it's important to ease baby's head out slowly to avoid tearing your internal tissues or your perineum. You will be told when to stop pushing and to blow out instead (it's nearly impossible to push while breathing out). A few more contractions with maybe a push or two for the shoulders to emerge and the baby wonderfully and beautifully glides out into the hands of your birth attendant or right onto the bed. You will feel the most glorious and remarkable relief that you have your baby out — your body's supreme effort has reached its goal, and you won't know whether to laugh or cry. Your eyes will be riveted on your baby, and you will sink back onto the bed or into your husband's arms and share a special moment.

Your birthcare provider will suction mucus out of baby's nose and mouth if necessary, rub baby's back to stimulate a breath (you'll then hear baby's first cry!), and then drape baby on you, tummy to tummy. While you both say "Hello, baby," oblivious to all else, a quick checkup is done. The cord will be cut after a few minutes so that the baby has an easier transition and gains the reserve blood from the placenta (some dads want to do the honors).

Some babies may need special care, such as suctioning meconium, stimulating respirations, or administering whiffs of oxygen, in order to make a healthy transition into life outside the womb. Please note: Most, if not all, of these simple procedures can be done with baby on your tummy — his safe place.

The Third Stage of Labor: Delivery of the Placenta

What you may feel. At this point you'll probably be exhausted after the work you have done and amazed at the miracle of new life. While you and Dad behold your baby and wonder over his tiny body, your birth attendant will go on working and so will your delivery system. You still have a small job left to do — deliver the placenta.

You may be so engrossed in your baby that you are oblivious to the placenta being delivered. But most women find that their family bonding time is interrupted by discomfort as uterus and birth attendant remind you that your job is not quite finished. You will feel some cramping and even a weak pushing sensation as somewhat milder contractions help deliver the placenta. Then, if you had an episiotomy or have a tear, your birth attendant will have a bit of stitching to do. As the local anesthetic is being injected in preparation for the suturing, it may sting a bit. The minor discomforts of the third stage of labor are overshadowed by the relief that birth is over and you are finally holding your precious baby.

The sudden changes in your body may cause you to have chills and shiver. Uncontrollable shakes can be quite unnerving, distracting, and uncomfortable. Ask for some warm blankets and use your deep breathing to physically relax yourself as much as possible.

What's happening in your body. Your uterus continues contracting, both to expel the placenta and to clamp down on uterine blood vessels to stop the bleeding. If there's a problem, you may receive an injection of Pitocin to help contract the uterus and stop the bleeding more quickly. If you have an IV, the Pitocin will be put in the tubing. You may not even know that this is happening as you will not be asked. A birth attendant may massage your uterus to help it contract and make sure it stays firm, since bleeding stops sooner when the uterus stays firm. This is usually pretty uncomfortable, but not always necessary. Delivery of the placenta may take from five to thirty minutes.

What you can do. Enjoy your baby. Hold, love, and caress this little life that you have labored for so hard. Keep your baby skin-to-skin on your abdomen. The warmth of your body will help keep baby warm. (A birth attendant will cover him with a warm towel.) In unmedicated births the baby is alert and aware. His instinct is to make crawling movements to propel himself in the direction of your breasts. He will find a nipple (the enlarged, darkened areola is his target) and lick and mouthe and eventually latch on to the nipple and start sucking, all on his own. Try not to help him too much. It's good for him to self-attach without interference from gowns and blankets, and without being hurried or prodded. His sucking on your nipple, coupled with the rush of motherly feelings as you see and touch your baby, release the hormone oxytocin, which naturally helps your uterus contract, helping to expel the placenta and stop the bleeding. (See the related section on the "birth crawl" in "The Hormonal Symphony of Birth," page 324.)

Each time you breastfeed your baby during the first week after birth, you will feel uterine cramps called afterpains. These are more intense in second and subsequent pregnancies than they are for first-timers. Don't let this discomfort discourage you or cause you to put off a feeding. If the afterpains bother you a lot, ask your practitioner if you can take acetaminophen or ibuprofen. Cramping means that the uterus is returning to its normal size. The cramping will be gone before you know it. Deep breathing helps you relax through it.

When it's Dad's turn to hold his new little person, he too can do it without his shirt on so they can be skin-to-skin for a while. If your baby must go to the nursery for routine checking (which can be done right there in your room, and with baby right on your tummy) or for a medical concern, send Dad with your little one. Insist that baby be brought back to you as soon as possible.

There is no reason for baby to cry after the first time. A newly born baby will be alert for about an hour, which provides a wonderful time for bonding. Then she'll sleep for a long stretch, and you can all take a well-earned snooze. Keep baby with you! She came from a warm, secure place and needs to feel that the world is safe and loving. (See page 330 for a discussion of bonding.) This is why most hospitals don't have newborn nurseries anymore. All healthy babies need to stay with mother from birth straight through to discharge from the hospital. Even cesarean-born babies can stay with mom if there's someone else in the room to help.

amniotic fluid

membrane

mucous plug

cervix

bladder

vagina

rectum

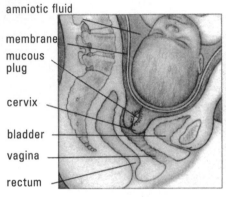

Prelabor.

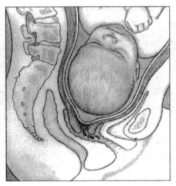

Bloody show; cervix dilating.

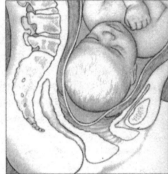

Membranes bulging; cervix effaced..

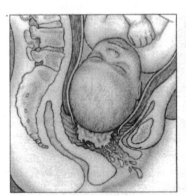

Membranes ruptured.

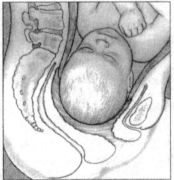

Transition; dilatation complete; pushing.

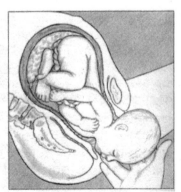

Delivery of baby.

MY PREGNANCY JOURNAL: NINTH MONTH

Emotionally I feel:

_____

_____

_____

_____

_____

Physically I feel:

_____

_____

_____

_____

_____

My thoughts about you:

_____

_____

_____

_____

_____

What I imagine your birth will be like:

_____

_____

_____

_____

_____

My weight:

_____

_____

_____

_____

_____

My blood pressure:

_____

_____

_____

_____

_____

My top concerns:

_____

_____

_____

_____

_____

My best joys:

_____

_____

_____

_____

_____

Visit to My Healthcare Provider

Questions I had; answers I got:

_____

_____

_____

_____

Tests and results; my reaction:

_____

_____

_____

_____

How I feel when I feel you move:

_____

_____

_____

_____

_____

How Dad feels when he feels you move:

_____

_____

_____

_____

_____

How I felt when labor began:

_____

_____

_____

_____

_____

Photos of birth, baby, new family together:

Comments:

_____

_____

_____

_____

_____

_____

_____

_____

_____

POSTPARTUM CHECKUP WITH YOUR HEALTHCARE PROVIDER

Depending on your birth circumstances, your healthcare provider will most likely see you within the first week after birth to check:

- Whether you are still having contractions

- How any surgical incisions (from surgical birth or episiotomy) are healing

- Questions you may have about postpartum adjustments

- Whether you are experiencing persistent bleeding or vaginal discharge

- Urinary problems

- Perineal discomforts, such as vaginal discharge, vaginal swelling, or hemorrhoids

- How breastfeeding is going

- Stress management suggestions

- Child-spacing options (most likely at a later checkup)

- Blood pressure and pulse check

- Possibly a hemoglobin check

- Healthy diet and lifestyle postpartum

- Palpation of your uterus to tell whether it's returning to its prepartum size

20

The Week After

Hi, Mom!" may be just the opening salvo from your long line of cheerleaders. After your baby's birth, your mind and body will remind you of the intense work you've just completed and of the major changes that are now taking place in your life. You have two tasks to complete: recovering from the birth and adjusting to motherhood. Even though holding your baby will more than compensate for the aches and pains throughout your body, there are still a few annoyances to cope with.

If you thought pregnancy was an amazing emotional experience, prepare yourself for the whirlwind of postpartum feelings. All of a sudden your life is no longer your own — you jump at your baby's every sound. Your body is going through another set of changes, and your hormones are shifting radically. In a month or two, you'll feel more in control, but for now you may feel joyful and fulfilled one moment and frightened and worried the next.

HOW YOU MAY FEEL

Thrilled. You've just survived the rigors of labor, and your baby is finally here. This is a big moment in your life, a natural high. You may find it hard to sleep, to think of anyone or anything but your baby. You may feel compelled to tell your birth story to anyone who will listen.

Overwhelmed. The full-time care of a tiny baby is a 24/7 job, and it's yours now, even though you may have had no previous training. The job begins when you're already worn out from labor and birth, and it may be months before you get more than three or four hours of sleep at a stretch. Of course you feel overwhelmed.

Need to rest. Your birthing hormones will prompt you to take what experienced moms call a "babymoon," where you block out disturbances not pertinent to baby care.

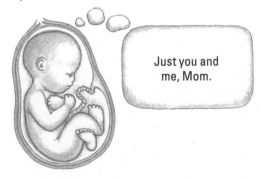

Just you and me, Mom.

Ups and downs. Lows often follow emotional highs. For months you've been preparing for your baby's Birth-Day, and now the big event is over. It's natural to feel a letdown, especially with the new challenges you're facing. You may also feel a fleeting twinge of sadness about no longer being pregnant. You are no longer the center of attention — your baby is.

You may even feel unsatisfied. If events occurred during your labor and delivery that led to a less-satisfying birth than you'd hoped for, talk them over with your doctor or midwife so you don't blame yourself for situations that were beyond your control. After all, you did birth a baby.

"Beat up." You've just been through the most strenuous work of your life. Nearly every muscle, joint, and organ of your body has worked overtime to push the baby out. It's no wonder you feel the effects from head to toe. Depending on the length and intensity of your labor and whether you had a vaginal or surgical birth, expect your body to feel the effects of delivery for at least a few weeks. Your eyes may be bloodshot due to broken blood vessels from intense pushing. You may also have popped some blood vessels in your face. Your baby's face may have similar marks, but on baby's face, these "spider marks" will clear up within a few days; yours may take a few weeks. In the days after birth, you may look and feel washed out, pale, and exhausted.

During the first few weeks, or even longer, you may feel bone-deep exhaustion and overall achiness and stiffness. Walking may be a chore. Even taking a deep breath may cause those overworked chest muscles to ache. Besides the benefit of time, try these remedies for your postpartum soreness:

- Rest.

- Soak in a warm bath.

- Get massages, especially on sore muscles.

- Replenish your body's need for fuel by eating and drinking nutritious foods.

- Hold your baby a lot to get your mind off your body.

Afterpains. Even after you've given birth, your uterus must continue contracting to get back to its original size. Uterine contractions also help to pinch off the blood vessels in the uterine lining to control postpartum bleeding. For a few hours after delivery, these contractions will be regular and rather intense. They will decrease in frequency and intensity over the next few days and weeks. Afterpains may resemble painful menstrual cramps or Braxton Hicks contractions. They intensify at the start of a feeding, since your baby's sucking stimulates the release of the hormone oxytocin, which contracts the uterus and stops bleeding.

Afterpains are not usually very intense following a first delivery, but they can be quite painful after subsequent births. To cope with the sharp discomfort, use whatever relaxation techniques worked for you during labor. This will help make breastfeeding more comfortable. Ask your doctor about taking pain relievers to ease the discomfort; most of these medications are safe to take while breastfeeding. Above all, don't avoid putting baby to the breast just because you know the cramping will start.

Painful perineum. Your sensitive perineum has been stretched to the limit and it may have been bruised or torn. If it has been cut into, it's bound to smart. To ease discomfort, promote healing, and prevent infection of this area, follow these guidelines:

- Do all you can to avoid an episiotomy (see page 370). Many mothers report that the discomfort during the healing of an episiotomy is worse than labor, since the throbbing at the site of the incision can sometimes last for weeks.

- Ask your nurse or healthcare provider to instruct you on "peri-care." Heat increases blood flow and promotes healing; cold numbs pain and decreases swelling. Both measures are necessary to heal a traumatized perineum. The nurse will tuck an ice pack up against your perineum as soon as possible (it will feel *so* good). You can continue using a cold pack for a few days — a maternity-size sanitary pad wet with ½ cup of water then frozen works well. Keep several made up ahead. She will advise you about soaking in a warm bath and show you how to squirt warm or cool water over your perineum, using a "peri-bottle" (plastic squeeze bottle). Try placing cool witch hazel pads between your perineum and the sanitary pad.

- Sit or lie in whatever position is comfortable. Leaning to one side may hurt more than sitting straight on a firm surface. If no position is bearable, try a rubber or inflatable "doughnut" to take pressure off your perineum. To prevent infection, change your sanitary pad every few hours and always wipe yourself from front to back to avoid dragging rectal germs across your perineum.

- Instead of wiping yourself with toilet tissue, clean your perineum after urinating or having a bowel movement by squirting a stream of warm water from your peri-bottle over the area. Blot dry with a soft towel. Wiping with tissue may be painful to sensitive tissues.

- If your perineal pains persist, your doctor may prescribe an analgesic that is safe to take while breastfeeding.

Bleeding and vaginal discharge. For days or sometimes weeks after birth, your uterus continues to discharge leftover blood and tissue, called lochia. In the first few days the lochia is red, in an amount comparable to a heavy menstrual period, and it may contain a few clots. Toward the end of the first week, the amount of lochia should decrease and become reddish-brown and thinner. In the next few weeks, this discharge changes from reddish-brown to pinkish, eventually to yellowish-white, and you will find yourself changing fewer pads. Any activity that increases the emptying of the uterus, such as standing, walking, or breastfeeding, will also increase the amount of discharge.

Continued vaginal bleeding can be frightening if you are not sure what's normal and what's not. Here are signs of possible trouble — situations in which you should call your doctor:

- Bleeding continues to be bright red and copious. With each day postpartum, the amount of your vaginal discharge should decrease, and its consistency should become less bloodlike. If after the first few days you are still soaking a sanitary pad with blood every hour for more than four hours at a time, call your doctor. Tampons are a no-no until you get clearance from your healthcare provider.

- You pass large clots or gushes of bright red blood. Many women will experience an occasional gush or golf ball–size clot after breastfeeding, but the bleeding should soon stop. Passing clots the size of a grape is normal for the first few days.

- The lochia has a persistent foul-smelling odor. It should either have no odor or smell like menstrual blood.

- You're experiencing increasing faintness and paleness, feel cold and clammy, and your heart is racing.

If the bleeding worries you, don't hesitate to call your healthcare provider. As you are healing postpartum, it's your job to notice the changes in your body; it's your healthcare provider's job to determine whether these changes are normal.

If you experience heavy and worrisome bleeding, lie flat and place an ice pack over your uterus just above the center of your pubic bone while waiting for a return call from your doctor or while en route to the emergency room. Or place the ice pack against the episiotomy site if the pain and bleeding seem to be coming from there. Usual causes of bleeding are failure of the uterine muscles to contract sufficiently, retained fragments of placenta, or infection. Your doctor will examine you to see whether any of these problems have occurred or whether what you are experiencing is just normal postpartum vaginal discharge.

Feeling faint. For a day or so after delivery, it's normal to feel light-headed and dizzy, especially when changing position from lying to sitting or from sitting to standing. You may feel woozy and wobbly when you walk. The end of pregnancy brings a sudden shift in blood volume and total body fluid; it takes a while for your cardiovascular system to adapt and to compensate for changes in position. Change positions slowly and gradually. Until this light-headed stage subsides (usually after a day), you may want to seek assistance when getting out of bed or walking, especially while holding baby.

Difficulty urinating. During the first day postpartum you may feel no urge to urinate, have difficulty passing urine when you do feel the urge, or feel a burning sensation while urinating. The bladder and urethra are right next to the delivery path, so it's no wonder these tissues are feeling squeezed, stretched, and bruised. Bladder function is suppressed by epidural anesthesia and may not recover until the effects of the drug wear off. An episiotomy or even a small tear can make it difficult to urinate, since the raw skin burns when urine touches it. You can see why it may take some time before you feel at ease in the bathroom. Urinary retention is so common after delivery that the nurse will repeatedly ask you, "Have you urinated yet?" Be prepared for her to check your bladder by palpating your lower abdomen to see whether it's distended. Here are ways you can get your urinary system working again:

- Drink lots of fluids, at least two 8-ounce glasses of liquid (water or juice) immediately after delivery.

- Run the water in the sink. Hearing running water gives your system the same idea.

- Stand or walk around rather than staying in bed. Allow gravity to help you urinate.

- Try to relax your pelvic-floor muscles, in fact your whole body, as you try to urinate.

- Soak in a warm tub, and urinate right there if that's more comfortable for you.

- The nurse may massage your bladder (if it's distended) to get it going.

- If your perineum has raw spots from a cut or a tear, fill your peri-bottle with warm water and squirt it onto your perineum as you urinate. The water will dilute the urine and lessen the burning.

Sometimes the bladder becomes full but won't empty despite all the effort from you and your nurse. If you haven't urinated by eight hours after delivery, your doctor may recommend a urinary catheter to empty your bladder and relieve the discomfort of its fullness. Retaining urine too long sets you up for cystitis, an infection of the bladder.

Problems with urinary retention end after a day or two, but expect a week or two of frequent trips to the bathroom. This is your body's normal way of getting rid of the extra fluid that has accumulated during the past nine months.

Leaking urine. It's normal, but annoying, to leak a few drops of urine when you cough, sneeze, or laugh. This "stress incontinence" is a temporary nuisance that occurs while your bladder and pelvic organs are rearranging themselves back to their pre-pregnancy positions. You'll be wearing a sanitary pad for the first few weeks anyhow, after which this annoyance will subside.

Profuse sweating. Another way that your body gets rid of the excess fluids accumulated during your pregnancy is by perspiring more, especially at night. For the first night or two wear cotton clothing to absorb the perspiration, and cover your sheet and pillow with a towel to absorb these night sweats. Excessive sweating or "hot flashes" are most prominent during the first week and gradually subside by the end of the first month.

Constipation. Your bowels may be as reluctant to work as your bladder, and for similar reasons.

The muscles involved in passing a stool may have been traumatized during passage of the baby. Drugs and anesthetics temporarily cause the intestines to be a bit sluggish. Besides these physical causes of constipation, many mothers have a psychological reluctance to do any pushing against their perineal muscles, either for fear of hurting these tissues or even because of a desire to rest them. Yet the sooner you get your intestines moving, the better you will feel. (See constipation care tips, pages 22 and 150.)

Painful hemorrhoids. Easing constipation relieves hemorrhoid irritation. (See hemorrhoid healing, page 227.)

Gas and bloating. The bowel sluggishness that contributes to constipation can also make you feel gassy, especially if you are recovering from a cesarean birth. Drinking and eating frequently, but in smaller amounts, and getting your body moving again will ease these discomforts. Rocking in a rocking chair is especially helpful for anyone recovering from abdominal surgery.

FEEDING THE POSTPARTUM MOTHER

While most hospitals get an A in safe medical childbirth practices, many get a failing grade in nutrition for their healing mothers. Considering the energy-draining feat you've just accomplished, you need — and deserve — to be served the most nourishing food. That being the case, either you'll have to make some special postpartum nutritional requests as you enter the hospital or, most likely, you'll have to order in and be served by friends and family. Prepare ahead of time a list of the nutritional requests they can bring to you during your postpartum stay in the hospital. One good item to have them bring is a homemade supersmoothie (see the recipe on page 24), preferably one that you enjoyed during your pregnancy. Sipping on your favorite smoothie is especially intestinal-friendly and healing if you've had a surgical birth. During your postpartum hospital stay, and certainly in the early weeks at home, try to follow the Healthy Pregnancy Plan that you learned in chapters 2 and 3.

Making Milk for Your Baby: Breastfeeding Starter Tips

You've just accomplished the most important job any human being can do: birthing another human being. Now you'll start the next most important job: nurturing your little human being. The breastfeeding starter tips you're about to learn are based upon Martha's nineteen years of experience breastfeeding our eight children, including two challenging babies (one with Down syndrome and the other adopted), as well as our combined forty-plus years of experience counseling breastfeeding mothers in pediatric practice and witnessing what works.

1. Get a professional start. How mother and baby get started with each other will set the tone for a successful breastfeeding relationship. While you may think that breastfeeding should come naturally and easily, it can be challenging at first. It is important to have good, up-to-date information and access to a professional

lactation consultant in case you have trouble. Prior to birth, you can attend a breastfeeding class where you will receive a list of reading materials and pictorials, particularly on proper latch-on. You can read *The Breastfeeding Book: Everything You Need to Know about Nursing Your Child from Birth through Weaning* (William Sears and Martha Sears). The 2013 edition of *The Baby Book: Everything You Need to Know about Your Baby from Birth to Age Two* (William Sears, Martha Sears, Robert Sears, and James Sears) also has a step-by-step pictorial. Most maternity wards have lactation consultants and knowledgeable nurses who can help you and your baby learn about the techniques on your first day together. If this help is not available, it's wise to line up a lactation consultant ahead of time and have her visit you with a hands-on demo during that first day. Of course, you probably had a breastfeeding talk during your childbirth class, but the details may lie buried somewhere in your mind, hard to remember when you have a squirming, hungry baby to feed.

2. Enjoy first feedings. Unless a medical complication prevents it, immediately after birth ask your birth attendant to drape baby over your chest and tummy, skin to skin, covered with a warm towel. Most newborn babies (of unmedicated births) are so eager to meet their new milk supply that they actually make crawling movements toward the breast, locate their target with very little help, and do what we call "self-attach." We have marveled at watching that little mouth root toward mom's nipple, as if drawn by some magic wave toward the breast. Don't rush this first introduction. Let baby simply lick and mouthe your nipple as you both enjoy these delightful moments. The sooner baby makes contact with your nipple and then actually starts sucking the better it is for both mommy and baby. Baby's sucking produces a hormone that stimulates the final stage of contractions, helping to expel the placenta. These sucking-induced contractions also control postpartum bleeding and hasten the return of your uterus to its pre-pregnant size. First feedings help ease the stress of birth for both you and baby.

It may help get him started to manually express from your nipple a few drops of the supermilk, colostrum, which is high in nutrients and immune-system boosters, exactly what baby needs. This "liquid gold" of first feedings is high quality, low quantity, so now is not the time to wonder how much baby is getting. At this point, your focus should simply be on understanding how this intimate relationship works.

3. Encourage correct latch-on. Babies (of most medicated births) who are unsure of what to do and don't self-attach will need guidance to find correct latch-on. The two magic phrases of latch-on are "wide open mouth" and "the lower lip flip." In the first couple of days when your breasts are still soft, teach baby to open her mouth wide as she takes the breast, so that her lips and

gums come far back on your areola, well past the nipple. Help her get a big mouthful of breast. Don't let baby suck on your nipple only, as you'll get sore very quickly. When baby attaches on the areola, she compresses the milk glands beneath the areola with her gums and draws the milk out. Be sure baby's lips, especially the lower lip, are turned out comfortably on your areola, instead of puckered in or tightened. If your baby tucks in her lip, gently pull it out with your finger as shown in the illustration.

Martha notes: My top breastfeeding tip? Babies suck on areolas, not nipples.

Dr. Bill notes: When I used to make obstetrical rounds with pediatric residents, the students would call these sessions "Dr. Sears's lower lip rounds." As we went from room to room showing first-time mothers how to get their newborns to latch on properly, I would use my index finger to gently press down on baby's chin, causing the lower lip to get a better grasp. Immediately mother would exclaim, "Oh — that feels better."

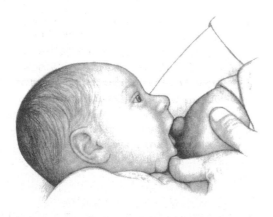

Open baby's mouth wide for proper latch-on.

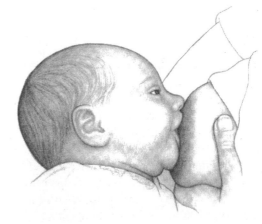

Lower-lip flip.

SCIENCE SAYS: BREASTFED CHILDREN TEND TO BE SMARTER AND HEALTHIER

A 2010 study found that children at five years of age who had been breastfed for at least four months showed a 30 percent lower risk of behavioral issues. These children were also less anxious and less clingy, and generally had better social relationships compared to their formula-fed peers. In our review of recent scientific studies, science agrees with what moms have always suspected: the more frequently and longer babies are breastfed, the more emotionally and intellectually healthy they are. Science shows that breastfed babies tend to:

- Have higher IQs
- Have fewer behavior problems
- Suffer from fewer allergic illnesses
- Be leaner as they grow up
- Have a lower rate of diabetes
- Score higher on tests in reading, writing, spelling, and math at age ten

4. Keep baby close. Unless a medical complication prevents it, have your baby room in with you so that she is always close to the breast. Remember, mothers and babies should remain close together from birth to discharge from the hospital. Of course, if you give birth at home or in a birthing center, this togetherness goes naturally with the territory.

Concerns You May Have about Breastfeeding

Engorged breasts. In the first couple of days postpartum you will notice only slight changes in your breasts. You may even wonder where all the milk is supposed to come from, as you produce only small amounts of the first milk, called colostrum (which is power-packed with nutrition and immune-boosting factors). But then, around the third day, you will be amazed to find that your breasts have taken on a life of their own; you seem to have grown two cup sizes.

Some mothers' breasts become suddenly and painfully engorged. Others, especially those whose babies have been nursing frequently, effectively, and throughout the night since birth, experience only a gradual increase in breast fullness. Your hormones are at work again: as estrogen and progesterone levels drop in the days after birth, prolactin — the milk-making hormone — takes over. As the breasts begin to do their work, the tissues swell. These dramatic changes may not have been part of the lovely, peaceful breastfeeding experience you envisioned during pregnancy. Your newborn may still be struggling to latch on. Your job is to stay calm — the best is yet to come. After your baby learns to latch on well and your breasts settle into a comfortable balance of milk production where supply equals demand, you will be well on your way to a gratifying, nurturing experience. Realize that some breast discomfort is common, especially for first-time mothers, but it will resolve. While breast fullness is inevitable, you need to take action to ease the discomfort and minimize the swelling. Prolonged engorgement sets you up for breast infections and other nursing difficulties.

- Help baby learn to latch on properly, *before* engorgement occurs.

- Use the "lower lip flip." Be sure baby's lower lip is everted (see the illustration on page 388).

- Rather than applying warm compresses, which can increase the swelling of breast tissue, apply cold compresses or packs of crushed ice to hard, painfully swollen breasts.

- Standing in a warm shower can trigger the milk-ejection reflex and help soften your swollen breasts. Let the water flow over your breasts and try some gentle massage and milk expression while standing in the shower to soften the areolas so baby can get a good latch.

- With engorgement, the nipple tissue flattens and the areola hardens, preventing baby from getting enough of your breast into her mouth to compress the milk sinuses, which are under the areola, beyond the nipple. She won't get much milk sucking only on the nipple, but she will stimulate your body to produce more milk, increasing the engorgement. If your breasts seem too full for baby to latch on well, use a breast pump or express some milk by hand, just enough to soften your areola enough that your baby can latch on to more than just your nipple. Don't pump or express too much, though, or else your body will mistake this for a change in baby's demand — and dramatically increase supply!

Nothing relieves breast fullness as quickly as a baby who is latching on and nursing well. Frequent feedings will eventually bring your milk supply in line with your baby's demands. Encourage your baby to nurse often. If he sleeps for long stretches during the day, wake him up to nurse after a couple of hours go by.

Sore nipples. Most sore nipples result from baby not latching on to the breast correctly. When your baby latches on and sucks effectively, your nipple goes to the back of his mouth, away from the tongue and gum action that would cause friction on tender nipples. Sore nipples are *not* an inevitable part of breastfeeding. If your nipples are starting to get sore, you need to pay attention to what's going on during feedings. Part of your job as a mother in the first few days is to help your baby learn how to breastfeed. You can do this, even if you're a first-time mother. While you may want to call in some helpers for expert advice (a knowledgeable nurse, a lactation consultant, an experienced friend, or a La Leche League leader), you are the expert on your baby. Stay calm, be patient, and the two of you will soon work it out. Here's what to do to relieve nipple soreness:

- Be sure to break the suction before removing baby from your breast by sliding your index finger inside his mouth between his gums. "Popping" a baby off the breast hurts!

- Nurse on the least sore side first. Nipple pain usually lessens as the milk begins to flow. Switch to the other side when you notice signs of the milk-ejection reflex: milk dripping from the other nipple, a tingling sensation in your breasts, a change in the baby's suck-and-swallow rhythm.

- Try stimulating the milk-ejection reflex before you put your baby to the breast, using warm compresses, massage, or gentle pumping.

- Breastfeed frequently — every two hours or so during the day. This will reduce engorgement and make it easier for baby to latch on.

- Let your nipples air-dry between feedings. Express a few drops of milk and let it dry on the nipple, which will help heal your skin.

- Use a purified lanolin product (such as Lansinoh) on your nipples between feedings to keep the skin moist so it will heal more quickly. Avoid using preparations that must be wiped off (ouch!) before feeding the baby.

- Wear an all-cotton bra that fits well, or go braless under a cotton T-shirt. Avoid bras with plastic or synthetic linings that hold moisture against the skin.

- Nursing pads with plastic inside will aggravate sore nipples. If a pad sticks to your breast, moisten it with water to release it and avoid skin irritation.

Most breastfeeding problems can be solved in a matter of days. If you are not getting the help you need and you believe your baby isn't getting enough milk, ask your doctor to refer you to a lactation specialist or contact La Leche League International (LaLecheLeague .org) for the name of a leader in your area. Breastfeeding is worth the effort.

Tongue-tie. Tight tiny tongues are one of the most common, undetected causes of poor or painful latch-on and insufficient milk delivery. Tongue-tie means that the frenulum, the membrane that attaches the tongue to the floor of the mouth, is shorter than normal, preventing the tongue from effectively cupping the areola and pressing out the milk. Once upon a time, newborn tongue-tie was ignored, since it doesn't seem to bother bottle feeders. It was simply passed off as one of those "he'll grow out of it" things. In our practices, we have discovered that untreated tongue-tie is one of the most common causes of early breastfeeding problems. So, we have become "clippers." Clues that your baby's tongue is tight enough for the frenulum to be clipped are:

- When baby opens her mouth to cry, a dent forms at the tip of the tongue, resembling the dip in the top of a heart shape.

- Baby's tongue cannot protrude past the lower gum.

- Your nipples are sore and latch-on is painful.

- Baby seems not to be getting enough milk, tires easily during feedings, and seems to gnaw on the nipple.

Clipping of the frenulum is a quick and painless procedure that your baby's doctor can do in the office. Clipping is best done in the early weeks when the frenulum is simply a thin membrane, and usually there is little (a few drops) or no blood. When baby's mouth is wide open, the doctor holds the tip of the tongue with a piece of gauze and uses scissors to clip the frenulum back to where it joins the base of the tongue. It should be done early on, as soon as the problem has been identified, rather than waiting to see whether things will get better. Waiting only puts mother through a lot of pain, and both of the nursing pair can get so frustrated that the decision is made to give up breastfeeding.

Dr. Bill notes: The procedure is so quick, easy, and painless that I tell the obviously anxious mother not to blink or she may miss it. The longer the tongue-tie is left unclipped, the more muscular the frenulum tether, and the more difficult the surgical procedure.

Breastfeeding after surgical birth. If you've had a surgical birth, you're doing double duty: healing yourself and feeding your baby. Try these time-tested strategies for successful breastfeeding:

- Pain suppresses milk production and makes it harder for you to enjoy your newborn. To decrease postoperative pain, talk to your anesthesiologist about using medications that will help you feel the most comfortable, yet alert, after the surgery.

- Ask your lactation consultant or attending nurse to show you how to breastfeed in the side-lying and clutch-hold positions. These positions keep baby's weight off your incision.

- When nursing in the side-lying position, surround yourself comfortably with pillows. Place one or two pillows between your back and the raised bed rail, another pillow between your knees, another under your head, and one behind baby. To support your incision while lying on your side, wedge a tummy pillow (a small foam cushion or even a folded bath towel) between the bed and your abdomen.

- Have the nurse or your partner bring baby to you and help you position her body and mouth for good latch-on.

- Be sure your mate watches how the professionals help you breastfeed. Encourage them to show him how to help you in the hospital and later on at home. It's especially important for dads to learn how to help you with the lower lip flip (see page 388).

- As much as possible, arrange to keep your baby with you in your room after a cesarean. Get help from dad, grandma, or a friend — someone who can be with you much of the time in the hospital and lend a hand with the baby.

Depending on the type of anesthesia and your recovery time, it may take a bit longer for you to begin breastfeeding and for your milk to come in. This can be a direct result of the medications or because mothers who have cesareans have fewer opportunities for early and frequent breastfeeding. The good news is that studies show that mothers who have surgical births are just as successful at breastfeeding as mothers who deliver vaginally, as long as their commitment to breastfeeding remains high, and they get the help they need.

Breastfeeding special needs babies in special circumstances. If your baby needs newborn special care — for example, if she was premature, has breathing difficulties, or has a genetic or developmental condition that requires extra medical care — it is even more vital that you breastfeed. The millions of immune-boosting white blood cells in each drop of that liquid gold will be one of the best medicines you can give your baby. Using the breastfeeding resource we list on page 431, you will learn how breast milk helps your baby in special circumstances.

As an example of how nature endows the mother to make just the right milk for her baby's needs, consider this. Suppose you birth your baby preterm. Mothers who deliver preterm babies also deliver milk that is higher in the nutrients premature babies need, such as calories, protein, and fats, especially the brain-building fats that you learned about on page 30. The immature intestines of premature infants have difficulty absorbing fat, especially formula fat. Again, enter mother's milk, which is rich in the enzyme lipase, which breaks down fat so that it is more digestible. Preterm milk is also higher in growth-building and immune-boosting proteins. In a nutshell, preterm babies need extra nourishment and protection. Mother's milk provides both.

If you are adopting an infant, instead of selecting a formula, consider feeding your baby donor milk from breastfeeding friends or a milk bank. The next best thing to mother's milk is another mother's milk. (See resources on page 425.)

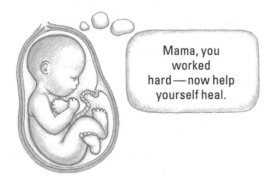

Mama, you worked hard—now help yourself heal.

How to Help Your Body Heal from Childbirth

Most of what you've learned in our Healthy Pregnancy Plan could be appropriately termed "the healthy maternity plan to help your body heal." Mustering your own internal medicines is how to help yourself heal. (Reread the section on why and how you tap into your pharmacy, page 59.)

During pregnancy and especially childbirth your tissues have *s-t-r-e-t-c-h-e-d*. For tissues to heal better and hurt less they need:

- Nutrients to repair and grow

- Adequate blood flow to deliver these nutrients

- A strong immune system to prevent and fight infection

- Protection from "antimedicines" — chemicals in food or the environment that hinder healing

The following tools will help your body use these four avenues of healing.

1. Eat healing foods. The twelve pregnancy superfoods you learned about on page 29 contain the main nutrients your tissues and immune system need. You'll notice that these superfoods have many nutrients in common and are colorful. Remember your grandmother saying, "Put more color on your plate"? Think: "White is wrong for healing." Instead of white bread, eat 100 percent whole grain. Instead of white rice, eat wild or brown rice. Instead of white or milk chocolate, eat dark chocolate.

2. Eat the five S's of healing foods: seafood, salads, smoothies, spices, and supplements. These are the food categories that should make up around 90 percent of your diet. They contain protein, calcium, probiotics, vitamins and minerals, omega-3s, and antioxidants, which are the main nutrients your body needs to heal. They also help you take advantage of a valuable healing perk called synergy. When you mix a lot of fruits, vegetables, seafood, and oils together, the nutrients work together for maximum healing effect. Review pages 28–50 and enjoy healing meals full of pregnancy superfoods.

3. Graze and sip. The smaller the meal, the faster you heal. Three important healing words are *stable insulin levels.* Grazers are more likely to keep their insulin levels stable;

gorgers are more likely to have erratic insulin levels. When insulin is too high and erratic, you get poor tissue healing, a weakened immune system, increased inflammation, and a decrease in tissue blood supply. (Review the grazing tips on page 21.)

4. Eat more seafood and/or take omega-3 supplements. Seafood is a top healing food. Omega-3s nourish healing tissues by helping the tiny oxygen-carrying red blood cells flow more quickly to deliver needed oxygen and nutrients to these tissues. The other main healing nutrients found in seafood are protein, vitamin D, antioxidants, and astaxanthin (the pink pigment in salmon) — one of nature's most powerful germ fighters and healing tissue protectors. (See AskDrSears.com/seafood.)

5. Avoid antihealers. Chemical food additives are antimedicines and delay healing, unlike real foods, which enhance healing. Your immune system identifies fake food as foreign food that doesn't naturally belong in your body. Over time, your immune system works on the fake food to build up biochemical debris that collects in tissues and prevents them from optimal healing. We constantly emphasize real foods, especially during pregnancy and postpartum. For better healing, go green before, during, and after your pregnancy (see pages 87–104).

6. Laughter is the best medicine. Humor heals by perking up the healing effects of the immune system and quelling the heal-harming effects of stress. Laughter raises the blood level of circulating germ-fighting soldiers called T cells, in addition to lowering the blood level of stress hormones. Children's hospitals are discovering the healing power of humor by providing caring clowns. May you never outgrow your kid-like appreciation for humor. (See page 78 for more on laughter.)

7. Enjoy the healing power of touch. If laughter is the best medicine, touch runs a close second. Hands heal, especially hands that care. Scientific research shows that touch heals by increasing natural killer cells, the body's most powerful weapons against foreign invaders such as germs. Touch also reduces stress hormones, which delay healing and increase pain. So, enjoy plenty of skin-to-skin time with baby and cuddle with hubby. (See page 60 for more touch tips.)

8. Listen to healing music. Music is a time-tested healer that works by reducing biochemicals that slow healing and increasing those that hasten healing. Put together your favorite medley of tunes and replay them often. (See page 77 for listening tips.)

9. Move your healing body. Movement heals by increasing the natural healing biochemicals in your body and decreasing those that impede healing. Not only does movement help heal the body, it heals the mind by releasing natural antidepressants. Movement also triggers the release of appropriate doses of natural pain relievers. Review how movement opens your body's natural pharmacy on page 59.

10. Sleep heals. Melatonin, the natural hormone that increases during sleep, has tremendous healing properties as an antioxidant. Sleep also heals your mind. Sleep deprivation increases anxiety and depression, which both delay healing. (See page 82 for sleep tips.)

11. Don't worry, be happy. Happy thoughts hasten healing. Unresolved stress delays healing. (Read some strategies for managing postpartum depression on page 75.)

Making the Transition into Motherhood

Many years ago we (Dr. Bill and Martha) began having babies, caring for babies in our medical practice, and then writing about babies. We started off only slightly informed, and as novice parents our wonders and worries were similar to yours. I (Dr. Bill) remember after the birth of our first child a friend said to Martha: "You're so lucky to have married a pediatrician!" Martha quickly replied, "Oh, he only knows about sick babies." She was right. When I started pediatric practice in 1972, even as a father of two, I was still in my learning phase. I decided to use my practice as a laboratory to learn more about well babies. I would observe savvy parents who seemed connected to their children, able to instinctively read the needs of their babies and children and know how to properly respond. They seemed to enjoy parenting more. There was a mutual trust between these parents and their children, and I observed fewer discipline issues. I kept careful notes about what these parents did, and over the next ten years I started to understand that most of these parents practiced what we call the Baby Bs:

- Bonding

- Breastfeeding

- Baby wearing

- Belief in the need to respond to baby's cries

- Bedding close to baby

- Beware of baby trainers

- Balance

As I learned from my patients, I also learned from my wife, a highly intuitive mother who trusted her gut instinct about the right parenting style for her and our children. One day as our youngest was having a temper tantrum, I watched as Martha handled it calmly and easily. I asked Martha how she had handled that tantrum so well. She said, "I got behind the eyes of Lauren and asked myself, 'If I were my child, how would I want my mother to respond?' and that's what I did." That has got to be one of the most useful nuggets of advice I have ever heard, and one I have also used as a general lesson in life.

Attachment parenting. What goes into raising a happy, healthy child? We looked at our own parenting experience, observations from my medical office, and scientific research, and formulated what we call *attachment parenting*.

Parents often ask me about attachment parenting. I tell them this: Suppose you birthed and raised your baby on a remote island without the influence of any baby books, in-laws, doctors, psychologists. All you had to use as your guide was your own personal intuition as parents. Attachment parenting is what you would naturally do.

The long-term effects of attachment parenting. When new parents would come into my office for their baby's checkups, I would write down their parenting style. Certainly, because of medical and lifestyle circumstances, not all parents could practice all the Baby Bs all the time, but those babies and parents who began life with many of the Baby Bs would merit a blue dot on the top of their chart. Over the years, I noticed that these "blue-dot babies" were not sick as often. And, when they did get sick, their parents instinctively knew what was a serious illness and what wasn't, and were able to seek proper medical care sooner. They had fewer discipline issues. Attachment parenting is an exercise in baby reading, and these parents knew their children so well that they naturally developed a style of discipline that fit their children's temperament. Because there is so much mutual trust between parent and child, a simple look of disapproval could redirect the child into more desirable behavior. As these children went to school, I noticed they had fewer of what I call the Childhood Ds that now infect our schools — ADHD, OCD, BPD, ASD. Wow! What a difference that first year of parenting makes.

More connected children. We became true believers in this style of parenting when we saw the differences in children whose parents had followed a more distant style of parenting: rigid schedules, let-'em-cry-it-out, not being responsive to baby's cries. These babies had a more distant look about them. They didn't study me during exams. They were "good babies" because they didn't cry much. Of course they didn't cry much, because they had been trained to fit conveniently into a parent's lifestyle, so that their cries fell on deaf ears. These less connected babies didn't thrive as well as attachment-parented babies. They didn't develop to their optimal potential intellectually, emotionally, and physically.

The main quality we noticed in our observational research over forty years was attachment-parented children had the quality of empathy. Isn't that one of the main qualities all parents want in their children? We have never yet seen an attachment-parented child who became a school bully. These "kids who care" are kind and compassionate.

Here's a summary of our advice to help you transition into parenthood:

1. Read *The Baby Book,* the companion to *The Healthy Pregnancy Book.* It begins with the birth of your baby, and even slightly before. Part I takes you from the events surrounding birth through the first few months of life with your new baby. If you want to go deeper into the seven Baby Bs of attachment parenting, also read *The Attachment Parenting Book* (all by William Sears and Martha Sears).

2. Surround yourself with savvy parents who seem to enjoy their parenting. Join the valuable support resource, Attachment Parenting International (see attachmentparenting.org).

3. Trust your intuition. This is your baby, and you are his parents. If some trusted friend or wannabe baby expert offers you a piece of parenting advice that does not feel right to you and doesn't fit the temperament of your baby, don't use it. In a nutshell, parenting means giving your children the tools to succeed in life. Attachment parenting gives you the tools to help you build more trust in your own intuition and help your child develop the tools to succeed in life.

4. Based upon your reading and the information you've gleaned from trusted friends and support groups, formulate your own parenting style even before birth. Then have the wisdom and flexibility to adapt your chosen style to the individual needs of your baby and realities of life after birth. After several decades of practicing, teaching, and learning about attachment parenting, the number one nugget of feedback we get about the Sears Parenting Library is: Thank you, Dr. Sears, for validating my own intuition!

III

If You Have a Challenging Pregnancy

We downplay the medical classification "high risk." While this term is often needed in medical charts to alert the medical staff to possible complications, a mother should never fearfully feel "high risk." Remember, one of the central messages of our book is to take the fear out of childbirth. Instead, we use terms of empowerment, such as "challenging," and any labor language that conveys to the mother that because of special obstetrical circumstances she needs to take extra care of herself to birth a healthy baby. In the following chapters we discuss the most common challenges and complications of pregnancy and provide mothers with the necessary tools to lower their risk of complications.

If you have been labeled "high risk," you need to be more informed, more responsible, more empowered, and more involved in the decision-making than the average mother. The first question you should ask yourself after you are classified as "high risk" is "What healthy changes can I make to lower my risk?" Even with special pregnancies, modern obstetrical innovations increase the chances of most of these babies turning out just fine.

21

Special Pregnancies

With technological advances in fertility and prenatal diagnoses also come challenging pregnancies and parenting.

HAVING A BABY AFTER AGE THIRTY-FIVE

If you're pregnant and over age thirty-five, congratulations! You are in the fastest-growing age group of American women having babies. In the past couple of decades more and more women have been having babies later. In fact, the number of women having babies over the age of thirty-five has doubled. And in our experience, this maturity trend has more positive than negative consequences. On the one hand, the worries you hear and read about do have some scientific basis. Statistically women over age thirty-five do have a slightly increased chance of having medical complications during pregnancy, such as:

- High blood pressure

- Gestational diabetes

- Miscarriage

- Chromosomal abnormalities

- Multiple pregnancies (because of the popularity of in vitro fertilization, or IVF)

- Placenta previa

- Preeclampsia

- Breech presentation

- Prematurity

Now the good news. While you may read that mothers over the age of thirty-five have "more difficult deliveries," in our medical practices this has not been our experience. We've noticed that women who have babies when they are thirty-five or older have certain advantages. A more mature woman is likely to take better nutritional care of herself, make wiser choices in assembling her birth team and choosing a birth place, and ask more insightful questions during interviews to select an obstetrician, midwife, and pediatrician. She may also choose a parenting style more carefully and deliberately. Our conclusion: While these more mature mothers may need extra obstetrical care, a healthy thirty-five-year-old mother should expect to carry and deliver as healthy a baby as a younger mother would. Except for the increased risk of chromosomal abnormalities, in general, the older mother's wiser birth choices more than make up for her statistical increase in complications.

If you're over the age of thirty-five and have already given birth in your younger years, you have the benefit of hindsight: You know what pregnancy is like, how to take better care of yourself, how to position yourself for easier labor and birth, and how to better deal with the stresses of pregnancy and early motherhood.

HAVING A BABY WITH DOWN SYNDROME

With increasing age comes increased risk of birthing a baby with a chromosome problem, most commonly one called a trisomy, meaning that most of baby's cells have three, rather than two, copies of a chromosome.

While there are other chromosomal abnormalities, such as trisomy 13 and trisomy 18, the most familiar is trisomy 21, or Down syndrome. Babies with trisomy 13 or 18 rarely survive. Babies with trisomy 21 not only survive but, with early intervention and guidance, become more of a blessing than a burden. Today's parents of children with Down syndrome have many more resources available to them: early intervention programs, expert medical care, government-funded programs, and more informed and available support groups.

If you're thirty-five to forty and pregnant, should you worry about birthing a baby with Down syndrome? We don't think so. If you look at the statistics, they're not so scary:

You will notice that between the ages of thirty-five and forty, your chances of having a baby with perfectly normal chromosomes is at least 99.5 percent. Very few risks in life have such good odds in your favor. But as you see from the statistics above, the risks go way up after age forty.

Discuss with your healthcare provider the benefits and risks of prenatal screening tests.

Mother's age	Risk of Baby with Down Syndrome	Risk of Baby with Any Chromosomal Disorder
20	1:1,667	1:526
30	1:952	1:385
35	1:378	1:192
40	1:106	1:66
45	1:30	1:21

Don't feel you are being discriminated against just because of your age if your doctor pushes the tests. A doctor is legally obligated to inform a woman over age thirty-five of the availability of prenatal screening tests for birth defects. Since the choice is up to you, consider these factors:

- Would the results of the test cause you to change the course of your pregnancy?

- Would knowing about a chromosomal defect beforehand help you adjust and prepare to parent a special needs baby?

- Would not knowing such important information cause you to have a worry-filled or less joyful pregnancy?

- Should you have an amniocentesis if you're thirty-five? Ponder these considerations: For mothers below age thirty-five, the risk of miscarriage resulting from amniocentesis may be similar to the risk of having a baby with a chromosomal defect. How do the risks compare with the benefits of the test in your particular obstetrical circumstances? Discuss the statistics with your doctor. Ask about the complication rate (especially the miscarriage rate) of amniocentesis in the hands of the doctor performing the procedure. The average risk of miscarriage following amniocentesis is 1 in 200. Your doctor's risk rate may be higher or lower than this, so you need this valuable information in making your decision about whether to have amniocentesis. With new screening tests, such as the Quad test, some mothers may elect not to have an

amniocentesis. This test, done between the fifteenth and twentieth weeks, measures the levels of four biochemicals in mother's blood that are markers for having an increased chance of having a baby with a genetic abnormality or structural abnormalities of the brain and spine. It is around 80 percent accurate in correctly identifying babies with Down syndrome (with a "false positive" rate of about 5 percent) and fails to detect around 15 percent.

Our seventh child, Stephen, has Down syndrome, something we did not know about beforehand (we elected not to have prenatal screening even though Martha conceived at age forty-four). Stephen has been a blessing to our family and has provided challenges that have made our lives richer. In some ways children with Down syndrome have fewer abilities than other children, but in many ways they have more. Stephen is perceptive, resourceful, lovable, and loving, and he has taught us a view of what's important in life that we would never have had without him. With the medical support, social services, and public education available for special needs children today, they are no longer the burden they were once considered to be. Instead, they are a blessing — just as any child is a blessing.

GENETIC TESTING

There are few areas as controversial or as complicated as screening for birth defects and inherited diseases. You may or may not want to avail yourself of available technology, but your healthcare provider will discuss your options. Here is an overview of the genetic tests that are currently available and some guidelines to help you select which ones are right for you and your family.

One perfectly reasonable approach is to simply not do any testing at all. Many pregnant couples are uncomfortable with the concept of testing and the implicit assumption that they would consider terminating the pregnancy if the baby had a serious condition. Some couples want to be tested in order to be able to prepare themselves and their families for the birth of a child with a defect. Many couples proceed with testing without being certain what they plan to do with the information. Fortunately the vast majority of couples will get good news on the results and have one less set of issues to worry about with the pregnancy.

Before or during early pregnancy: screening for "carrier" status. The mother and the genetic father of the baby can choose to be tested themselves for a variety of diseases. Your healthcare provider will normally take a family history and health history of the couple and may offer a variety of tests based on these histories and your "gene pool" background. For example, people of dark-skinned African descent will be tested for sickle cell trait. Individuals of eastern European Ashkenazi Jewish background will be offered testing for diseases such as Tay Sachs, since there is a high incidence of carrier status in this disease and others. Caucasian couples can be offered testing for cystic fibrosis, a disease that can cause serious lung problems in children. These diseases are all caused by recessive genes, which a healthy person may have and not know about because a single gene causes few or no symptoms, while getting two of them, one from each parent,

can cause significant disease. If both parents are carriers of the same gene, there is a one in four chance that a fetus will inherit the disease in question.

Genetic mutation screening. Babies can also have abnormalities in the number of chromosomes or the structure of chromosomes. The most commonly known condition associated with an abnormal number of chromosomes is Down syndrome, or trisomy 21, in which there are three rather than two copies of the twenty-first chromosome. Less common problems include trisomy 13 and 18; Turner syndrome, in which a girl only has one X rather than two X chromosomes; and Klinefelter syndrome, in which a boy has one Y chromosome and two X chromosomes rather than an X and a Y. All of these have significant health repercussions for the baby. The risk of abnormalities is sometimes random but often increases with maternal age.

This blood test detects the usual fetal chromosomal abnormalities and correlates 99 percent with amniocentesis results, thus often making an amniocentesis unnecessary. Currently technology exists to actually culture fetal cells out of the maternal bloodstream by the tenth week, which allows genetic testing of the fetus with a simple maternal blood draw. There are very real benefits to knowing in advance whether there is a problem, since the timing of delivery, the place of delivery, and the rapid initiation of treatment in specialized perinatal centers can give the baby a better chance. Some defects require surgical correction, and if the parents know about a problem in advance they can identify the center in their area with the most experience treating their baby's specific health challenges.

The science and technology of more precise genetic testing are steadily evolving. For updates, consult: AskDrSears.com/genetictesting.

MOTHERING MULTIPLES

The cliché of "more challenges, but more fun" certainly applies to carrying and birthing multiples. Not only do you feel one feisty kickboxer in there, you get to feel siblings jockeying for position.

How multiples are suspected and detected. Your obstetrician or midwife may suspect you're carrying multiples by the size of your uterus. Naturally, more babies need more room, so your uterus is likely to feel bigger at your early checkups than if it were housing only one occupant. An ultrasound may confirm a multiple pregnancy, although even experienced hands and high-tech ultrasound can miss it until around twelve weeks. Growing more babies requires making more growth hormones, although detection of higher levels than usual is not a reliable indicator of multiples. The Quad screen during genetic testing may give a hint that mom is housing multiples.

What you may feel. If you're carrying more than one baby, the typical feelings of pregnancy, both pleasant and unpleasant, are likely to be magnified. While how mothers show and feel varies with multiples just as it does with singleton pregnancies, many mothers of multiples have more morning sickness and tummy troubles. When your body has to work twice as hard, it may get twice as tired. And, if you're carrying more than one baby, you're going to need more rest, more nutrition, more medical care, and more support and help at home. Fathers of multiples take note: If your wife's body is doing double duty to birth more than one of *your* babies, she will need more help from *you*. Think, *we're* having twins! Or more!

WHY SO MANY MULTIPLES?

The number of twin births has more than doubled in the past decade, and triplets and more have quadrupled. While around 3 out of every 100 pregnant women have a double or triple blessing (95 percent of multiples are twins), more and more women are carrying more and more babies for these reasons: More women are having babies at an older age. Older moms may ovulate more than one egg at one time, probably because of the higher level of hormones that stimulate ovulation. Another boost to the mushrooming multiple baby boom is the increasing use of fertility technology to assist parents who want babies but aren't able to conceive in the conventional way. When you implant a bunch of fertilized eggs into a long-awaiting and willing uterus hoping that at least one will take, chances are great that you're going to birth more than one. Another reason for multiples is the rising obesity epidemic, because the hormonal fluctuations that accompany obesity slightly increase the chances of multiple births.

What you can do to birth healthier babies. Expect your healthcare provider to predict the possible challenges you might have when carrying multiples. That's her job. The more babies you carry, the higher your chances of preterm labor, preeclampsia, a surgical birth, and even the possibility of one baby not surviving the pregnancy or the birth. Here are some ways you can help your chances of having a healthy multiple pregnancy:

Choose your healthcare provider more wisely. In fact, the term "more" summarizes everything you need to do to have a healthier pregnancy. Depending on how your pregnancy progresses, your obstetrician may invite a specialist, or a perinatologist, to co-care for you during your pregnancy. If you're primarily under the care of a midwife, she will likely transfer your care to an obstetrician to assist in your care and birth. Your provider will discuss with you the possibility of preterm delivery and assist you in choosing a hospital that has optimal newborn-care facilities, since the chances of neonatal intensive care go up proportionally to the number of babies you are carrying. And, since there is only so much room in the womb, the more babies you need to birth, the sooner they need to get out and the more premature they will be.

Practice the Healthy Pregnancy Plan more diligently. As outlined on pages 28–72, you will need to be more careful about what you eat, how much weight you gain, and the type of exercise you do. The more babies you carry, the bigger you will get. And the bigger your babies get, the smaller and more frequent your meals get, since that extra need for womb room leaves less food room in your stomach and intestines. No, you do not need to eat twice as much, but you are likely to need around an extra 300 nutritious calories a day, 25 grams of protein, 20 milligrams of iron, and extra folic acid. (These nutrients are in addition to the extra ones you need to grow a singleton baby.) Yes, obviously, you will gain more weight because you are growing more babies along with more uterine tissue. A healthy weight gain for a mother who began her pregnancy at an optimal weight would be around 35 to 45 pounds with twins, and as much as 50 pounds with triplets.

Regarding exercise, the more babies you are carrying, the more wisely you have to carry yourself when moving. Since those babies are eager to get out and the risk of preterm delivery goes up, discuss with your healthcare provider what exercises you should avoid, usually jogging, jumping, and any movements that trigger those eager babies to push down on your already pressurized cervix. Since you're naturally carrying more weight on your joints, be more protective of them during exercise. Again, swimming wins out as the best exercise for mothers of multiples.

Do multiple networking. You will need multiple help, and here's where social networking really shines. Try the National Organization of Mothers of Twins Clubs (NOMOTC.org) and Mothers of Multiples Society (MothersofMultiples.com).

HOW MULTIPLES ARE MADE

Usually when one sperm reaches one egg, they make one baby. When two different eggs are fertilized by two different sperm, you get two different babies, or *fraternal* twins. Fraternal twins look somewhat alike, like other siblings, and they can be boy and girl, two boys, or two girls. Less commonly, one egg is fertilized by one sperm and then it divides into two, resulting in *identical* twins. They will look alike and be the same gender.

Double your enjoyment of sex? Yes? No?
Unless advised by your healthcare provider, you don't have to worry about enjoying sex just because you are carrying twins. Because women carrying multiples have an increased risk of delivering prematurely and because orgasm can stimulate uterine contractions, conventional wisdom had been that these women should abstain from orgasm during the third trimester. Recent studies, however, have shown no relationship between intercourse and the premature delivery of twins.

Yes, there is more labor involved in carrying multiples, but there can also be more joy. After you've survived the first-year blur of the exhaustion of caring for two or more babies, you can sit back and have double the fun as you watch these babies crawl after, and then run after, each other, and this makes it all worthwhile. Please don't worry about the double college tuition just yet.

22

If You Have Medical Complications

ather than clutter this book — and your already overworked mind — with a discussion of the things that may go wrong during pregnancy, we have put all of the possible complications of pregnancy into one chapter here in the back of the book, because for the great majority of mothers pregnancy goes right. Some women experience minor and temporary complications. Some experience major ones. Use this chapter as a reference to read about only those problems that you know you have. If you don't have them, don't worry or read about them. When your energy is so rightly focused on growing a baby, the last thing you need is to worry about problems you are not likely to have. If you do have a complication, we want to empower you to work in partnership with your healthcare provider to manage it as much as possible. Remember what we've said many times: you are first, a participant in your healthcare, and second, a patient.

ANEMIA

Anemia is a less than optimal level of red blood cells. Most anemia during pregnancy is due to a deficiency of iron in your diet. Iron is necessary to make the extra blood you need to nourish yourself and to make the billions of red blood cells your baby needs. Insufficient iron or "tired blood" makes for a tired mom. Around 20 percent of pregnant women are iron deficient, and it occurs most often during the second half of pregnancy when the extra iron you eat doesn't keep up with the extra blood cells you need to make for you and baby. You may have difficulty determining whether you are anemic, since the symptoms of iron deficiency — fatigue, tired muscles, irritability, and poor concentration — can occur simply from being pregnant. During pregnancy your healthcare provider routinely checks your blood count (hemoglobin and hematocrit), yet you can still be iron deficient even if your "blood count" is normal. Another reason the hemoglobin and hematocrit are not a true reflection of your iron status is that they may reflect that you are anemic when you aren't. Because of a process called hemodilution, your hemoglobin and hematocrit may reflect lower values than before you were pregnant, but you may not have symptoms of anemia. This is known as the "physiological anemia of pregnancy." If you suspect that you are anemic, ask your healthcare provider to check the *ferritin level* in your blood, which is a more accurate measure of the iron stores in your tissues. A low ferritin level (less than 20) is a sign that your tissue stores of iron are being depleted. Not only is iron deficiency tiring for mother, it's unhealthy for baby. Anemic mothers are more likely to deliver low-birth-weight or premature infants.

How to be sure you are getting enough iron. Most women need to double the amount of iron in their diet when they're pregnant, eating at least 30 milligrams of elemental iron each day, more if anemic or carrying multiples. This means that most women need to take an iron supplement during pregnancy. Even though nature gives your iron levels a boost by increasing absorption of iron from foods when you are pregnant, it's challenging to consume enough dietary iron without eating excess calories. It's best to begin taking iron supplements early in pregnancy or, even better, before you are pregnant in order to store extra iron. Try these tips to be sure you're getting sufficient iron for you and baby:

- See page 47 for a list of the best sources of iron.

- Eat foods high in vitamin C (citrus fruits, kiwi, strawberries, and green peppers), which, when eaten along with iron-containing foods, increase the intestinal absorption of the iron. Drinking milk, tea, coffee, and antacids inhibit the absorption of iron. Instead, drink orange or grapefruit juice to absorb the most iron from your meals, and drink those other beverages between meals.

- If iron upsets your already upset stomach, ask your healthcare provider whether you can safely delay taking iron supplements until after your morning sickness subsides, since the greatest demand for iron occurs in the second half of your pregnancy. Even better, try taking them in small doses throughout the day and eat iron-rich foods.

- Be label savvy. The amount of iron listed on a supplement bottle label may be misleading. Look for the phrase "elemental iron," which indicates the amount of iron that is available for absorption. For example, a "300 milligram ferrous sulfate tablet" contains 60 milligrams of elemental iron. If the iron supplement you are taking doesn't reveal the amount of elemental iron, ask your pharmacist how much it contains.

BED REST PRESCRIBED

Around 20 percent of expectant mothers need to take some of their pregnancy lying down. At any time during pregnancy, complications can confine you to your bed for days, weeks, even months. While the occasional woman may welcome this doctor-mandated time off her feet, for most all rest and no work or play is no vacation.

Complications that banish a pregnant woman to bed in the first half of pregnancy are unexplained bleeding and the threat of an impending miscarriage. In the second half of pregnancy, the most common reason for bed rest is the threat of preterm labor. Other reasons for prescribed bed rest later in pregnancy include high blood pressure, preeclampsia, incompetent cervix, premature rupture of membranes, and chronic heart disease.

Obstetricians prescribe bed rest (medically termed "therapeutic positioning") if there is a concern that being up and active could harm the health of baby or mother. The less active mother is likely to have a less irritable uterus for several reasons:

- Bed rest decreases the pressure of baby on the cervix, thus reducing the likelihood of premature cervical stretching and contractions.

- Rest increases blood flow to the placenta and thus improves the delivery of nutrients and oxygen to help baby grow.

- Rest is also likely to reduce a mother's high blood pressure.

SCIENCE SAYS: "THERAPEUTIC BED REST" OFTEN UNNECESSARY.

A 2013 article published in *Obstetrics and Gynecology* concluded that there is insufficient science to recommend strict bed rest for complications such as threatened miscarriages, high blood pressure, or preeclampsia. These researchers also pointed out the potential risks, such as vein thrombosis, bone and muscle weakness, and psychological trauma. This research is leading many birthcare providers to ease off prescribing strict bed rest during pregnancy.

Eleven Top Tips to Make the Best of Your Rest

While some women gladly abide by the doctors' orders for bed rest, for most it's an unwelcome inconvenience. There are always so many other things to do in addition to growing a baby. Yet, when you consider that you will have plenty of other chances to do those things but only one chance to complete this pregnancy, being in bed for nearly 24 hours a day can be managed. Here are some ways to cope with your confinement.

1. Knowledge is restful. Know exactly what you can and cannot do. Be sure you understand what your healthcare provider means by "bed rest." You can pretty much figure that bed rest means refraining from the more "active" activities that go on in bed — sex and orgasm. But check to be sure you understand whether your doctor recommends total bed rest, which means sponge baths in bed and bedpans, or whether you get the luxury of bathroom privileges and an occasional walk to the kitchen. Ask whether you can slowly walk up and down stairs or are instead confined to one floor. Bear in mind that most doctors overprescribe the degree of bed rest, realizing that most human beings do not easily adapt to such a drastic change in lifestyle and will occasionally cheat. Find out whether your doctor thinks that mental stress is a problem. Some women need to rest their minds in addition to their bodies. Can you deal with office work over the phone? While you won't want your older children using your bed as a trampoline, can they stay in the room with you for much of the day?

2. Make a nice nest. If you have to stay in bed, you might as well create a comfortable bed you like to stay in. Have your bed placed near or facing a window so that you have fresh air and a view. Put anything you'll need within arm's reach on a table next to your bed. Keep your journal and all kinds of reading material on an adjacent table. Move the television or the sound system into the bedroom. Buy or rent a small refrigerator for your bedside snacks. Be kind to your recumbent body: place a foam "egg crate" pad on top of your mattress.

3. Don't worry, be happy. Sure, you are missing your job, your kindergartener's school play, and the simple pleasure of strolling through the park. And a person can take only so much downtime, especially if you have been used to being busy; you can read only so many novels, watch only so much TV, and meditate on your baby for only so long. But rather than dwell on what you're missing, think about what you are enjoying. Even if you find yourself feeling bored, listless, and depressed, these feelings will eventually subside, and you will have happy days again. Focus on what you are doing for your baby and on the benefits to you of resting and relaxing. The good thing about the emotions of pregnancy is that downs are usually followed by ups. Think positive.

I lay there imagining what my life would be like if I didn't have to stay in bed. I had to stop thinking about that since it served no purpose and only made me more depressed.

When you have so much time to just sit and think, your emotions are likely to run wild. You may worry about the baby's health and survival, fret about how your husband and kids are coping, be bored with too little to do, feel anxious about things you should be doing, and dislike feeling dependent. You may feel angry and disappointed about the course of your pregnancy. You may grow impatient as each day seems to get longer and longer. You'll probably feel tempted to cheat and get up for a while. Each day in bed will bring on new emotions to work through, yet continuing to focus on the goal of delivering a healthy baby can help you overcome these feelings and keep you in bed as long as you need to stay there.

4. Designate Mr. Mom. Seek your mate's help. This may be the first time in your life that your mate waits on you and seems to get very little in return — except, of course, that you are growing his baby. Prolonged bed rest during pregnancy can bring couples closer or put them at a distance. Abstaining from sex and curtailing the activities that you usually do together may be difficult in a marriage that may already be stressed. In addition, your husband is now holding down two jobs, taking care of you and bringing home the bacon, and this can add to the stress. Yet, if you are creative, a lot of bedside romance can take place: candlelight dinners followed by a video, breakfast in bed, and daily massages that promote circulation and feel so good. Being cared for by a sensitive mate can add new depth to your relationship. And for a spouse turned cook, waiter, masseur, and entertainer, this could be the first time in his life that he has had to put someone else's needs ahead of his own — good preparation for becoming a father.

Now that my husband is being mom, shopper, and housekeeper, he realizes how tough my job is and has quit making cracks about how I have an easier job than he does. While I'm in bed, he has to cover all the bases.

If you have older children, get used to issuing orders from your bed or the couch. On the day you begin bed rest, call a family meeting and, together with your spouse, lay down the house rules, telling your children the importance of your resting in bed, being waited on, being served, and being loved. Your husband should take the lead and show your children how he expects them to behave toward you and tell them that they should avoid disturbing you. Be sure that they understand that you welcome their company, but that doesn't mean that they can just run in and jump on your bed anytime they wish.

With children younger than four or five, you'll probably need some babysitting help if you are to get any rest. When you don't have another grown-up around, welcome your children around your bed, but on peaceful terms. You might even enjoy having a daily tea party there with your three-year-old. Have your bed or couch set up so that the DVD player, snacks, and children's books are within your reach. Make sure that there are lots of toys around, too. But don't forget that even an eighteen-month-old toddler can follow simple instructions to get himself a tissue or pick out a book. Expect cooperation and you will get it.

5. Enjoy your new "office." Work from your bed. While you can't be physically active, you can usually do mental work while lying in bed — balance the checkbook, make appointments, write shopping lists, help with the children's homework, or work on a laptop computer (use a lap desk: a cushioned, protective board that you place on your lap to hold your computer). If the doctor permits, you can also keep up with your job by teleconferencing or doing paperwork. If you need to go on disability leave, be sure to apply for it.

6. Keep your blood moving. Keep fit while in bed. With your doctor's OK, do some simple exercises in bed, such as leg lifts and ankle flexing, calf stretches, and upper-arm exercises with light weights. Exercising helps promote circulation and keeps your muscles (including your heart) in shape.

7. You deserve extra touches. Pamper yourself. Staying in bed does not mean denying yourself all of the pleasures of life. Hire a massage therapist (or ask a friend) to give you a head-to-toe massage once a week. Find out whether your hairdresser will come to your bedside.

YOUR DAILY REMINDERS

Put this list on a big card next to your bed and add your own. Read it when you need a perk up.

- I may never get this much rest for the next few years.

- My husband just got upgraded to Mr. Mom.

- Don't worry, be lazy.

- I don't have to be anywhere at any time.

- My to-do list is the shortest it will ever be.

- I can enjoy breakfast in bed.

- I now have more time in bed with my mate than I ever had.

- Imagine the precious gift I'll get when I get out of bed.

8. Bond with your baby. Many women on prolonged bed rest face a dilemma: though this would seem an ideal time to contemplate the miracle of pregnancy and to bond with the baby, the usual reason for being on prolonged bed rest is the very real possibility of losing the baby. So some women find that even though they have plenty of time to think about and plan for the baby, they are afraid to invest much emotional energy. Without the usual distractions and tasks of daily life, it's easy to worry that every spot of blood is going to be the end of your baby, or that each contraction may be the one that sets off premature labor. Remember that the vast majority of women who are confined to bed go on to delivery healthy babies.

9. Make downtime catch-up time. This may be the only time in your adult life that you will have so much time to do just what you want to do, provided you stay in bed. There are many activities a bed-rester can enjoy. Read the classics you've been too busy for. Catch up on sports. Get that box of photos into albums. Write that article you've been meaning to write, or get on the Internet. Write letters. Create art. Study a language using audiocassettes. Learn about real estate, teaching, or some other field you've been too busy with your real job to explore. Hand-piece a quilt. Read to your kids. Laughter makes boring bed rest tolerable: treat yourself to joke books and comedies on DVD. Don't watch the news. You get the idea.

I had to really work at it, but after a week or so I came to enjoy being waited on a little. It had been years since I'd been on the receiving end of so much loving attention.

10. Enjoy funny friends. Choose your visitors carefully. Lying in bed for long periods of time can make you crave adult conversation. Invite over friends who are good listeners. It is likely that many of your friends will not understand your feelings about staying in bed. Be prepared to hear, "You are so lucky. I'd love to stay in bed for two months." Other friends may be more empathetic and realize that continued bed rest isn't all that natural or enjoyable. Pick out a friend who makes you laugh and invite her over frequently. Be sure it's someone who brings her own treats and doesn't expect you to play hostess.

Some people felt that I was so lucky to just sit there and watch TV and rest all day, but it's not that simple. I couldn't get up without feeling guilty and wondering if this was the trip to the bathroom that would push me into a miscarriage or a preterm delivery. It really helped when my friend came by and did my hair and then just sat and listened.

11. Ease into life out of bed. Don't overdo it when you come off bed rest. When you finally get out of bed, it's easy for your mate, kids, and everyone else around your house to feel that you are suddenly available to them again full-time. Serve notice that you are going to ease back into the household routine and will still be needing a lot of help and rest. When you do stand up after lying in bed for a long time, you may feel that parts of your insides aren't quite with you. The aches and pains from being in bed will gradually ease over the next few days, and your body will accustom itself to being active again.

When I did get the green light to get out of bed occasionally, I didn't push it. I didn't want to blow three months in bed in one day. I kept focusing on my goal: to bring my baby to term.

ONLINE SUPPORT FOR COOPED-UP MOMS

Ask your practitioner to give you the phone numbers of other mothers similarly confined to bed. Sometimes you can talk each other through a particularly dull day. Or contact Sidelines (Sidelines.org), a support group that maintains a national hotline of volunteers who offer support and match you with other bedridden moms-to-be. This group is the brainchild of a California mother who was confined to bed during her high-risk pregnancies and figured out a way to use her free time for the good of other women in her circumstances. Ask these experienced bed-resters for practical suggestions on what helped them cope. Mothers who have lain in bed for six straight weeks or more will give you ideas on how to pass the time.

A volunteer at Sidelines suggested that since I had so much time on my hands to connect with my baby, I might want to ask to find out its sex so that I could better connect. Previously, I hadn't wanted to know the sex — I wanted to be surprised — but I took her advice. Using this time to bond more specifically with my son meant that I wasn't just sitting there twiddling my thumbs. There was something special about calling our baby by the name we had chosen. This suggestion helped me a lot.

BETA STREP INFECTION

Because Group B Streptococcus (GBS) is a common bacterial inhabitant of the vagina, many women unknowingly carry GBS and have no symptoms. Yet, they run the risk of passing on this germ to their baby during delivery. GBS can cause a serious infection in your baby soon after birth, so your healthcare provider is likely to test you for it by a cervical swab at around thirty-seven weeks or when you begin labor. If you test positive for GBS in your urine, your healthcare provider may treat you with intravenous antibiotics. If you test positive for GBS when you go into labor, you will be given an intravenous antibiotic to lower the chances of transferring this germ to your baby.

FIFTH DISEASE

This viral infectious disease, so named because it was the fifth of the viruses discovered to cause fever and rash, is a common childhood illness that is very contagious but seldom harmful to children or adults. It is characterized by fever, a red rash on the face (looking like "slapped cheeks"), and a lacy red rash on the legs and trunk of the body. Adults with this illness may also have sore joints, and people with some types of hemolytic anemia may experience flare-ups. Fifth disease is contagious for up to a week before the facial rash appears, so people are often exposed to the virus unknowingly. Although this virus is usually harmless to children and nonpregnant adults, there are special concerns for pregnant women. If you are not already immune to the virus (most adults are) and are exposed during the first trimester of your pregnancy, you have a slightly higher risk of miscarriage (1 to 2 percent higher than normal). Infection of the baby during the latter part of pregnancy can break down baby's blood cells, causing anemia. If you have been exposed to fifth disease, your healthcare provider may perform a blood test to see whether you are already immune. If you are, you do not need to be concerned. If not, or if another blood test shows that you have recently been infected with the virus, your healthcare provider may monitor you more closely.

GENITAL HERPES

If you had a previous infection with genital herpes, the stress of pregnancy can cause even an old infection to flare up. A newborn baby can acquire the herpes infection during passage through an infected birth canal. If a mother gets a new herpes infection or a flare-up of a previous infection just prior to labor, it is now standard obstetrical procedure to protect baby from getting infected with the active herpes infection by performing a surgical birth. If you've had genital herpes in the past but the sores do not flare up prior to birth, chances are that you've developed enough antibodies to the herpes infection and have passed these antibodies on to your baby. If this is the case, or if cultures are negative, it's unlikely your baby will be infected and, therefore, your healthcare provider is likely to recommend that you go ahead with a vaginal birth.

GESTATIONAL DIABETES

Mothers are diagnosed with gestational diabetes if they had normal blood sugars before their pregnancy but experience higher than normal blood sugars during their pregnancy. While around 5 percent of mothers develop gestational diabetes during pregnancy, the good news is that it is one of the most preventable on the list of pregnancy complications. Your healthcare provider will test you for gestational diabetes sometime around the twenty-eighth week, especially if you have these risk factors:

- A family history of diabetes

- Greater than healthy weight gain for your body type

- Gestational diabetes in a previous pregnancy

If your healthcare provider presents you with this diagnosis, first be sure that this is based on the proper blood tests and not just an oral glucose tolerance test (read about which blood tests to get, page 211).

How to prevent and control gestational diabetes. Here's our five-step program for preventing and controlling gestational diabetes:

1. Eat real foods, especially the top twelve pregnancy superfoods (see page 29).

2. Graze according to the rule of twos: eat twice as often, eat half as much at a time, chew twice as long, and take twice the time to dine. (Read about

the blood sugar benefits of grazing on page 21.)

3. Gain the amount of weight that's right for you and baby (see page 51).

4. Move! (Reread chapter 5 for information on how movement keeps your blood sugar and blood insulin levels from spiking too high.)

5. Reduce stress. Unresolved stress raises stress hormones, which raise blood sugar. (Review the stressbusters on page 75.)

While most mothers can either prevent or control gestational diabetes using these five methods, if your blood sugar remains too high, your doctor may prescribe medication to keep your blood sugar in the optimal range. The reason your healthcare provider will screen you carefully for high blood sugar is that the longer your blood sugar remains too high, the higher your risk of complications, such as:

- An extra-large baby, prolonged labor, and a more complicated birth

- An increased chance of cesarean

- An increased chance of baby developing low blood sugar or hypoglycemia within hours after birth

- An increased chance of baby developing obesity and blood sugar problems as a child

- An increased chance of developing gestational diabetes in your next pregnancy

- An increased chance of developing type II diabetes later in adulthood

Remember an important health tip we emphasized in our Healthy Pregnancy Plan in Part I: *stable insulin levels* are three magic words for a healthier mother and baby and a less complicated delivery. Gestational diabetes is much like type II diabetes, both of which can usually be prevented and controlled by making healthier diet and lifestyle choices. Blood sugar levels usually return to normal right after delivery.

TYPE 1 DIABETES

Being pregnant may be just the motivation a mother needs to get her type 1 diabetes under control. Uncontrolled diabetes during pregnancy can lead to:

- Prematurity

- Miscarriage

- A large baby and difficult delivery

- Newborn hypoglycemia

- An increased chance of needing a cesarean

- Birth defects

The good news is that many women with type I diabetes deliver healthy babies. But because the normal hormonal fluctuations of pregnancy often require diabetic mothers to take more insulin during pregnancy, stabilizing insulin levels becomes even more challenging — yet more necessary — than before you were pregnant. To help you control your diabetes as best you can, try these tips:

Select the right doctors. Consult your diabetes specialist about management while pregnant, since the complications of diabetes, such as kidney problems and high blood pressure, can increase during pregnancy. Select an obstetrician who specializes in challenging pregnancies. Your doctor will go over a program of blood sugar regulation and insulin usage. To help control your diabetes and increase your chances of having a healthy delivery and healthy baby, your obstetrician may partner with a perinatologist, who has extra training in caring for mothers with complicated pregnancies or where problems are anticipated at birth. The perinatologist may co-manage a mother's labor and delivery along with her regular obstetrician. If your diabetes is difficult to control during your pregnancy, it is wise to birth your baby in a hospital with a neonatal intensive care unit.

Read Part I of this book. It's especially important for you to follow the diet and lifestyle tips given in chapters 2 through 6. This advice could have been entitled "Tips for Diabetes Control during Pregnancy." While these tips are necessary for all pregnant women, they are even more necessary for mothers with diabetes.

While insulin doesn't cross the placenta, blood sugar does. So if your blood sugar is too high, baby will be overdosed with sugar and required to produce more insulin to handle the extra sugar. The extra insulin stores the excess sugar as fat, and this accounts for the large size of babies born to mothers with diabetes.

Because newborns of diabetic mothers are often born in a state of high blood sugar, which may fall quickly after birth (known as neonatal hypoglycemia), they need to be monitored for blood sugar in a special care nursery for the first day or two after birth.

It is particularly important to control diabetes in the first month of pregnancy, when baby's organs are developing, and during the last month, when the risk of prematurity and neonatal hypoglycemia is highest. Be especially diligent during the week prior to delivery; this will increase the chances of your baby being born with more stable blood sugar.

While infants of mothers with diabetes have a greater chance of being premature, your doctor may elect to do a preterm induction ahead of your due date, since uncontrolled diabetes can affect the blood vessels of the uterus so that they become insufficient to nourish a baby.

HELLP SYNDROME

This syndrome is a severe form of preeclampsia. The diagnosis is made by the following blood test indicators, which led to this acronym: **h**emolysis (the breakdown of red blood cells), **e**levated **l**iver enzymes, and **l**ow **p**latelet count (the blood cells involved in clotting). This unusual complication of preeclampsia requires hospitalization for blood pressure monitoring and blood tests, and nearly always results in elective preterm delivery. The abnormalities in platelets, blood cells, liver enzymes, and blood pressure return to normal shortly after delivery.

HEPATITIS B

It's important for mothers to be tested for hepatitis B during pregnancy since women can carry the virus but not have any symptoms and, therefore, not know they are infected. Hepatitis can be transmitted from an infected mother to her baby during birth, since baby is exposed to mother's blood and body fluids. (The placenta protects baby during pregnancy.)

Newborn infection with this virus is preventable with detection and treatment, yet if undetected or untreated, baby may get infected, become a hepatitis B carrier, and go on to develop chronic liver disease. If you do test positive, your newborn will be given a shot of the hepatitis B immunoglobulin within a few hours of delivery and the hepatitis B vaccine prior to discharge from the hospital.

SHOULD BABIES ROUTINELY GET THE HEPATITIS B VACCINE?

Some healthcare providers believe that all newborns should routinely be given the hepatitis B vaccine within a day or two of delivery, followed up by two booster shots by the baby's primary care doctor within the next six months. Giving hepatitis B vaccine to healthy newborns whose mothers test negative for hepatitis B is controversial. We believe that the hepatitis B vaccine should not be given routinely to a newborn if the mother tests negative. There is little medical reason to give every newborn the hepatitis B vaccine. Doctors like to give the shot while baby is in the hospital in case mother doesn't bring baby back for routine vaccines. Obviously, this isn't true for most parents. Also, we and other doctors have seen many newborns develop a fever shortly after getting the hepatitis B injection. Fever in a newborn is a serious concern requiring blood tests and prolonged hospitalization because of the uncertainty of whether the fever is due to a reaction to the shot or baby has acquired another type of unrelated infection. Because newborns do not have strong enough immune systems to fight bacterial infections, they are often given antibiotics while waiting forty-eight hours for the culture reports. To avoid opening up the baby — and the doctor — to this therapeutic and diagnostic dilemma, many healthcare providers have stopped recommending routine hepatitis B vaccines to newborns of mothers who test negative. Instead, they give the three doses of hepatitis B vaccine at the two-month, four-month, and six-month checkups, or according to the current vaccine schedule recommended by the American Academy of Pediatrics.

Since some hospitals give the first hepatitis B shot while baby is still in the hospital without discussing it with the parents, here is our recommendation: If you test negative for hepatitis B, make it known to the nurses, and be sure it's recorded in your chart, that *you do not wish your baby to get the routine hepatitis B vaccine.* Let the medical staff know that instead you will get the hepatitis B vaccine in your doctor's office according to the schedule that your doctor judges is right for your baby. If you don't let your requests be known, you run the risk of your baby getting the hepatitis B vaccine as a newborn without your consent.

HIGH-RISK PREGNANCY

We prefer the term "high-responsibility" pregnancy. Our term goes beyond using specialized medical care and a high-tech hospital; it implies that *you* must take greater responsibility for your own care and your own birth decisions. Instead of resigning yourself to the high-risk label, becoming a passive patient, and leaving all birth decisions up to your doctors, become a high-responsibility mother. Take an even more active role in your birth partnership; cooperation between you and your care providers is essential. You need to be more informed and more involved in decision-making than the average mother, and you need to take better care of yourself. The first question you should ask your doctor after you are classified as high-risk is what specific things you can do to lower that risk.

The label "high-risk" is unnecessarily scary. Hearing the term naturally makes you wonder, "Risk of what?" "High-risk" is just a medical term that obstetricians use to describe mothers who have a higher than average risk of experiencing health problems during their pregnancy or birth, or of delivering a baby with issues. Common risk factors are insulin-dependent diabetes, high blood pressure, or signs of premature labor. Remember, this term reflects only a statistical probability that a problem may occur in your pregnancy or with your baby; it is not an absolute prediction, and you, in fact, may have no problems at all.

HYPEREMESIS GRAVIDARUM

This scary term simply means that your nausea and vomiting in early pregnancy are so persistent and severe that you get dizzy, weak, and dehydrated, often requiring temporary hospitalization for intravenous rehydration. Certainly, contact your healthcare provider if you find that, despite all the natural methods you've tried, your vomiting is getting worse, or you're feeling increasingly dry, weak, and lightheaded. A few hours of intravenous rehydration and complete rest of the intestines in the outpatient department of a hospital may be just what your wretched intestines need.

If you are experiencing the following signs of dehydration, call your doctor:

- You're urinating less and your urine appears darker in color.

- Your mouth, skin, and eyes feel dry.

- You feel increasingly tired.

- You become lightheaded and your thinking is foggy.

- You feel increasingly weak and faint.

- You haven't been able to keep any food or drink down for twenty-four hours.

INCOMPETENT CERVIX

This is another one of those not-so-nice medical terms that simply means that your cervical muscles are unable to hold your baby inside long enough. When the cervix begins to dilate and thin out prematurely, there is a risk of miscarriage or premature delivery. This may result from a congenital weakness in the cervix or from extreme stretching from previous deliveries or cervical surgery. Incompetent cervix occurs in varying degrees in 1 to 2 percent of all pregnancies, yet with proper diagnosis and management, most mothers go on to deliver healthy babies. Cervical incompetence may be diagnosed during a miscarriage, during a routine examination for spotting or bleeding, or after premature passing of the mucous plug. If cervical incompetence is suspected, your doctor may elect to perform a cervical cerclage, which involves suturing the cervix to keep it closed. Whether or not cervical suturing is needed depends on whether the ultrasound or visual vaginal exam shows that the cervix is opening prematurely. Suturing is usually done around the eighteenth or twentieth week of pregnancy, and the sutures are removed close to the due date. In addition to performing a cerclage, your healthcare provider may recommend bed rest and medication should contractions begin prematurely. About 25 percent of women with cervical incompetence will deliver prematurely, but the majority of these babies are healthy.

INTRAUTERINE GROWTH RESTRICTION (IUGR)

Your healthcare provider may suspect that your baby is not growing optimally based on measurements of the growth of your uterus during routine prenatal visits. This suspicion can be confirmed by ultrasound. If you have none of the risk factors for IUGR — smoking, excessive alcohol or drug use, undernutrition — IUGR may be due to insufficient placental nourishment, which might happen for no apparent reason. Although rare, IUGR could indicate a genetic

problem. If your healthcare provider suspects IUGR, it's likely that he will carefully review your eating habits, overall health, lifestyle, stress level, and any other habits that could affect your baby's growth. Your healthcare provider will carefully review these factors in case there are things you could be doing to boost your baby's growth. Another reason that it's important to know about IUGR before birth is that it alerts the medical team to take proper precautions after the baby is born. Due to less than optimal body fat, babies with IUGR have difficulty maintaining stable body temperature and are prone to unstable blood sugars. These babies are likely to need a couple of days of observation in a special care nursery. In addition, after birth it's important for mother to get extra breastfeeding help to be sure baby gets adequate nutrition for catch-up growth.

MISCARRIAGE: FEARING AND GRIEVING

You may find yourself checking for bleeding or spotting every time you go to the bathroom. This is a normal reaction for women who have had previous miscarriages.

Why do miscarriages occur?

At least half of all early miscarriages (those occurring before twelve weeks) are due to chromosomal abnormalities in the fetus so severe that growth cannot continue. Your body's immune system recognizes this genetic problem and triggers a miscarriage. Other less common causes of early miscarriages include infections, hormonal deficiencies (especially progesterone), rare immune system abnormalities (e.g., mother makes antibodies against the placental tissue), and exposure to environmental toxins, drugs, or cigarette smoke.

Late miscarriages (those occurring after twelve weeks) are more likely to be due to structural abnormalities of the uterus (for example, a uterus divided by a wall of tissue) than genetic abnormalities in the baby. Fortunately, these abnormalities affect less than 1 percent of women. Other causes of late miscarriages are abnormal attachment of placenta, uterine fibroids (benign tumors), an incompetent cervix, or infections. For around a third of all miscarriages, the cause is unknown. Miscarriages are *not* caused by sexual intercourse, safe exercises, heavy lifting, hanging pictures, doing your usual amount of work and play, a minor fall or accident, or stress or emotional upsets.

When are miscarriages most likely to occur?

Most miscarriages occur before the eighth week of pregnancy. As your pregnancy progresses, the chance of miscarrying decreases.

How common are miscarriages?

Most pregnancies begin with a healthy fetus, growing in a normal uterus, and result in a healthy baby. Studies have shown that around 10 percent of confirmed pregnancies end in miscarriage. However, an unusually heavy, late menstrual period may indicate a pregnancy and very early miscarriage. Therefore, the general figure for miscarriages is thought to be closer to 20 percent.

Is there anything a mother can do to lower her chances of miscarrying?

In most cases there is nothing you can do to prevent miscarriage, as most miscarriages are caused by factors outside your control. There are, however, a few things that might help: give your baby a healthy womb environment by following the guidelines in our Healthy Pregnancy Plan, pages 9–104; refrain from smoking (even exposure to secondhand smoke puts you at higher risk for having a miscarriage), harmful drugs, and excessive alcohol; and avoid exposure to environmental toxins.

If you have had several miscarriages, your doctor will probably want to do special tests to see whether a cause can be found. In many cases, she can help you achieve a pregnancy that goes to term. Structural abnormalities can be corrected by surgery. Hormone deficiency can often be compensated for by hormone therapy. Medical science has solutions for many of the common — and not so common — causes of repeated miscarriage.

How will I know if I had or am about to have a miscarriage?

These are the signs that a miscarriage has occurred or is under way:

• Bleeding, either bright red or dark brown, depending on how recently the miscarriage began. As many as 20 percent of women with healthy pregnancies may have one or two episodes of spotting or light vaginal bleeding early in pregnancy, so a bloody discharge from the vagina does not necessarily mean that a miscarriage has occurred or will occur. Bleeding that is as heavy as a menstrual period or that continues for several days is more likely to be associated with a miscarriage.

- Cramping abdominal pain, similar to menstrual pains, and/or a low backache.

Late miscarriage is more obvious than early miscarriage. The bleeding is heavier and often includes the passage of clots. Uterine contractions can become very intense. Sometimes these signs and symptoms signal an impending miscarriage — called a "threatened miscarriage" — rather than a completed one. In general, the longer the bleeding occurs and the greater the accompanying symptoms of pain, the more likely the pregnancy will end in miscarriage. If you suspect a threatened miscarriage, your doctor will, of course, do a vaginal exam. (This exam does not increase the chances of a miscarriage.) By using repeated ultrasound examinations and by monitoring the HCG hormone level in your blood, your doctor can determine whether this pregnancy is likely to continue or end in a miscarriage. If ultrasound examinations show that baby is growing and the hormone levels stay high, chances are high that the pregnancy will continue.

What should I do if I suspect I'm having a miscarriage?

Call your healthcare provider immediately, especially if you are passing clots or grayish-pink tissue. If your bleeding is heavy and persistent or your pelvic pains intensify, go to your nearest emergency room. (Try to collect what has come out in a jar. It can be examined to determine whether the genetic makeup of the baby is normal, and also the sex of the baby.)

If you suspect you have miscarried, your practitioner will perform a vaginal examination or ultrasound to determine whether the miscarriage is complete (i.e., you have passed the fetus and the supporting tissues) or incomplete (i.e., some of it still remains in your uterus). Miscarriages that occur prior to eight weeks are usually complete. The later in pregnancy a miscarriage occurs, the more likely it is to be incomplete. If your healthcare provider determines that your miscarriage is incomplete, she will probably want you to have a D&C (dilation and curettage). Since there are many other reasons for vaginal bleeding, *your doctor should do an ultrasound to confirm the diagnosis of miscarriage before doing a D&C.* You may need to request this. In a D&C, while you are under general or local anesthesia, your cervix will be dilated and any retained placenta will be removed from the uterus. During this procedure the doctor may attempt to determine the possible cause of the miscarriage by examining your uterus for any structural abnormalities.

I'm so glad I had an ultrasound before I had a D&C because the ultrasound showed the problem was placenta previa and not a miscarriage. I think of this now as I hold my baby in my arms — what might have happened if they had acted on a misdiagnosis?

If you have not miscarried, your doctor or midwife may monitor you with ultrasound and blood tests.

If I have already had one miscarriage, does that mean I am more likely to have another?

Not necessarily. If this was your first known miscarriage, your risk of having a second one is only slightly higher than if you had never had a miscarriage, especially if your first miscarriage showed a chromosomal abnormality or occurred very early in pregnancy, or you have previously given birth to a healthy baby. Even after experiencing two miscarriages, your chances of having a third one are not much higher than if you had never had one. If you have had two miscarriages, you have a 65 percent chance of carrying your next baby to term; a woman who has never miscarried or who has had only one miscarriage has roughly an 80 percent chance of carrying to term. After three miscarriages, however, your chances of carrying your next baby to term go down to 50 percent. After three consecutive miscarriages, you would be wise to have a complete obstetrical evaluation to see whether there are any underlying medical reasons that could cause you to have future miscarriages. If no reason can be found, you may reasonably assume that you still have an excellent chance of carrying a baby to term.

It's important to do all you can to work through your feelings and not let the visions of your previous miscarriage dampen the joy of your present pregnancy. Even so, some women who have had multiple miscarriages report not being able to fully overcome their fear until the moment they hold their healthy baby in their arms. It's normal for a woman who has experienced previous miscarriages to want to keep the news of her pregnancy private as long as possible (at least past the point when the previous miscarriage

occurred), for fear of having to go through the trauma of "untelling." She may even subconsciously suppress her excitement, delay choosing names, and even wait until the very last minute to decorate baby's nursery. It's important to bond with your baby in the womb even when you face the risk of losing your baby. While it's normal to fear that this pregnancy may also end in a miscarriage, chances are greater than not that you will go on to give birth to a healthy baby. It is our belief that both the very young infant in the womb and the mother of that infant need that sense of belonging, to honor the life they share. We believe that it benefits both of them during the pregnancy, no matter how brief it may turn out to be.

I'm afraid to get my hopes up for fear of losing you before you are born. I have been afraid to get to know you for fear I will lose you, because I have already lost one baby. But I know that I'm only cheating both of us out of the joy of bonding.

Grieving after a miscarriage. People who have never had a miscarriage may not understand the loss of a pregnancy. Their attitude may be "It's no big deal; you can have another baby." But for you it is a very big deal, and it may take a long time to get over it. Everyone celebrates the news of a pregnancy, but few know how to acknowledge and help to grieve the end of one. It may help to name the baby you've lost if you haven't already and have a private time of saying "We'll always remember you." Don't immediately try to "replace" this baby with another before you have worked through the grieving process and can truly let this baby go. Discuss with your practitioner when you can safely try to conceive again.

PLACENTA PROBLEMS: PLACENTA PREVIA, PLACENTA ACCRETA, PLACENTA ABRUPTIO

Placenta Previa. Sometimes a normal placenta develops in an abnormal location and partially or completely covers the cervix. Called placenta previa, this quirk occurs in around 1 out of 200 pregnancies. With *marginal* placenta previa, the edge of the placenta is near the margin of the cervix. As the uterus grows, the low-lying placenta may move away from the cervix and present no problem. If the placenta partially or totally covers the cervical opening — preventing a vaginal delivery — baby will probably require a surgical birth. Placenta previa is usually discovered early in pregnancy on a routine ultrasound. If it's simply a low-lying placenta or marginal placenta previa, it's important that mother approach this finding as "no problem, no worry," since the placenta can migrate upward away from the cervix as the uterus grows. Sometimes placenta previa is suspected when a woman has painless bleeding anytime during the second half of pregnancy, especially during the final month. Your healthcare provider may prescribe bed rest or limited activity if there is a danger of bleeding, since the goal of treating placenta previa is to prevent bleeding and lower the risk of premature delivery. Health-threatening bleeding from placenta previa is uncommon, especially if the precautions recommended by your healthcare provider are followed. Mothers who have placenta previa have a slightly increased chance of having it again, a complication your healthcare provider will be alerted to.

Placenta Accreta. In this rare condition (occurring in approximately 1 in 2,500 pregnancies) the placenta attaches so deeply to the wall of the uterus that it doesn't automatically detach during delivery, and it needs to be removed surgically after delivery. The risk of placenta accreta increases if you've needed a surgical birth for previous placenta problems.

Placenta Abruptio. This placental problem occurs in slightly less than 1 percent of pregnancies and is most commonly detected in the third trimester. In this condition the placenta partially or completely detaches from the uterine wall before or during labor. Here are the clues to this problem:

- Sudden onset of profuse bleeding

- Sudden onset of unusual back or abdominal pain

- Uterus is unusually tender when examined by your healthcare provider

While ultrasound may detect the separating placenta, often it does not. Premature separation of the placenta is usually a medical emergency, requiring emergency delivery if the baby's blood supply is compromised or bleeding continues. If this problem is suspected, your doctor will probably put you in the hospital and monitor your baby's well-being and the degree of bleeding. If the bleeding stops, you are not in labor, and baby is in no distress, your doctor may recommend bed rest at home. If only a slight placental separation occurs and baby is in no distress, a vaginal birth may be possible. Yet, if the bleeding continues or baby's health is threatened, emergency cesarean may be performed. If abruption of the placenta occurs, there is an increased chance that it will recur in subsequent pregnancies, and your healthcare provider will monitor you closely.

PREECLAMPSIA

Also known as pregnancy-induced hypertension, preeclampsia occurs in around 7 percent of all pregnancies and is most likely to occur later on in pregnancy. It is most common in first pregnancies. Risk factors for preeclampsia include carrying multiples, previous history of high blood pressure, and diabetes. Your healthcare provider is likely to make this diagnosis if you have:

- Protein detected in your urine test

- Extreme swelling of hands, face, and ankles

- High blood pressure

- Headaches and blurred vision

- A sudden spurt in weight gain (more than 2 pounds in a week or 6 pounds in a month) due to excessive retention of fluids

The most important goal for you and your healthcare provider is to control your blood pressure, since untreated, prolonged high blood pressure can compromise uterine blood flow, leading to premature delivery. In fact, because of the increased risk of compromised blood flow to the baby, healthcare providers often elect to do a preterm induction or surgical birth. If mother's high blood pressure can't be managed with relaxation and bed rest, the doctor may give intravenous medications to lower the blood pressure and increase uterine blood flow.

The high blood pressure of preeclampsia nearly always returns to normal within a few weeks after delivery. Keep in mind that once you've had preeclampsia, your chances of having it in subsequent pregnancies are low. One of the best home remedies to control blood pressure and prevent preeclampsia is to follow the diet and lifestyle tips of the Healthy Pregnancy Plan in Part I.

PREMATURE LABOR: BIRTHING A PRETERM BABY

Around 90 percent of mothers carry their babies to maturity, defined as thirty-seven weeks or more. With the increasing availability of expert neonatal care units, even the majority of premature babies do quite well. While some of the causes of premature birth are due to quirks beyond your control, such as placental abnormalities, structural problems in the uterus, uterine fibroids, early rupture of the membranes, an incompetent cervix, or multiple births, there are many diet and lifestyle choices that you can make to greatly lower your chances of delivering a baby prematurely. Among them:

- Don't smoke.

- Don't take illegal drugs.

- Get good prenatal care.

- Gain the optimal weight for you.

- Reduce prolonged, unresolved stress.

The best way to lower your chances of birthing your baby prematurely is to faithfully follow the Healthy Pregnancy Plan in Part I.

Even though 37 weeks is the current norm for "maturity," recent studies show that an extra two weeks matures baby's brain development. These findings are prompting many birthcare providers to consider 39 weeks as a healthier definition of maturity.

To become an informed and valuable member of the medical team caring for your premature baby, read *The Premature Baby Book: Everything You Need to Know about Your Premature Baby from Birth to Age One* (William Sears and Martha Sears). Also see *Hold Your Premie: A Workbook on Skin-to-Skin Contact for Parents of Premature Babies* (see resources, page 426).

RH INCOMPATIBILITY

Early in your pregnancy, your healthcare provider will test your blood to see whether you are Rh positive or Rh negative. Eighty-five percent of mothers are Rh positive. This percentage is slightly higher among African Americans, and nearly all Asians are Rh positive. If you are Rh positive, you do not need to be concerned. If you are Rh negative, you will need some special care. The Rh factor is a protein on the surface of red blood cells. You and your baby inherit genes that make these cells either have this Rh factor protein (Rh positive) or not (Rh negative). If your blood type is Rh negative and baby's father is Rh positive, baby could have Rh-positive blood, and some of the baby's Rh-positive blood can leak into your circulation during pregnancy, at birth, or following a miscarriage. Consequently, your immune system will interpret these Rh-positive cells as "foreign" and produce antibodies against the Rh factor in baby's blood. This leads to breakdown of these blood cells, causing anemia in baby. Even though Rh incompatibility sometimes does not present a problem in the first pregnancy, RhoGAM (see below) is usually still given at 28 weeks even in these first pregnancies if the father's blood type is either Rh positive or unknown.

If you test Rh negative and baby's father is also Rh negative, you needn't be concerned. If baby's father is Rh positive, your healthcare provider will monitor your Rh status. If you tested Rh negative early in a subsequent pregnancy, your doctor will test for Rh antibodies around the seventh month of your pregnancy.

Around twenty-eight weeks, if an Rh incompatibility is suspected, your healthcare provider will give you an intramuscular injection of a vaccine called Rh immunoglobulin (RhoGAM) to keep you from forming Rh-positive cells and antibodies to them. This also keeps the antibodies from crossing over into baby. If within a couple of days after birth baby tests Rh positive, baby may also be given an injection of RhoGAM. If an Rh incompatibility is suspected, RhoGAM is also given following a miscarriage if you are Rh negative to reduce the chances of your body and your next baby being sensitized to the Rh factor.

Dr. Bill notes: Before we had such diligent prenatal monitoring and the use of RhoGAM, babies affected with Rh antibodies would often need blood transfusions, which, fortunately, is now rarely necessary.

Besides Rh incompatibility, there are a few other rare incompatibilities. This is why you will have your blood type and antibody screens checked during routine prenatal tests.

Resources for a Healthier Pregnancy

Books

The Baby Book: Everything You Need to Know about Your Baby — From Birth to Age Two, by William Sears, Martha Sears, Robert Sears, and James Sears (Little, Brown, revised edition 2013). This useful companion to *The Healthy Pregnancy Book* begins with information about the postpartum period and is especially helpful in getting parents off to the right start with their newborns.

The Portable Pediatrician: Everything You Need to Know about Your Child's Health, by William Sears, Martha Sears, Robert Sears, and James Sears (Little, Brown, 2011). This book features timely and practical information on every childhood illness and emergency, including when to call the doctor, what reassuring signs can help you know your child is OK, how to treat your child at home, and much more — all in a convenient A-to-Z format.

The Birth Book: Everything You Need to Know to Have a Safe and Satisfying Birth, by William Sears and Martha Sears (Little, Brown, 1994). This book discusses events leading up to and surrounding birth and contains many birth stories to illustrate a wide variety of labors.

Baby on the Way, by William Sears, Martha Sears, and Christie Watts Kelly (Little, Brown, 2001). A short picture book to introduce baby to siblings during pregnancy.

Becoming a Father: How to Nurture and Enjoy Your Family (The Growing Family Series), by William Sears (La Leche League International, 2003). A collection of Dr. Bill's fathering tips on being the best dad you can be.

The Breastfeeding Book, by Martha Sears and William Sears (Little, Brown, 2000). Everything you need to know about nursing your child from birth through weaning.

Father's First Steps: 25 Things Every New Dad Should Know, by Robert W. Sears and James M. Sears (Harvard Common Press, 2006).

Gentle Birth, Gentle Mothering: A Doctor's Guide to Natural Childbirth and Gentle Early Parenting Choices, by Sarah J. Buckley, MD (Celestial Arts, 2009). This is one of the most scientifically referenced and informative books on pregnancy and parenting. We recommend it for expectant parents who want to be more empowered in their pregnancy and birthing choices.

The Hormonal Physiology of Childbearing, by Sarah J. Buckley, MD (Childbirth Connection, 2013). A scholarly text giving detailed explanations of the hormonal physiology of birth.

Hold Your Premie, by Jill and Nils Bergman (2010). Available from Geddes Productions, www.GeddesProduction .com. A must-read book on how parents can help their premature baby thrive; valuable tips on baby brain development.

A Child Is Born, by Lennart Nilsson (Jonathan Cape, fifth edition, 2010). This book is a masterpiece of fetal photography from one of the world's leading medical and scientific photographers. It takes expectant couples on a photographic journey from fertilization to delivery and helps them appreciate the miracle that is happening inside the mother's body.

The Joy of Natural Childbirth, by Helen Wessel (Bookmates International, fifth edition, 1994). This classic book portrays birth from a biblical perspective.

Childbirth without Fear: The Principles and Practice of Natural Childbirth, by Grantly Dick-Read (Pinter and Martin, 2013). This classic helps laboring mothers break the fear-tension-pain cycle.

Birthing from Within: An Extra-Ordinary Guide to Childbirth Preparation, by Pam England (Partera Press, 1998). A midwife's series of birthing classes to empower mothers to make wise birth choices.

Pregnancy, Childbirth, and the Newborn: The Complete Guide, by Penny Sinkin (Meadowbrook, 2010). Written by an experienced doula, this book helps mothers through a wide variety of birth choices.

25 Things Every New Mother Should Know, by Martha Sears with William Sears (Harvard Common Press, 2005).

DVDs

Grow Your Baby's Brain, by Jill and Nils Bergman, available from Geddes Productions, www.GeddesProduction.com. Shows what parents and birthcare providers can do at birth and in the newborn period to help babies grow smarter.

Relaxation Music

Heartstrings, by Jason and Nolan Livesay, available at iTunes. Music composed by the artist to help his wife relax during her pregnancy and the birth of their first child, the Searses' sixth grandchild.

Educational Materials

L.E.A.N. Expectations. Online interactive workshops that teach expectant mothers the best health and nutrition habits for their family. Examine this prenatal course at DrSearsWellnessInstitute.org.

Geddes Productions, www.Geddes Production.com. Peruse this website and you will find a list of insightful books and DVDs on getting the best start with your baby immediately at and after birth. We personally know many of the authors and highly recommend their instructional resources.

Attachment Parenting International (API), AttachmentParenting.org. By joining this network of like-minded and experienced parents, you will find tools and resources to help you get the best start with your baby and find an AP support group.

Apple Tree Family Ministries, www .appletreefamily.org. Biblically based education about God's design in pregnancy, childbirth, breastfeeding, and early parenting.

Professional Labor Assistants

Doulas of North America, DONA.org. A resource to help find a labor support person in your area.

Breastfeeding

La Leche League International (LLLI), LaLecheLeague.org. The most experienced and trusted resource and support group for breastfeeding mothers.

Baby Carriers

Balboa Baby, BalboaBaby.com. A collection of baby carriers, nursing pillows, and other helpful items that babies love and make life easier for parents.

Bedside Sleepers

Arm's Reach Co-Sleeper, ArmsReach.com. A must-have bedside bassinet that enables baby and mother to sleep close to each other for easier nighttime comforting and feeding, yet allows each to have their own bed space.

Resources for Twins and Multiples

National Organization of Mothers of Twins Clubs: nomotc.org. A mother-to-mother network providing valuable resources and support to parents of multiples.

Down Syndrome

National Down Syndrome Society, ndss.org. The National Down Syndrome Society is the national advocate for the value, acceptance, and inclusion of people with Down syndrome.

National Down Syndrome Congress, ndsccenter.org. Provides information, resources, support, and education, as well as teaching advocacy and networking opportunities.

Additional Online Resources

Coalition for Improving Maternity Services (CIMS): www.motherfriendly.org.

"Our Moment of Truth." From the American College of Nurse Midwives, this article discusses midwifery care with information for consumers. Free document available for download at: ourmomentoftruth.midwife.org.

"Birth in Action." A DVD from Dr. BJ Snell that incorporates preparation for birth and includes her birth center: www.midwife .org/Birth-in-Action-An-Autobiographical-Documentary-of-One-Family-s-Journey.

"Perineal Massage in Pregnancy." A handout from the *Journal of Midwifery & Women's Health,* Volume 50, No. 1, January/February 2005. Available free online at: onlinelibrary.wiley.com/ doi/10.1016/j.jmwh.2004.09.013/pdf.

Safe Seafood Sources

www.Vitalchoice.com, our top choice for wild seafood

www.MontereyBayAquarium.org, a trusted educational resource for updates on safe and sustainable seafood

Acknowledgments

The biggest "thank you" goes to the mothers in our practices who shared their pregnancy and birth stories and became our "board of advisers" for how to write this book. A special thanks to our literary adviser, Denise Marcil, and to our editor, Tracy Behar, and copyeditors Peggy Freudenthal and Karen Wise, for their diligent advice on how to improve this book. We also thank Tracee Zeni, our dedicated assistant of twenty-five years. And thanks to our LEAN Expectations coaches, especially Lisa Devine, for giving us valuable feedback from their students on what pregnant mothers like to read. Thanks also for Kathy Nesper's help in fine-tuning our sections on childbirth education for parents. And last, and most, we thank our own children for the birth memories we cherish.

Index

abdominal discomfort, 115, 155

abdominal muscles separating, 228

acupressure, 123

adrenaline, 97, 326–27, 336

air travel, 229–32

alcohol use, 4, 90, 92–93

allergies, 15, 27, 30, 178–79

American College of Nurse-Midwives, 136, 139, 242–43

American Congress of Obstetricians and Gynecologists (ACOG), 93, 135, 140, 156, 242–43, 272, 278–79

amniocentesis, 155, 156, 210, 401

amniotic fluid, 228, 338, 345

analgesics, 104, 282, 291, 307–09, 312

anemia, 179, 406–07

anesthesia, 281, 348. *See also* epidurals

anxiety

  in first month, 111–12

  Bradley Method and, 139

  due date and, 126

  electronic fetal monitoring and, 269

  fear-tension-pain cycle, 235, 306–07, 326, 363, 365

  labor and, 137, 349, 361

  miscarriages and, 112, 166–67, 174

  pain-management techniques and, 294–95, 297, 300

  what-ifs, 259–60

aspartame, 83, 94–95

attachment parenting, 395–96

Attachment Parenting Book, The (William Sears and Martha Sears), 396

Attachment Parenting International, 234, 396

Baby Book, The (William Sears, Martha Sears, Robert Sears, and James Sears), 387, 396

baby kicking

  in fifth month, 199–200

  in sixth month, 218–19

  in seventh month, 258

  in eighth month, 289, 290–91

  in ninth month, 342

  children feeling, 205, 206, 218, 291

  fathers and, 209, 218, 219, 258

  quickening, 175

  sleep difficulties and, 80

Baby on the Way (William Sears, Martha Sears, and Christie Watts Kelly), 128, 205

backache, 166, 222–25, 258, 315, 358

balance, 61, 65, 257, 342

bed rest, 407–12

belly button changes, 204

Bergman, Jill, 328, 335

Bergman, Nils, 328, 329, 330, 335

beta strep infection, 359, 412

beverages, 43, 44–45, 56, 64, 67, 80, 98

birth attendants, 130, 133, 238, 277–78, 329, 330

birth balls, 241, 354

Birth Book, The (Williams Sears and Martha Sears), 268

birth centers, 139, 240–42
birth defects
    excess weight gain and, 53
    genetic screening for, 155–56, 174, 401–03
    green environment and, 87–88, 90, 93, 100, 101, 114
    medications and, 104
    ultrasound and, 156
birthing bed, 239
birthing centers, 139–40, 364
birth plan, 262, 267–68, 294
birth stories, 111, 130, 208, 235, 259, 295, 349
birth team, 128–30, 135, 239
birth weight, 88, 89, 91, 92
bladder infections, 150
Blaylock, Russell, 17, 94
bleeding
    in second month, 154–55
    bloody show, 358, 376
    car accidents and, 234
    contacting healthcare provider about, 155, 364, 384, 385
    implantation, 109, 115, 127, 154
    miscarriages and, 419–20
    placenta previa and, 165
    postpartum care and, 384–85
    ultrasound for evaluation of, 156
bleeding gums, 177–78
bloating, 115, 151, 230, 341, 386
blood-brain barrier, 17, 41, 74, 94
blood clots, 37, 230
blood sugar
    exercise and, 59, 64
    feeling faint and, 179
    gestational diabetes and, 211
    grazing and, 21, 75, 180
    overdue and, 345
    pregnancy-induced nausea and, 117, 120–21
    sipping solution and, 23
blood tests, 106, 127, 134
blood vessels, 59–61
bloody show, 358, 376
body aches and pains. *See also* headaches
    in sixth month, 219–25
    in seventh month, 258
    in eighth month, 290
    in ninth month, 341–42
    backache, 166, 222–25, 258, 315, 358
    groin pains, 258
    joint pain, 53, 61, 64, 66

postpartum period, 383
    sleep difficulties and, 80
body fat
    grazing and, 21
    harmful chemicals stored in, 17–18
    high-fructose corn syrup and, 95
    postpartum body fat, 52
    preconception planning and, 6–7
    shedding excess "mommy fat," 53, 61
    sipping solution and, 23
    weight gain during pregnancy and, 52
bonding
    cesarean births and, 281–82
    childbirth classes and, 236
    children and, 206, 207
    delivery and, 375–76
    fathers and, 209, 281, 282
    fetal heartbeat and, 161–62, 176
    hormonal harmony and, 327–28, 329, 336
    knowing baby's gender and, 210
    labor and, 280
bone density, 61
BPA (bisphenol A), 98, 100, 101
Bradley Method, 138–39, 237–38, 260, 274
brain development
    in third month, 160
    in seventh month, 254
    in eighth month, 288
    alcohol use and, 93
    cholesterol-lowering drugs and, 104
    cigarette smoke and, 89
    fetal origin of diseases and, 12–13, 17
    food chemicals and, 94
    omega-3 fats and, 30–33
    organic foods and, 41
    premature pruning and, 94
    right-fat diet and, 19, 39
    seafood and, 29
bras, 149, 162–63
Braxton Hicks contractions
    in sixth month, 219
    in seventh month, 258–59
    in eighth month, 290
    in ninth month, 339
    massage during, 304
    oxytocin and, 324
    prelabor and, 358
    relaxation during, 290, 298, 342
breast changes, 115, 148–49, 162, 164–66, 204, 341
breastfeeding

afterpains and, 375
bonding and, 327–28, 329
breast changes and, 149
carpal tunnel syndrome and, 221–22
cesarean births and, 392
childbirth classes and, 236
choosing pediatrician and, 263, 266
cigarette smoke and, 91
colostrum, 204, 325, 388, 389
engorged breasts, 389–90
epidurals and, 314
hospitals and, 240
latch-on, 388, 389
lower-lip flip, 388, 390, 392
postpartum body fat and, 52
preventing allergies and, 27
prolactin and, 327, 336, 389
sore nipples, 390–91
special needs babies, 392–93
starter tips, 387–89
taste shaping and, 217
tongue-tie, 391–92
vegetarian diet and, 35
Breastfeeding Book, The (William Sears
    and Martha Sears), 387
breathing
    in seventh month, 255–56
    in eighth month, 289
    in ninth month, 342, 344
    Bradley Method and, 238
    deep breathing, 219
    imagery and, 299
    pain-management techniques and, 305–06
    shortness of breath, 256
    sleep and, 84
    stressbuster for, 76–77
breech position, 135, 272–74, 288–89, 371, 399

caffeine, 80, 96–97, 120
calcium, 29, 39, 48, 177, 221
calorie requirements, 26, 29, 47
cardiovascular disease, 12, 14–15, 95
carpal tunnel syndrome, 221–22
car travel, 100, 233–34
catecholamines, 326–27
cat-litter boxes, 99, 118
cell membranes, 17, 30, 324
cell phones, 99, 141
Centers for Disease Control and Prevention (CDC),
    14, 18, 231

cephalopelvic disproportion (CPD), 271–72, 276–77
cervix
    bloody show and, 358, 376
    dilation of, 291, 295, 302, 309, 313, 326, 347, 351,
        352, 359, 363, 366
    effacement of, 351–52, 361, 363, 376
    incompetent cervix, 417–18
    inducing labor and, 346
cesarean births. *See also* vaginal birth after
        cesarean (VBAC)
    breastfeeding and, 392
    childbirth philosophy and, 129
    cycle of, 275–76
    epidurals and, 317
    excess weight gain and, 53
    exercise and, 61, 281
    healing after, 280–81
    liability issues and, 269–70, 273
    making best of, 281–82
    prevention of, 274–76
    rate of, 135, 237, 241, 268–70, 274
    reasons for needing, 270–73
    scheduled, 278–79
    vitamin D and, 34
checkups with healthcare provider
    first-month visit, 106, 133–34
    second-month visit, 145
    third-month visit, 159
    fourth-month visit, 173
    fifth-month visit, 196, 211
    sixth-month visit, 216
    seventh-month visit, 252
    eighth-month visit, 287
    ninth-month visit, 337
    postpartum visit, 381
    preconception checkup, 5
childbirth. *See also* cesarean births; delivery; due
        date; labor; pain-management techniques;
        postpartum care
    birthcare reform, 273
    birth plan, 262, 267–68, 294
    complications of, 53, 61, 136, 137, 189
    descent, 352
    exercise and, 59, 61, 68–72
    increasing chances of vaginal birth, 274–76
    Kegel exercises, 68–70
    "natural" childbirth, 239
    packing and preparing for, 343–44
    pharmacological birth, 239, 241, 326, 331–35
    philosophy of, 129–30, 131, 132, 139, 235, 240

childbirth *(Cont.)*
  physiological birth, 239, 241, 326, 328, 331–35
  progress of, 351–52
  stretching exercises, 70–72
  technological interventions in, 135–36, 138, 239, 240, 241, 269
childbirth classes, 131, 138, 208, 234–38, 281, 307
childbirth educators, 235, 236–38, 239, 262
Childbirth without Fear (Dick-Read), 235, 306
children
  baby's heartbeat and, 161
  fatigue and, 149
  feeling baby kicking, 205, 206, 218, 291
  mothering while pregnant, 205–07, 340
  pregnancy announcement and, 128
chiropractic care, 166
chocolate, dark, 44, 58, 97, 124, 125, 150–51, 393
cholesterol-lowering drugs, 104
chromosomal abnormalities, 399, 400, 401, 402, 418
chronic illness, 4, 5
cigarette smoke, 4, 8, 88–92, 98, 116
clean fifteen, 41–42
clothing, 62, 64, 122–23, 151, 162, 180, 184, 226
Commission for the Accreditation of Birth Centers (CABC), 241
congestion, nasal, 178–79
constipation
  in second month, 150–51
  in ninth month, 341
  exercise and, 61, 151
  grazing as relief for, 20–21, 151
  greens and, 39
  postpartum care and, 386
  pregnancy-induced nausea and, 120
  prevention of, 227
  sipping solution and, 23, 150
contact lenses, 201
contraception methods, 3, 4
contractions. *See also* Braxton Hicks contractions; labor; pain-management techniques
  breathing during, 305–06
  car accidents and, 234
  length of, 300
  prelabor contractions, 359
  rest and release during, 298
  resting between, 296, 297, 298, 306, 347, 350, 351, 363, 367
  rhythm of, 301
  true contractions, 359–60
cord blood, 18, 88, 267

cortisol, 16, 57, 78, 82, 83, 326–27, 336
counterpressure, 292, 304
couvade syndrome, 228

dark chocolate, 44, 58, 97, 125, 150–51, 393
dehydration, 117–18, 120–21, 125, 150, 179, 232–33, 348
delivery
  bonding and, 375–76
  cortisol and, 326–27, 336
  crowning, 372, 374
  episiotomies and, 370–71, 372
  forceps or vacuum delivery, 273, 274, 365–66, 370, 371
  tissue healing, 37
dentist, 5, 161, 177–78
diabetes. *See also* gestational diabetes
  fetal origins of disease and, 13, 14, 16, 21
  high-fructose corn syrup and, 95
  planning for pregnancy and, 4
  preconception checkup and, 5
  sleep deprivation and, 79
  type 1, 414–15
diarrhea, 232–33, 358
Dick-Read, Grantly, 235, 306
Dick-Read, Jessica, 235
digestive problems, 23. *See also* bloating; constipation; heartburn
dilation, of cervix, 291, 295, 302, 309, 313, 326, 347, 351, 352, 359, 363, 366
dirty dozen, 41–42
dizziness, 63, 179–80, 231, 233, 385
doctor. *See* health-care provider
doulas, 131, 137, 138, 261–62
Down syndrome, 400–401, 402
dreams, 81–82
dropping (lightening), 289, 341, 358
Drugs in Pregnancy and Lactation (Briggs, Freeman, and Yaffe), 104
drug use, 4, 90, 92
dry cleaners, 99
dry eyes, 37, 201
due date
  accuracy of, 126
  checkups with healthcare provider and, 134
  conception dating, 125, 126
  menstrual dating, 125, 126
  overdue, 345–46
  simple do-it-yourself method, 126
  ultrasound dating, 126, 156, 345

eating habits. *See also* pregnancy superfoods
  childbirth classes and, 236
  eating outside, 122
  5-S diet, 44–45, 183, 280, 393
  grazing and, 6, 20–22, 55, 75, 103, 116,
    120–21
  labor and, 347–48, 355
  nutrition questions, 25–27
  optimal weight gain and, 54–58
  postpartum care and, 386–87, 393
  preconception planning and, 6
  prenatal supplements and, 22, 25, 26
  sipping solution, 22–23, 55, 121
  sleep and, 79, 83
  traffic-light eating, 35, 45–46
  white-out your diet, 44
ectopic pregnancy, 154
eggs, 39, 42, 83
electrolytes, 150, 220–21, 233, 348
electronic fetal monitoring (EFM)
  cesarean births and, 269, 275
  epidurals and, 311, 317
  healthcare provider's views on, 132
  hormonal harmony and, 331, 333
  intermittent, 347
  pitocin and, 333
  pushing stage and, 373
  rise in, 135
  telemetry and, 240, 347
  vaginal birth after cesarean and, 276
elevator (Kegel exercise), 69–70
emotional/physical issues. *See also* mood disorders;
    stress
  in first month, 110–16
  in second month, 148–54
  in third month, 162–64
  in fourth month, 175–79
  in fifth month, 198–99, 204–05
  in sixth month, 218–25
  in seventh month, 254–58
  in eighth month, 289–91
  in ninth month, 339–42
  advice and, 198–99
  exercise and, 61, 66, 75
  fetal origin of disease and, 16
  grazing and, 21
  mothering feeling, 204–05, 260
  omega-3 fats and, 32–33, 37
  postpartum period, 382–87
  preconception planning and, 4

sipping solution and, 23
sleep difficulties and, 81, 82
employment
  environmental toxins in, 100, 190
  fatigue and, 113, 149
  maternity leave, 111, 185, 186–90
  pregnancy announcement and, 128, 185–88
  working while pregnant, 185–91, 342–43
endocrine system, 12, 21
endorphins, 61, 292, 296–98, 316, 325–26, 349
endothelium, 59–61
energy level, 176, 254. *See also* fatigue
Environmental Health Perspectives, 99–100
environmental issues. *See* green environment
Environmental Working Group, 41, 101
epidurals
  administration of, 310–11
  cesarean births and, 268–69
  epi-lite, 312
  home births and, 244
  hormonal harmony and, 331, 332, 333
  pain-management techniques and, 309–17
  safety of, 314–17
  timing of, 313–14, 347, 368
  types of, 311–13
epigenetics, 9–10, 325–26
epinephrine, 78, 297, 326
episiotomies, 131, 138, 370–71, 372, 375, 384, 385
estrogen, 104, 109, 117, 152–53, 181, 201, 323–24, 339
excitotoxins, 17, 94
exercise
  anytime-anywhere exercises, 66
  for back, 225
  benefits of, 59–61
  cesarean-birth healing and, 61, 281
  childbirth classes and, 236
  clothing for, 62, 64
  constipation and, 61, 151
  for easier childbirth, 59, 61, 68–72
  failure to progress and, 275
  fathers and, 209
  for feet, 202, 220, 224, 257
  getting overheated, 68
  hemorrhoid prevention and, 227
  intensity level, 62–63
  internal medicines and, 59–61
  keeping off your back, 65
  Kegel exercises, 68–70, 227, 228, 371, 372
  knowing limits, 63, 67
  for leg cramps, 220–21

exercise *(Cont.)*
  leg-pumping exercises, 226, 230
  no-no exercises while pregnant, 65
  optimal weight gain and, 57, 61
  postpartum care and, 394
  precautions for, 64
  preconception planning and, 7-8
  self-help skills, 103
  sleep and, 61, 82
  stress and, 75, 77
  stretching exercises, 70-72
  swimming as ideal exercise, 66-67
  in third trimester, 63-64, 66
  tips for, 61-65
  twenty pregnancy perks of, 61
eyeglass prescription, 201
eyes. *See* vision

Facebook, 141
faintness, 63, 179-80, 231, 233, 385
fathers
  in first month, 118-19
  in second month, 153-54
  active labor and, 363, 365
  baby kicking and, 209, 218, 219, 258
  baby's heartbeat and, 161
  Bradley Method and, 237-38, 260
  cesarean births and, 281
  childbirth classes and, 236
  childbirth philosophy and, 129
  childcare and, 207
  delivery and, 330
  early labor and, 362
  fears of childbirth pain, 295
  feeling pregnant, 228
  involvement in pregnancy, 207-10
  labor coaches and, 260, 262
  massage and, 209, 223
  pregnancy announcement and, 127
  pregnancy-induced nausea and, 118
  prolactin and, 327
  sex and, 164-68, 259
  transition stage and, 367-68
fatigue, 23, 112-14, 115, 149, 219
fats, 33, 37, 42. *See also* omega-3 fats
FDA (Food and Drug Administration), 93, 94, 95, 314
fear. *See* anxiety
feet
  in fifth month, 201-02

  elevating, 179, 202, 220, 226, 230, 257
  exercises for, 202, 220, 224, 257
  massage, 202, 304
fertility, 3, 4, 136, 238, 273, 403
fertilization, 108
fetal alcohol syndrome (FAS), 93
fetal development. *See* brain development; growth of baby
fetal distress, 271
fetal effect, 11-12
fetal heart beat, 147, 160-62, 176, 269, 271, 314
fetal heart rate, 63, 97, 271, 345, 365, 370. *See also* electronic fetal monitoring (EFM)
fetal hiccups, 197, 258
fetal movement
  in fifth month, 197, 199-200
  in sixth month, 218-19
  in seventh month, 258
  in eighth month, 288-89
fetal stress response, 279-80
fever, 104, 314-15
fiber, 22-23, 36-37, 39-40, 43-44, 56, 120, 151
fifth disease, 412-13
fish. *See* seafood
5-S diet, 44-45, 103, 183, 280
flaxseeds, 35, 40, 43
flexitarian diet, 25
fluid requirements
  air travel and, 230
  constipation and, 151
  dizziness and, 179
  for labor, 347, 348, 355
  postpartum care and, 385
  skin care and, 183
  thirst signals, 150, 256
  water and, 43, 150
folate/folic acid, 29, 38-39, 47
F.O.O.D. (fetal origins of diseases), 11-19, 21
foods. *See also* eating habits; pregnancy superfoods
  aversions to, 116
  blended foods, 23, 121
  chemicals in, 93-96, 394
  chewing, 57, 152
  common gassy foods, 151
  cravings, 54-58, 115, 124-25
  nutrient-dense foods, 28, 36, 38, 39, 44, 56, 58, 120, 125

genetics, 9-10, 13-14, 325-26
genetic screening, 134, 155-56, 174, 401-03

genital herpes, 272, 276, 413
gestational diabetes, 14, 21, 59, 61, 79, 211, 399, 413–14
gravity edema, 256
grazing
    in first month, 116
    air travel and, 230
    blood sugar levels and, 21, 75, 180
    constipation and, 20–21, 151
    heartburn and, 20, 152
    for hemorrhoid prevention, 21, 227
    labor and, 348
    optimal weight gain and, 55
    postpartum care and, 393–94
    preconception planning and, 6
    pregnancy-induced nausea and, 120–21
    self-help skills, 103
    snacks, 22
green environment
    alcohol use and, 92–93
    caffeine and, 96–97
    cigarette smoke and, 88–92
    drug use and, 92
    environmental toxins, 97–101
    fetal origin of disease and, 17–18
    first trimester and, 87, 89, 92, 93
    food chemicals and, 93–96
    pollutants' effects on baby, 87
    preconception planning and, 7, 90, 114
    pregnancy-induced nausea and, 116
    sensitivity to toxins, 87
green-light eating, 35, 45–46, 58, 161
growth of baby
    1–4 weeks, 107–10
    5–8 weeks, 146–48
    9–12 weeks, 160–61
    13–16 weeks, 174–75
    17–20 weeks, 197–98
    21–25 weeks, 217–18
    26–29 weeks, 253–54
    30–33 weeks, 288–89
    34–40 weeks, 338–39
guilt feelings, 114–16, 154
gut brain, 20, 122

hair, 99–100, 203–04
Hale, Thomas, 104
hands
    numbness/tingling in, 221–22
    swelling in, 256

Hathaway, Jay, 237
Hathaway, Marjie, 237
headaches, 63, 179, 201, 257, 364, 423
healthcare provider. See also checkups with
        healthcare provider
    childbirth philosophy, 129, 131, 132
    choosing hospitals/place of birth, 139–40, 238
    choosing midwife, 135–39, 238
    choosing obstetrician, 130–34, 135, 137, 238, 274
    choosing pediatrician, 263–66
    exercise and, 61–62
Healthy Pregnancy Plan
    and conception, 3
    eating habits, 20–27
    L.E.A.N. and, 4
    motivation and, 11–19
    multiples and, 404
    nine top tips, 10
    pregnancy superfoods, 28–50
    vaginal births and, 274
heartburn
    in second month, 151–52
    in eighth month, 289
    in ninth month, 341
    chewing and, 57
    positions for, 124
    pregnancy heartburn, 20
    pregnancy-induced nausea and, 121, 122, 149
    sipping solution and, 23
    sleep and, 80
heart rate
    in second month, 149
    in seventh month, 255
    caffeine and, 97
    drug use and, 92
    exercise and, 62, 63
    postpartum care and, 385
    sleep and, 79, 84
    stress and, 78
hemorrhoids, 21, 85, 226–27, 341, 386
heparin lock, 309, 347
Hepatitis B, 415–17
high blood pressure, 37, 201, 256, 262, 317, 399
high-fructose corn syrup (HFCS), 22, 40, 95–96
high-risk pregnancies. See special pregnancies
high satiety factor, 37, 40, 54
home, detoxifying, 98
home births, 139–40, 242–45
hormonal harmony
    in second month, 152–53

hormonal harmony *(Cont.)*
  birth bonding, 327–28, 329, 336
  cesarean-birth healing and, 281
  of childbirth, 323–36
  exercise and, 59, 68
  finale, 335–36
  grazing and, 21
  grow-and-prepare hormones, 323–24
  labor and, 327–28, 339, 347
  performance-enhancing hormones, 326–27
  pharmacological versus physiological birth, 326, 328, 331–35
  power-and-process hormones, 324–25
  produce-milk and bond-with-baby hormones, 327
  relieve-and-relax hormones, 325–26
  supportive birthcare attendants, 330
hormones
  body fat needed for, 7
  breast changes and, 148
  constipation and, 150
  contraception methods and, 3
  exercise and, 64
  frequent urination and, 115
  heartburn and, 152
  labor and, 339
  pain-management techniques and, 294
  placenta producing, 323–24, 325
  preconception checkup and, 5
  pregnancy-induced nausea and, 116, 118, 149
  pregnancy's effect on, 4, 112, 152–53, 198
  relaxation and, 297
  sex and, 164–65
  skin changes and, 181–82
hospitals
  "baby-friendly," 240
  childbirth classes, 235, 237, 238
  choosing, 139–40, 239–40
  labor tubs and, 303
  timing of arrival, 364
  vaginal birth after cesarean, 135–36, 139–40, 270, 277–78
household tasks, priorities for, 113, 118
human chorionic gonadotropin (HCG), 109, 116, 127, 134
hyperemesis gravidarum, 117, 125, 417
hyperinsulinism, 211

imagery, 292, 299–300, 351
immune system
  exercise and, 61

fetal origin of diseases and, 12, 15
  implantation and, 109
  laughter and, 78
  omega-3 fats and, 32–33
  postpartum care and, 393, 394
  seafood and, 34
  stress and, 74
immunizations, 5, 266
implantation, 108–09, 115
incontinence, 68, 69
infertility treatments, 136, 268, 273
inflammation, 3, 23, 177
insect repellents, 101
insulin, 21, 61, 95, 211
insurance plans
  for baby, 264–65
  choosing birth center and, 241, 242
  choosing doctor and, 130, 133
  choosing hospital and, 139, 239
  choosing midwife and, 137
  choosing pediatrician and, 264
  labor coaches and, 261
  maternity leave and, 187
  vaginal birth after cesarean and, 275–76
International Cesarean Awareness Network (ICAN), 193, 234, 277
International Childbirth Education Association (ICEA), 236–37
intestinal gas, 151, 230, 386
intrauterine growth restriction (IUGR), 418
iodine, 29, 49
iron, 29, 47–48, 180, 406, 407
itchy skin, 154

journaling, 76, 133–34, 140–41

Kegel exercises, 68–70, 227, 228, 371, 372
Kitzinger, Sheila, 368

labor. *See also* pain-management techniques; pushing stage
  active labor, 359, 362–63, 365, 376
  advantages to baby, 279–80
  analgesics and, 208–09
  back labor, 223, 296, 302, 304
  childbirth classes and, 236
  delivery of placenta, 374–75
  encouragement during, 331
  excess weight gain and, 53, 54
  exercise and, 61, 67

failure to progress, 270–71, 275, 277, 316, 317, 331
4-1-1 formula, 259, 364
healthcare provider interview and, 131, 132
ideas and devices for, 355
inducing, 346
irritability during, 304
Kegel exercises, 69
labor tubs, 239, 241, 244, 301–04, 347, 351, 367
midwives and, 136–37, 138, 242, 269, 273
mobility during, 350
music and, 77, 348, 349, 350
oxytocin and, 324–25
packing and preparing for, 343–44
peaceful environment for, 348–49
positions for, 241, 271, 275, 277, 292, 308, 312–13, 350, 351, 353–57, 367
prelabor, 355, 358–59, 376
progress in, 346–51, 354
risk factors for premature labor, 165, 167, 229
stages of, 355, 358–76
terminology of, 351–52
transition stage, 303, 309, 314, 347, 366–68, 376
trial of labor after cesarean, 274, 278–79
vocalizing during, 350
labor coaches, 129, 131, 137, 260–63, 275–76, 295–96, 350
lactation consultants, 240, 387
La Leche League International, 234, 236, 390, 391
Lamaze International, 237
laughter, 78, 168, 349, 394
L.E.A.N. (lifestyle, exercise, attitude, and nutrition) habits, 4, 13, 14, 58
leg cramps, 152, 219–21
lochia, 384–85

marriage, 81, 82, 86, 88, 111. *See also* fathers; sex
Martha's Pregnancy Salad, 38
massage
  in first month, 115, 119
  in fourth month, 175
  backache and, 222, 223
  breast massage, 149
  fathers and, 209, 223
  foot massage, 202, 304
  labor and, 349
  leg cramps and, 220
  pain-management techniques and, 292, 298, 304–05
  perineal massage, 138, 372
  scalp massage, 203

for skin care, 185
maternity leave, 111, 185, 186–90
meconium, 345
medical complications
  anemia, 406–07
  bed rest, 407–12
  beta strep infection, 412
  fifth disease, 412–13
  genital herpes, 413
  gestational diabetes, 413–14
  HELLP syndrome, 415
  Hepatitis B, 415–17
  high-risk label, 242, 417
  hyperemesis gravidarum, 417
  incompetent cervix, 417–18
  intrauterine growth restriction, 418
  miscarriages, 418–22
  placenta and, 422–23
  preeclampsia, 423
  premature birth, 423–24
  Rh incompatibility, 424
medications. *See also* pills-skills mindset
  analgesics, 104, 282, 291, 307–09
  cautions concerning, 104, 114
  for diarrhea, 233
  for pain management, 307–17
  preconception planning and, 4, 7
Medications and Mothers' Milk (Hale), 104
meditation, 77–78
melanin, 181, 183
membranes, rupture of
  active labor and, 363, 364, 376
  artificially rupturing, 346
  early labor and, 361
  labor tubs and, 303
  prelabor and, 358–59
memory lapses, 74, 199, 255
metabolism, 6, 15–16, 43, 53, 62, 79
midwives
  as birth attendants, 130, 330
  birth centers and, 240–42
  choosing, 135–39, 238
  in hospitals, 240
  labor sitting and, 136–37, 138, 242, 269, 273
Midwives Alliance of North America, 139
miscarriages
  amniocentesis and, 401
  anxiety concerning, 112, 166–67, 174
  caffeine and, 96–97
  causes of, 418–19

miscarriages *(Cont.)*
  cigarette smoke and, 88, 91
  drug use and, 92
  environmental toxins and, 100
  grieving after, 421
  preconception checkup and, 5
  previous miscarriages, 421
  signs of, 419–20
  special pregnancies and, 399
  waiting for pregnancy and, 3
"mommy brain," 74, 199, 255
monosodium glutamate (MSG), 83, 94, 120
mood disorders, 5, 7
morning sickness. *See* pregnancy-induced nausea
    (PIN)
motherhood transition, 395–96
mothering feeling, 204–05, 260, 288, 297
multiple births
  cesarean births and, 268, 272–73
  infertility treatments and, 136, 268, 273, 403
  pregnancy-induced nausea and, 117
  rate of, 403
  sex and, 405
  special pregnancies and, 399
  ultrasound and, 126, 403
  weight gain during pregnancy and, 51
music
  labor and, 77, 348, 349, 350
  pain-management techniques and, 292, 298–99
  postpartum care and, 394
  sleep and, 83, 84
  as stressbuster, 77

nails, 99, 101, 204
napping, 82, 114, 207
narcotic pain relievers, 307–09, 312
National Institutes of Health, 33, 94, 96–97
nausea. *See* pregnancy-induced nausea (PIN)
neonatal intensive care, 217, 240
nesting, 199, 290, 340–41, 360
neurotoxins, 17, 94
nipples
  in first month, 115
  in third month, 162, 166
  in fifth month, 204
  birth crawl and, 328, 336, 375
  labor tub and, 303
  sore nipples, 390–91
  stimulation for inducing labor, 346, 349
nosebleeds, 178

nutrigenetics, 13–14
nutrition. *See also* eating habits; pregnancy
    superfoods
  baby's birth weight and, 13
  nourishing nine nutrients, 29
  nutrient-dense foods, 28, 36, 38, 39, 44, 56, 58,
    120, 125
  pregnancy nutrition at a glance, 47–50
  questions concerning, 25–27
  synergy of nutrients, 38, 45
nuts, 36–38

obesity
  birth complications and, 136
  exercise and, 61
  failure to progress and, 271
  fetal origin of diseases and, 12, 16
  grazing and, 21
  high-fructose corn syrup and, 95
  weight gain during pregnancy and, 51, 53
odors, 115, 116, 122
oil change, 33, 37
Omega-3 Effect, The (William Sears and James
    Sears), 33, 34, 37
omega-3 fats
  health benefits to pregnant mothers, 37
  oil change, 37
  postpartum care and, 394
  premature birth prevention and, 161
  recommended intake of, 29, 33, 47
  scientific evidence on, 31–32
  in seafood, 29, 30–36
  for skin care, 183
  supplements, 34
oral glucose tolerance test (OGTT), 211
organic foods, 41–42
orthostatic hypotension, 179
orthotic inserts, 202
oxytocin, 278, 316, 324–25, 327–36, 368, 375

pain-management techniques
  analgesics, 104, 282, 291, 307–09, 312
  balanced mindset and, 294
  Braxton Hicks contractions and, 290
  breathing and, 305–06
  causes of pain, 291–92
  cesarean births and, 268–69, 282
  childbirth classes and, 235, 236, 237, 307
  distraction and, 292, 300, 305
  epidurals and, 309–17

fear and, 294–95
hypnobirthing, 274, 306–07
labor coaches and, 260, 295–96
labor tubs, 301–04
massage and, 292, 298, 304–05
medications for, 307–17
midwives and, 244
music and, 292, 298–99
options for, 291–92
pain rating scale, 294
pain receptors, 292
pain tolerance and, 293
perspective on pain, 300–301
purpose of pain, 293
relaxation and, 292, 296–98
transcutaneous electrical nerve stimulation
    (TENS), 296
parasympathetic nervous system (PNS), 76, 77
parenting philosophy, 263–64, 266, 395, 399
pelvic discomfort, 115, 152, 163, 258, 341–42
pelvic floor muscles, Kegel exercises for, 68–70, 227,
    228, 371, 372
pelvic rock exercises, 71
pelvic tilt exercises, 71
perineum, 368, 372, 373, 383–84
periodontal disease, 5, 178
persistent organic pollutants (POPs), 98
personal care products, 101, 184, 185
pesco-vegetarian diet, 25
photographs, 166, 208–09
pills-skills mindset, 7, 8, 102, 103, 104
pitocin, 291, 316, 331–35, 375
placenta
    in first month, 109
    in fifth month, 198
    caffeine and, 96
    car accidents and, 234
    cigarette smoke and, 88
    delivery of, 374–75
    drug use and, 92
    environmental toxins and, 100
    epidurals and, 314
    fetal origin of disease and, 16, 17, 18
    hormones produced by, 323–24, 325
    stress and, 74
    sucralose and, 95
placenta abruptio, 422–23
placenta accreta, 422
placenta previa, 165, 399, 422
plastic containers, 98, 101

positions
    avoiding lying on back, 85, 179, 257, 271, 275, 367,
        372, 373
    for back massage, 223
    changing positions slowly, 179, 225, 255, 385
    epidurals and, 311
    for heartburn, 124
    knees-to-chest position, 72, 222, 223, 227
    for labor, 241, 271, 275, 277, 292, 308, 312–13,
        350, 351, 353–57, 367
    for lifting, 224, 225, 257
    for pregnancy-induced nausea, 124
    for pushing stage, 353–54, 372, 373
    for sexual intercourse, 168, 259
    for sitting, 223–25, 230, 256
    for sleep, 84–85, 179, 222, 226, 256, 257
    for standing, 223
positive self-talk, 74–76
postpartum care. See also breastfeeding
    afterpains and, 375, 383
    checkup, 381
    childbirth classes and, 236
    healing from childbirth, 393–94
    midwives and, 138
    perineum and, 383–84
    urination and, 385–86
    vaginal discharge and, 384–85
postural hypotension, 179
posture, 223, 225
potassium, 152, 221
preconception checkup, 5
preconception planning, 3–8, 90, 114
prediabetes, 53–54
preeclampsia, 256–57, 276, 364, 399, 423
pregnancy. See also special pregnancies
    early signs of, 114–15
    risk and, 242
    sharing news of, 127–28
    tests for, 127
pregnancy brain, 74, 199, 255
pregnancy-induced nausea (PIN)
    in first month, 107, 115, 116–24
    in second month, 146, 148, 149
    exercise and, 61
    food cravings and, 124–25
    positions for, 124
    questions concerning, 117–19
    stomach-friendly tips, 119–24
    stomach-soothing favorites, 121
    triggers for, 120

pregnancy superfoods
  avocados, 39
  beans and lentils, 40
  blueberries, 40
  cesarean-birth healing and, 281
  characteristics of, 28
  eggs, 39
  5-S diet, 44–45
  flaxseeds, 40, 43
  greens, 38–39
  nutrition at a glance, 47–50
  nutrition questions and, 25, 26
  nuts, 36–38
  oatmeal, 44
  olive oil, 43–44
  postpartum care and, 393
  preconception planning and, 6
  seafood, 29–36
  tofu, 44
  top twelve foods, 28–29
  white-out your diet, 44
  yogurt, 39–40
premature birth
  cigarette smoke and, 89, 91, 161
  drug use and, 92
  exercise and, 61, 161
  medical complications, 423–24
  multiples and, 404
  periodontal disease and, 178
  prevention of, 161
  special pregnancies and, 399
prenatal supplements, 5, 22, 23, 25, 26, 120, 133
prescription drugs. *See* medications
Primetime Health (William Sears and Martha
    Sears), 103
probiotics, 40, 151
progesterone, 104, 109, 117, 152–53, 181, 323–24,
    339
prolactin, 91, 297, 327, 336, 389
prostaglandins, 104, 346
protein, 29, 50
pulse test, for exercise, 63, 67
pushing stage
  analgesics and, 309
  endorphins and, 297
  epidurals and, 269, 313, 314
  imagery and, 299
  positions for, 353–54, 372, 373
  techniques for, 369–70, 372
  transition stage and, 367, 376

real-food diet, 6, 54–55, 103
recipes, 24, 38
red-light eating, 35, 45–46, 58
relaxation
  in first month, 115
  in ninth month, 344
  Braxton Hicks contractions and, 290, 298, 342
  breathing and, 76–77
  childbirth and, 235
  childbirth classes and, 236
  exercises in, 298
  labor coaches and, 261
  labor progress and, 347, 361, 363
  music and, 77
  pain-management techniques and, 292, 296–98
  self-help skills, 103
  sleep and, 82, 84
relaxin (hormone), 64, 68, 201, 326
resources, 191, 425–27
Rh incompatibility, 234, 424
rule of twos, 21, 120, 227

salads
  5-S diet and, 45
  Martha's Pregnancy Salad, 38
saliva production, 149
salmon, 34, 35, 36
sciatica, 222
seafood, 29–36, 45, 394
secondhand smoke, 8, 88, 89
selective permeability, 17
selective serotonin reuptake inhibitors (SSRIs), 104
serotonin, 75, 83, 84, 124, 325, 339
sex
  in seventh month, 259
  abstinence recommendations, 165, 167
  episiotomies and, 371
  fear of miscarriage and, 166–67
  inducing labor with, 346
  mixed feelings about, 164–65
  multiple births and, 405
  myth of deprived man, 167–68
  redefining, 167
  spotting after, 154
shoes, 201, 202, 225, 257
shoulder dystocia, 371
sipping solution, 22–23, 55, 103, 121, 150, 152, 393–94
sitting positions, 223–25, 230, 256
skin care, 37, 101, 181–85
skin changes

in fourth month, 181–83
glow, 181
itchy skin, 154, 181–82
lines, 182–83
pigmentation, 183, 184–85
pregnancy acne, 182
pregnancy mask, 181
redness, 182
skin tags, 182
spider veins, 183
stretch marks, 181
sleep
in first month, 114
in sixth month, 219
in eighth month, 291
in ninth month, 344
baby kicking and, 80
before-bed rituals, 83
caffeine and, 80, 97
causes of wakefulness, 79–82
cesarean-birth healing and, 281
darkness for, 84, 114
deep (non-REM), 79–80
difficulty with, 79–80
eating habits and, 79, 83
eggs and, 39, 83
excess weight gain and, 53
exercise and, 61, 82
pillow placement, 85, 256
positions for, 84–85, 179, 222, 226, 256, 257
postpartum care and, 394
pregnancy-induced nausea and, 123
pregnancy sleep prescription, 82–86
REM sleep, 80, 81
sleep needs during pregnancy, 79
snooze foods, 83
temperature of bedroom, 84, 86
smoothies
Dr. Bill and Martha's Pregnancy Supersmoothie, 24
5-S diet and, 45
for labor, 348
postpartum care and, 387
pregnancy-induced nausea and, 120
snacking, 22, 56, 64, 83, 120–21
snooze foods, 83
social networks, 141
special pregnancies
defining, 397–98
having baby after age thirty-five, 399–400

hospital choice and, 139, 242
labor coaches and, 262–63
squatting
labor position and, 241, 271, 276, 303, 312–13, 353–57
pushing stage and, 353–54, 373
stretching exercises, 70, 71
starvation ketosis, 118
stem cells, 17, 267
stillbirth, 92
stress
caffeine and, 97
cesarean-birth healing and, 281
effect on baby, 73–75, 161
exercise and, 75, 77
fetal origin of disease and, 16
journaling and, 76, 140
optimal weight gain and, 57
overdue and, 345
postpartum care and, 394–95
preconception planning and, 7
pregnancy brain, 74
pregnancy-induced nausea and, 122, 124
sleep and, 81, 83–84
swimming and, 77
ten stressbusters, 75–78
unproductive worry cycle, 163–64
subsequent pregnancies
abdominal muscles and, 228
baby dropping and, 289, 341, 358
baby's kicking and, 199
growth of uterus, 175
having baby after age thirty-five, 400
pushing stage and, 368
replaying previous birth, 290, 295
sucking
for fluid intake, 150
for pregnancy-induced nausea, 121–22, 149
sucralose, 94–95
sudden infant death syndrome (SIDS), 8, 89, 91, 92
supplements
5-S diet and, 45
prenatal supplements, 5, 22, 23, 25, 26, 120, 133
support hose, 220, 226, 230
sweeteners, 40, 58, 94–95
swelling, 61, 67, 85, 220, 256–57, 290
swimming, 66–67, 77, 116, 180, 222, 257, 342
sympathetic nervous system (SNS), 76, 77

tailor sitting, 70, 71
tailor stretching, 70, 71, 72
talk test, for exercise, 63, 67
taste shaping, 6, 34, 43, 217
temperature, body, 68, 180, 222
thirst signals, 150, 256
thumb-sucking, 217, 338
thyroid hormones, 116
tiredness. *See* fatigue
toxemia, 53, 262–63
traffic-light eating, 35, 45–46, 58
trans fats, 33, 37, 93, 95
travel, 100, 229–34
treats, 45, 55, 56, 58, 97, 124, 125, 150–51
tryptophan, 83
Twitter, 141

ultrasound
    in second month, 147, 148, 156
    in third month, 160
    in fourth month, 176
    for calculating due date, 126, 156, 345
    fetal size and, 278
    gender of baby and, 210
umbilical cord, 267, 272, 328, 345
urinalysis, 106, 134
urination frequency
    in first month, 115
    in second month, 146, 150
    in fourth month, 176
    in eighth month, 289
    in ninth month, 341
    labor and, 348
    prelabor and, 358
    sleep difficulties and, 80
    triple voiding, 228, 230
urine
    color of, 43, 117
    difficulty urinating, 385–86
    leaking urine, 227–28, 289, 386
    pregnancy test, 127
uterus. *See also* contractions
    in fourth month, 174, 175
    in fifth month, 197, 204
    in sixth month, 217, 219, 226
    in seventh month, 254, 255–56
    in eighth month, 290, 291

vaccinations, for travel, 231
vagina, changes in, 164–65, 168

vaginal birth after cesarean (VBAC)
    healthcare provider choice and, 132, 274
    hospital policy and, 135–36, 139–40, 270, 277–78
    insurance plans and, 275–76
    labor coaches and, 261, 278
    motivation for, 276–77
    rate of, 273, 277, 279
    risks of, 278
    support groups for, 277
vaginal discharge
    in seventh month, 258
    postpartum care and, 384–85
    prelabor and, 358
    signs of infection, 176–77
varicose veins, 226–27
vegan diet, 25–26, 35–36, 37
vegetarian diet, 25, 35–36, 37
veins, enlargement of, 225–26
vernix caseosa, 198, 217, 338
vision
    in fifth month, 201
    eggs and, 39
    omega-3 fats and, 37
    seafood and, 29
    swelling and, 257
visualization, 299–300, 351
vitamin B$_{12}$, 29, 48
vitamin C, 49, 177
vitamin D, 26–27, 29, 34, 49, 177, 184
volatile organic compounds (VOCs), 98
vomiting. *See* pregnancy-induced nausea (PIN)

walking
    in ninth month, 341
    cravings and, 58
    exercise and, 66, 116
    labor progress and, 346, 350, 354
    to reduce swelling, 257
    as stressbuster, 77
    treading lightly, 225
weight gain
    distribution of, 52
    excess weight gain, 53–54
    exercise and, 61
    guidelines for, 51–52
    insulin and, 21
    pregnancy-induced nausea and, 117
    sipping solution and, 23
    strategies for optimal weight gain, 54–58, 61
    vaginal birth and, 274–75

weight loss, 344–45
What Babies Need (William Sears, Martha Sears, and Christie Watts Kelly), 205
white noise, 85–86
white-out your diet, 44
womb environment, 11–12, 16, 43, 217

work. *See* employment
worry. *See* anxiety; stress

yellow-light eating, 35, 45–46, 58

zinc, 49

About the Authors

William Sears, MD, and Martha Sears, RN, are the parents of eight children and the authors of more than forty bestselling books on parenting. They are the pediatric experts whom American parents increasingly rely on for advice and information on all aspects of pregnancy, birth, childcare, and family health. Dr. Bill received his pediatric training at Harvard Medical School's Children's Hospital and Toronto's Hospital for Sick Children. He has practiced pediatrics for more than forty years and is an associate clinical professor at the University of California, Irvine, School of Medicine. Martha Sears is a registered nurse, former childbirth educator, and lactation consultant. They live in Dana Point, California.

Linda Hughey Holt, MD, is a board-certified obstetrician/gynecologist and the mother of three children. She graduated from Yale, attended the University of Chicago for medical school and residency, and has served on the medical faculties at Northwestern University, Rush University, and the University of Chicago. She has authored and contributed to a number of books, including *The Pregnancy Book*. Linda is currently in an active full-range practice, teaches obstetrics at NorthShore University HealthSystem, an affiliate of the University of Chicago, and has participated in medical missions to Guatemala and Bolivia and done volunteer work with the Indian Health Service. Most important, she never ceases to wonder at the miracle of birth.

BJ Snell, PhD, CNM, FACNM, is the owner of Beach Cities Midwifery and Women's Health Care and the Beachside Birth Centers in Laguna Hills and Long Beach, California. She is also a professor at California State University, Fullerton, where she is the director of the Midwifery and Women's Health Care/Nurse Practitioner graduate program. A graduate of the Oregon Health and Science University midwifery program, she has birthed over 3,300 babies in her twenty-seven-year midwifery career and is a resource for many women and health professionals on the management of normal pregnancy, childbirth, and the early transition to parenthood. Married for thirty-five years and the mother of two sons, Dr. BJ remains in awe of the personal strength and trust that women have for labor and birth and how that is enhanced when they have support and guidance from their provider.

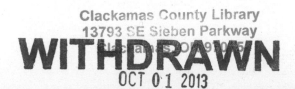